Manual Therapy
in Children

For Churchill Livingstone:

Publishing Director, Health Professions: Mary Law
Project Development Manager: Dinah Thom
Project Manager: Joannah Duncan
Designer: Judith Wright

Manual Therapy in Children

Edited by

Heiner Biedermann MD

Practitioner in Conservative Orthopedics, Cologne, Germany, and Member of the European Workgroup for Manual Medicine. Formerly Surgeon at the Surgical Department of the University of Witten-Herdecke and Schwerte Hospital, Germany

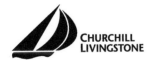
CHURCHILL
LIVINGSTONE

EDINBURGH   LONDON   NEW YORK   OXFORD   PHILADELPHIA   ST LOUIS   SYDNEY   TORONTO   2004

CHURCHILL LIVINGSTONE
An imprint of Elsevier Limited

First published 2004

ISBN 0 443 10018 7

British Library Cataloguing in Publication Data
A catalogue record for this book is available from the British Library

Library of Congress Cataloging in Publication Data
A catalog record for this book is available from the Library of Congress

Notice
Medical knowledge is constantly changing. Standard safety precautions must be followed, but as new research and clinical experience broaden our knowledge, changes in treatment and drug therapy may become necessary or appropriate. Readers are advised to check the most current product information provided by the manufacturer of each drug to be administered to verify the recommended dose, the method and duration of administration, and contraindications. It is the responsibility of the practitioner, relying on experience and knowledge of the patient, to determine dosages and the best treatment for each individual patient. Neither the publishers nor the editor and contributors will be liable for any loss or damage of any nature occasioned to or suffered by any person acting or refraining from acting as a result of reliance on the material contained in this publication.

The Publisher

Transferred to Digital Print 2009

Printed and bound in Great Britain by
CPI Antony Rowe, Chippenham and Eastbourne

Contents

Contributors

Lilia Babina, MD
*Professor, Neuropediatric Department, Pediatric
Rehabilitation Clinic, Pjatigorsk, Russia*

Heiner Biedermann MD
*Practitioner in Conservative Orthopedics, Cologne,
Germany and Member of the European Workgroup for
Manual Medicine (EWMM). Formerly Surgeon at the
Surgical Department of the University of Witten-
Herdecke and Schwerte Hospital, Germany*

Bodo E. A. Christ MD
*Professor, Institute of Anatomy and Cell Biology,
University of Freiburg, Germany*

Arnd Friedrichs
Friendly Sensors AG, Jena, Germany

Onur Güntürkün PhD(Psychol)
*Professor of Psychology, Faculty of Psychology,
Ruhr-University Bochum, Bochum, Germany*

Akira Hori MD
*Professor, Research Institute for Neurology and
Psychiatry, National Nishi-Tottori Hospital, Tottori,
Japan*

Ruijin Huang PD DrMed
*Institute of Anatomy and Cell Biology, University of
Freiburg, Freiburg, Germany*

Susanne Huber Dipl Phys Dr rer nat
*Research Fellow, Friedrich-Miescher Laboratory of the
Max-Planck-Society, Tübingen, Germany*

Freddy Huguenin MD
*Former Consultant at the University Clinic of
Physical Medicine and Rehabilitation of Geneva,
Switzerland*

Michael E. Hyland BSc PhD BCPsychol
*Department of Psychology, University of Plymouth,
Plymouth, UK*

S. Iliaeva MD
*Rehabilitative and Physical Medicine, Cologne,
Germany*

Bärbel Kahl-Nieke PhD DrMed(dent)
*Chair of Department of Orthodontics, College of
Dentistry, University of Hamburg, Hamburg,
Germany*

L. E. Koch DrMed
*General Practitioner and Member of the European
Workgroup for Manual Medicine (EWMM),
Eckernförde, Germany*

Heike M. Korbmacher DrMed(dent)
Associate Professor, Department of Orthodontics, College of Dentistry, University of Hamburg, Hamburg, Germany

Hanne Kühnen DrMed
Pediatrician, Kevelaer, Germany

H. Mohr
Physiotherapist and Member of the European Workgroup for Manual Medicine (EWMM), Manual Therapist and Lecturer, Ede, The Netherlands

R. Rädel MD
Orthopedic Surgeon, Herne, Germany

Jan-Marino Ramirez PhD
Professor of Anatomy and Neurosciences, Department of Anatomy, The University of Chicago, Chicago, Illinois, USA

Dorin Ritzmann DrMed FMH(Gynecology/Obstetrics)
CertMedHypnosisTraumaTherapy (EMDRFrancineShapiro)
Zürich, Switzerland

R. Sacher MD
Private Practitioner and Member of the European Workgroup for Manual Medicine (EWMM), Dortmund, Germany

Reinhard W. Theiler DrMed FMH
Pediatrician (neuro-rehabilitation) and Member of the European Workgroup for Manual Medicine (EWMM), Trimbach, Switzerland

Peter J. Waibel MD
Chief of Section, Radiology Department, Ostschweizer Kinderspital, St Gallen, Switzerland

Preface

'I don't like writing – I like having written' – Dorothy Parker once said. This holds true for almost every writer and certainly for me. To comprehend the pleasure felt at this moment (all the chapters have been sent to the publisher and the only thing left to do is to write these short lines) might be difficult for somebody who was not (yet) in this position.

It is more than five years since English and Dutch friends proposed writing a book on manual therapy in children. Soon it became clear that this rapidly developing field was too vast to be dealt with by one author alone. The search for contributors willing to share their competence began, and I am immensely grateful to all of those willing to sacrifice their rare spare time to write their chapters.

Almost as admirable was the patience of those on the publisher's side who waited unwearyingly while the complex material was rearranged over and over again to gain a satisfactory form and structure. Needless to say the initial deadline for this book was exceeded by many months.

During these years, several congresses brought countless discussions. All those questions and criticisms helped to create a coherent concept out of the observations of the practical work with children. The friends and colleagues of the European Workgroup for Manual Medicine are exemplary in that regard, but also all those pediatricians who took an interest in the potential of manual therapy without actually practising it. Some of them contributed material to this book, others offered valuable hints and pointed out weaknesses in the arguments.

The quest to be up to date is as unviable as the search for the end of the rainbow – but both may lead to insights not reached otherwise. The inevitable delay between the submission of the manuscript and the finished book has to be accepted stoically if one wants to avoid endless addenda.

The basic tenets of what is presented here have stood the test of time and in publishing these findings, we hope to encourage others to comment and criticize in order to use this as a base for further improvements.

All those around somebody working on a book suffer – from the different forms of neglect the concentration on such a long-term project implies. To thank one's wife and offspring for their comprehension is but a shallow recompense for it, and as formulaic as it may be, it inevitably opens the 'thank you' section.

All the colleagues who helped with their advice and criticism come a close second, to be followed by the team at Elsevier who endured the long delays and constant alterations. Representing the first group Editha Halfmann, Uli Göhmann and Bruno Maggi have to be mentioned; at Elsevier I want to thank especially Mary Law, Dinah Thom and Joannah Duncan for patience and the entire production team, encouragement and all their helpful remarks.

Jenny Fox rendered the text a bit more comprehensible with her 'native speaker' advice and her proofreading.

Last but not least I want to thank my young patients and their families for feedback, motivation and for making available all the material and photos used in this book – their book, in a way.

'Tritt frisch auf – tu's Maul auf!– hör bald auf!' Martin Luther once said; we tried to heed that advice.

Heiner Biedermann
Antwerp 2004

Chapter 1

Introduction: reviewing the history of manual therapy in children

H. Biedermann

'DO YOU HAVE TO KNOW PHILOSOPHY TO PLAY THE PIANO?'

'*No, but it helps*' might be an appropriate answer. And, translated into the lingo of manual therapy: You do not *have* to know about the history of our trade, about neurophysiology or anatomy to manipulate – but to reach a certain professional level, it helps – a lot.

Nobody with any knowledge of music doubts the idea that you need to understand the cultural and philosophical context of a piece of music you want to interpret. If playing music was as simple as copying the notes onto an instrument, you could feed a given score to the computer and – plop! – the perfect music is played. But it is the interpretation of the player which turns a sterile bit of notation into a work of art. And as the society in which one plays one's tunes evolves, so does the interpretation of the great compositions. There will never be the 'ultimate' interpretation of Beethoven's 9th or Schubert's Forellenquintett.

The same is true for manual therapy. The way we interact with our patients is crucially dependent on an exact appraisal of their physical and psychological condition. Techniques that were well established in the 1930s would be considered a bit brutal today.

With small children the situation gets even more complex, as we have to take into account an entire family, i.e. the parents and siblings present at the consultation. How much of a success an individual treatment will be depends at least as much on the good contact between therapist and family as on the technical know-how of the former.

Any contact between two individuals has effects on both of them. For the purposes of this book, we can limit the scope by defining manual therapy as the deliberate touching of the patient by a trained therapist with the intention of improving the patient's condition. Seen from close enough, manual therapy (and even more so *manual therapy in children* – MTC) is a simple mechanical procedure. One might be tempted to confine a treatise to the bare necessities, a 'how to' of the different techniques available. This approach would be an antidote to the sometimes lofty explanations offered for some of the methods available today. Quite a few books are organized according to such a scheme. The reader is offered a short introduction about the history of the specific method presented in the text, and then page after page showing a therapist, his/her patient and the different positions possible.

Such a Kama-Sutra of manual techniques has some merits – to remind the experienced of what is possible – but it cannot replace the real thing, i.e. learning by observing and in close contact with a proficient teacher. So we shall not avoid those 'how-to' pictures entirely, but these parts of the book are few and not the most important ones.

In teaching and demonstrating manual therapy in children, one encounters two principal reactions:

- One group of colleagues – the bigger one – watches and after an hour or two their body language expresses very clearly the idea that they have seen it all. As it looks so simple – just a little push on the side of the neck – why waste any more time! These guests leave the consultation and my address book equally quickly.
- A second, smaller group looks more closely and these colleagues more often than not start to ask a lot of questions about the details of the exam-

ination. This may get a bit tiring sometimes – but it is for them that this book is intended.

THE LESSONS OF MTC FOR MANUAL THERAPY IN GENERAL

What we find is what we are looking for – this is nowhere more true than in medical research. As a young student one enters the arena with the somewhat naive thought that what we are pursuing is the truth, and nothing but the truth. But we are condemned to deviate from this noble goal from the beginning, and have to embrace the constraints of our neurophysiological input capacity and the limits of our budget – to name but two of the more extreme obstacles on our way to 'the truth'.

When trying to present a paper about a medical problem, we end up more or less with the advice the *Economist*'s editor gave to a young employee 'Simplify, then exaggerate!'. There seem to be two ways out of this dilemma, and they have, almost always, opposite directions. The traditional 'scientific' approach is to partition the complexity of the clinical picture till we arrive at a level where the task seems to be clear enough to be cast into a linear question of 'what if'. This is basically the realm of the evidence-based medicine (Sackett et al 1997) so much in vogue now. This approach is an excellent tool to decide questions like 'If I want to treat cystitis with an antibiotic, which one would be best?'

One is reminded of the statement of the biochemist A. Szent-Gyorgyi (1972): 'I moved from anatomy to the study of tissues, then to electron microscopy and chemistry, and finally to quantum mechanics. This downward journey through the scale of dimensions has its irony, for in my search for the secret of life I ended up with atoms and electrons which have no life at all. Somewhere along the line life has run out of my fingers.'

When we try to simplify – and simplify we must in order to get to grips with the complexity of disease and disorder – we have to keep in mind what we do. And we have to keep in mind that the questions we can ask in a reductionist context are not necessarily the most relevant.

The second approach, as exemplified by manual therapy in the non-trivial sense (see Chapter 22), aims at re-establishing a functional equilibrium which renders its effects dependent on a multitude of other influences, psychological as well as physical. Such an approach has to be based on the results of reductionist research, but it takes into account the complex interaction with other levels of maintaining the homeostasis and these mechanisms are in most cases not quantifiable by 'hard' science. This is one reason why the treatment of small children is of such importance to us. Here we find a situation which we can define much better than the far more complex pictures in older children, let alone adolescents or adults. In babies we deal with a rather clear-cut pathology, the two main factors being genetic predisposition and the history up to the moment of the first examination – which means in almost every case the details of delivery, if we do not take into account the tiny number of cases with trauma after birth.

Therefore it is possible in these cases to bridge the gap between a rigorous enquiry on the one hand and the taking into account of all relevant factors on the other hand.

As soon as the individual history starts to diversify, such a synthetic view becomes almost impossible. In order to gain meaningful statements we have to simplify more than may be good for the task at hand. Take, for example, something as 'simple' as headache – an indication *par excellence* for manual therapy and excruciatingly complex in its web of causal dependencies.

If we were honest and serious we would have to take into account all the other contributing factors relevant for the development of these complaints. The professional and private situation is but the most obvious one of these contributing factors. Other medication, endocrinologic details and quite simply the age and type of the patient play a role, too. Last but not least we have to take into account that not everybody considers a given problem serious enough to go and see a doctor, so

what we are confronted with is not necessarily the whole spectrum of complaints. And – as stated in the beginning – the socio-cultural context we are working in plays an important role, too.

This dilemma occurs as soon as we look for long-term effects of any given therapeutic intervention. Maybe this is the reason why that kind of research has been so neglected. Applied to manual therapy this means that it is much easier to evaluate the effect of a lumbar manipulation on low back pain than that of a cervical manipulation on the wellbeing of a baby. But is it the most relevant question?

The first studies we shall be able to complete will be about problems that are suitable for a rather restricted protocol. And, yes, it is necessary to do such research – not because the questions we can answer in such a way are the most pressing ones, but because it helps to breach the wall of incomprehension that separates the majority of pediatricians from manual therapy. If we can demonstrate the efficiency of MTC in such a necessarily very restricted context, this first step opens the possibility of entering into a constructive discussion beyond those who are already convinced or at least interested.

In the context of manual therapy in children, two different but interrelated topics have to be dealt with. On the one hand, there is a clinical and pathophysiological concept which needs to be defined in order to become a useful diagnostic tool. To this end, the two acronyms of KISS and KIDD were proposed and will be discussed in Chapters 24 and 25. On the other hand, one has to choose the optimal method to deal with such a disorder once the diagnosis has been confirmed.

It seems to be useful to make it clear from the beginning that there is no stringent connection between the diagnostic and the therapeutic level. Most forms of manual therapy propose one method as the best (and only) solution, very often dismissing other, similar techniques as vastly inferior. For the naive observer it is sometimes astonishing to see that the methods proposed by the different schools are indeed very similar and that a distinction is sometimes a little bit artificial, to put it mildly.

There is – on the other hand – indeed a connection between the theoretical considerations and their practical realization inasmuch as certain procedures seem to be more promising than others. But the bottom line of all advice about the recommended techniques for manual therapy in children should be: *Do not touch the cervical spine too often!* The closer one gets to the occipito-cervical junction, the more time this highly volatile system needs to adapt to the – therapeutic, but nevertheless irritating – input. Speransky (1950) wrote extensively about the 'second hit phenomenon'. He pointed out that a sensitive structure – today we would talk about a network – can handle a quite severe trauma once, but decompensates if a similar second, much weaker trauma is encountered too soon afterwards.

THE ROLE OF THE THERAPIST

Observing different practitioners of manual therapy – be it chiropractors, doctors or physiotherapists – one quickly realizes that there are almost as many techniques as people practicing them. Apart from the purely physical level, there is the 'philosophical' level, too. A 2 meter tall man with a background of orthopedic surgery will use different techniques from a petite woman of 1.6 meters who trained initially as a neuropediatrician.

All these different people may pretend to follow the same procedures, but what a difference. And let us not forget that in order to succeed, manual therapy has to rest on a base of confidence and trust. The empathy necessary to achieve such a solid person-to-person contact should come spontaneously, but has to be fostered. It is better not to treat somebody where one senses a lack of trust. Already, therefore, it is indispensable to have more than MTC at your disposal. Such a situation arises only very rarely, but I consider it to be of paramount importance to be able to shrink from applying a manipulation when this basic trust seems to be missing. The empathy has to be

present on both sides – and it is a mistake to think one can empathize with everybody. Manual therapy necessitates an intimate bodily contact between two strangers and the therapist as well as the patient should have the right to refuse.

MTC INFLUENCES BODY AND SOUL

Since the famous 'je pense, donc je suis' of the seventeenth-century philosopher Descartes (1596–1650), exploration of the natural world has gradually been freed from the constraints of religious dogma, thus enabling the ever faster development of the natural sciences we see today. It is on the basis of this liberating Renaissance thought that all our research stands (and it should not be forgotten that even Newton, living a generation later than Descartes, still devoted the bulk of his writing to parts of science like astrology, i.e. topics we do not classify as such nowadays).

The liberating influence of the Renaissance on philosophy and science (till then considered as one) can hardly be overestimated. But it came at a price. As a preventive measure to avoid too much scrutiny from the church authorities, Descartes postulated the separation of the spiritual realm and the body – the latter being accessible to our investigation. The eternal soul was said to be disconnected from the body's function and thus beyond our reach. An invisible barrier fenced off everything connected to the 'soul'.

In the nineteenth century another boost to the scientific understanding of our body came with the ideas of Virchow (1821–1902), a German pathologist who founded *cellular pathology*, thus postulating a microscopically detectable alteration of cells as the basis of any pathological process (Virchow 1865). This approach led to enormous progress in hygiene and in the understanding of infectious and degenerative diseases – but again at a price: functional disorders had almost no place in this system.

An examination of these two milestones of Western thought regarding the health sciences is beyond the scope of this chapter, but it helps to be aware of the context we work (and argue) in. Repercussions of the separation of body and soul in Western thinking abound, and in connection with the postulate of a morphological pathology at the root of every medical problem this creates an unconscious censorship. 'Hardware problems' fit into this pattern of thinking, 'software problems' much less – and to accept that a functional disorder can lead to a morphologically fixed pathology requires an even greater effort.

A good example is the ongoing discussion about 'difficult' children. One indicator of the trickiness of this problem is the changing nomenclature applied to these children: an entire collection of three-and four-letter words has been proposed over the years (MCD – minimal cerebral damage, POS – psycho-organic syndrome, etc.). Now the fashionable label is ADHD (attention deficit hyperactivity disorder) and again we encounter a field much too big to be handled exhaustively here. But the problems associated with and labeled as ADHD have a close connection with many of the phenomena we observe in children with problems originating in functional spinal disorders. In treating these children successfully one can at least alleviate the situation and thus give the families a new perspective.

The appeal of seeing metabolic problems as the basis of these disorders can be traced back to the elegant possibility of not looking into the interdependence of mind and body, of individual and environment, of nature and nurture. This bigger view involves the observer in the process, be it the worried parents or the therapist trying to help.

As in the treatment of migraine, we cannot get to the structural roots of the problem – we influence trigger mechanisms and aggravating circumstances. But in doing so, manual therapy can more often than not help these children and their families and provide the leeway necessary for a turnaround. Theiler, in Chapter 12, deals with some of these observations.

THE LONG TRADITION OF MTC – AND WHERE WE ARE HEADING FOR

Manual therapy in children is an old craft and part of the caregiving in almost all cultures, albeit without explicit mention as a treatment of spinal disorders. Leboyer (1976) published a beautiful book about Indian baby massage where many treatments have a striking similarity to techniques of MTC or soft-tissue osteopathy. Andry's seminal book on orthopedics (published in 1741) contains entire chapters about the treatment of newborn babies with postural asymmetries and similar practices are documented in books about massage (Baum 1906) or general healthcare (Cramer et al 1990).

With the 'scientification' of medicine in the nineteenth century the earlier oral history of 'Behandlung' (the German word for therapy, literally translated: 'something done with the hands') in the sense of manual therapy began to be recorded in textbooks, albeit under various headings such as massage, kneading the nerves, improving circulation. At that time, most explanations were based on mechanical models. At the end of the nineteenth century the paradigms used to understand the effects of these therapies were based on hydraulic or electric schemas. In the second half of the twentieth century the accent shifted to cybernetic or rather 'informatical' models – small surprise. The *Zeitgeist* inspires fashion in science, too.

So if one looks hard enough, there are morsels of MTC to be found even a few centuries back, and these scattered pieces of a big mosaic have many resemblances to the kind of MTC we support today. The basic difference can be found in the conceptual frame. The idea of a certain subgroup of children tending to react distinctively to functional disorders of the cervical spine came only after observing many babies and their families and taking into account their long-term development. We realized that the same trauma does not at all cause the same reaction in every child (and even less so in adults). We called these babies 'KISS kids' to indicate that their problems were at least partly systematic. The patterns we found first took us back to the moment of birth as an important trigger for these pathologies. Later on we realized that to understand the situation fully, one has to go back further, i.e. take into account the prenatal development and the disposition inherited from the parents too – genetic or epigenetic.

Alerted by the early onset of vertebrogenic disorders, we started systematically to screen the case histories of older children. The picture that evolved led us to the formulation of KIDD, i.e. a sensorimotor disorder based on an early (and untreated) KISS pathology. As these children are of school-age and have encountered many more external influences than the babies suffering from KISS, their web of pathology is much more complex. Whereas the chapter about KISS (Chapter 24) deals with a rather well-defined symptomatology, the KIDD chapter (Chapter 25) discusses a much more complex *Gestalt*.

Two pieces of circumstantial evidence make us surmise that KISS and KIDD influence the later course, too. We see a lot of parents with their problems after the babies have been treated successfully, and we see the same patterns in these problems. It goes without saying that in adults the situation is even more complex and difficult to decipher than in adolescents, but with the knowledge of what we found in their children, some details are more evident than if the parents were treated independently.

The gender of the parent who comes to seek treatment is by no means accidental – which is the second clue. When the baby is a boy it is far more probable for the father to come later on, and the same is true for daughter and mother. Quite often this gender-related predisposition extends into the entire clan, viz. the uncle or the grandfather of a baby boy who shows up.

These interesting observations are very difficult to verify in the context of a private consultation. But they are so clear-cut that even then one cannot but notice them. Much research needs to be done along these lines and it seems more than probable that this might help us to align our indications for manual therapy in general and MTC more particularly with the framework of mainstream pediatrics.

MTC DEPENDS ON SUPPORTING THERAPIES

In the following chapters we try to present those parts of manual therapy in (small) children that are different from the manual therapy we know in adults and to develop the rationale for the conceptual framework we propose for MTC. The main emphasis is on the systemic impact of appropriately applied manual therapy, thus preparing the ground for (re-)educating the sensorimotor system by means of ancillary specialties such as speech therapy or 'classic' physiotherapy.

To a superficial observer this manual therapy does not look very different from other forms of *contact treatment*. We shall try to explain the crucial distinctions which necessitate, on one hand, a much more precise evaluation of the patient to be treated and, on the other hand, sufficient time for the patient to adapt to this therapeutic impulse.

There is no sharp distinction between this variety of manual therapy and other therapies dealing with small children and using the upper cervical spine as a primary starting point – quite a lot of what we have to say is valid for these methods, too. But it would be imprecise to put all these methods in one big bag and treat them as interchangeable options. One of the most important differences – not least from the viewpoint of the family concerned – is our intention to minimize the impact of manual therapy on the small children we treat as much as possible. Any therapist has to strive to be as unobtrusive as possible.

After more than 20 years of practical experience we can say with some confidence that in the great majority of cases very few treatments suffice (see Chapter 17). This does not mean that there is no additional therapy complementing the initial effect of manual therapy; but these therapies follow different procedures and are better summarized under the broad label of *re-education*. These approaches do indeed need frequent and long-term application. Often the parents (or to be more honest: the mothers) are trained to treat their children on a daily basis in order to make these approaches work.

The most important aspect of this is to keep in mind that the situation in newborn babies is fundamentally different from what we know about adults or even from the situation in adolescents or older children. We shall not be successful in the analysis and treatment of the problems of the newborn if we are not aware of this.

It is not only the anatomy that is radically different. The most important discriminating factor is the absence of all 'learned' patterns apart from the few acquired in utero and during birth. This clean slate is an opportunity and a threat at the same time, enabling the newborn infant to develop very rapidly – in both good and bad directions.

Neurophysiological research suggests that we start life with a far greater amount of neurons and synapses than those we use as an adult. The structuring depends on the appropriate use and non-use of these connections ('use it or lose it'), thus giving the newborn baby an amazing variety of possible developmental paths and the environment an equally amazing influence on the developing neuromotor organization. We are about to learn how much our epigenetic pattern is formed in the perinatal period and how these few months determine large parts of the biography of an individual (Lopuhaa et al 2000, Roseboom et al 2000). We shall have to go back to this phenomenon time and again, as it influences nearly all aspects of our interaction with these small human beings.

This book tries to bridge the gap between the 'small' push on one side of the upper cervical spine of a child and the vast effects triggered by this intervention at a crucial spot and an equally crucial point in time. The broad range of contributors should give the interested a firm foundation from which to get to grips with this complex situation. We leave a lot of loose ends, and in the 3 years it took to finalize the book, quite a few bits of new information and ideas turned up to complete – and sometimes even correct – the concept. In that sense we present 'work in progress' – but in medicine, who doesn't?

References

Andry de Boisregard N 1741 L'orthopédie ou l'art de prévenir et de corriger dans les enfants les difformités du corps. Vv Alix, Paris

Bum A 1906 Handbuch der Massage und Heilgymnastik. Urban & Schwarzenberg, Berlin/Vienna

Cramer A, Doering J, Gutmann G 1990 Geschichte der manuellen Medizin. Springer, Berlin

Leboyer F 1976 Shantala, un Art traditionel: le massage des enfants. Seuil, Paris

Lopuhaa C E, Roseboom T J, Osmond C et al 2000 Atopy, lung function, and obstructive airways disease after prenatal exposure to famine. Thorax 55:555–561

Roseboom T J, van der Meulen J H, Osmond C et al 2000 Coronary heart disease after prenatal exposure to the Dutch famine, 1944–45. Heart 84:595–598

Sackett D, Richardson W, Rosenberg W et al 1997 Evidence-based Medicine. Elsevier Science, New York

Speransky A D 1950 Grundlagen der Theorie der Medizin. Verlag Werner Saenger, Berlin

Szent-Gyorgyi A 1972 What is life? Biology Today 24–26

Virchow R 1865 Die Cellularpathologie in ihrer Begründung auf physiologische und pathologische Gewebelehre. A Hischwald, Berlin

SECTION 1

The theoretical base

SECTION CONTENTS

Sensorimotor development of newborn and children from the viewpoint of manual therapy

H. Biedermann

On oublie rien de rien,
on s'habitue, c'est tout ...

Jacques Brel

All neurological development falls into two broad categories: pattern generation and pattern recognition. Most of the internal processes are dependent on a base rhythm, be it breathing or digestion. These are two examples with extremely different frequencies, the latter being coupled with the diurnal pattern and the former dependent on an internally generated pattern which undergoes multiple adaptive influences until it is finally carried out.

It is of basic importance to come to grips with the complexities of such a system based on an internal pattern generator and the external modifiers acting on it. The chapter by Ramirez (Chapter 5) takes us to the cutting edge research of micro-neurophysiology, and tries to unravel some of the intricacies of pattern generation.

These mechanisms are very old and shared between most vertebrates with only minor differences. The contribution of Huber (Chapter 6) on the other side deals with the complexities of pattern recognition and the surprising proficiency of very small children in decoding complex visual clues. From Huber we learn how early these abilities are trained and how a basic pattern recognition is established quite early in childhood. It is not too surprising that the research group Huber belongs to has not yet taken into account the influence that

11

the proper functioning of the upper cervical spine has on proprioception and head movement – these insights have only just reached neuropediatric research. But Huber's chapter gives us some clues as to how disturbances in proprioceptive input complicate the computation of spatial information. In Chapter 25 we examine some of the implications of this concept for the treatment of behavioral and neuromotor problems in schoolchildren.

The basic phenomenon – and the reason why disturbances in the early stages of neuromotor development exert such a wide-ranging influence – lies in the realization that we rarely 'unlearn' an acquired pattern. As Jacques Brel says in his famous 'chanson', we don't forget anything, we just get used to it. So patterns acquired in early childhood can influence our behavior years and decades later. This makes the understanding of neuromotor development at the beginning of our life so important. The postnatal period is paramount for our understanding of this process, as it is the first time we are able actively and directly to influence these developments.

Onto this basic level of interaction many other influences are added, from the primal needs of food and drink, to warmth and support in the all-important immersion in a stable and loving atmosphere in the baby's home, with as much bodily contact as possible (Cattaneo et al 1998, Cleary et al 1997, Feldman et al 2002, Fohe et al 2000, Ludington-Hoe et al 1991, Simkiss 1999, Tessier et al 1998). To cast the net even wider, one has to evaluate the socioeconomic status of the family and its social integration in a local community (Wilkinson 1996, Wolf and Bruhn 1997) – a dimension of wellbeing often overlooked or underestimated.

Even if we were able to take these aspects into account when evaluating the child's future, we would not be in a situation to do much about it. The big advantage of manual therapy in early childhood is that it gives us an opportunity to improve the situation of a child without interfering with the other forms of help available and – last but not least – without a big investment in time and energy. We are able to help children even

in situations where other forms of therapy would not work because the amount of discipline and persistence they require is not likely to be forthcoming from the families concerned.

Immersed in the treadmill of our daily work we tend to forget what we learned during our studies – and are not even aware of all the new information produced since we left university. One motivation behind this part of the book was to help in overcoming this. The chapters by Huang and Christ (Chapter 3) and Hori (Chapter 4) present the state-of-the-art information concerning embryological development in the cervical area and the central nervous system and its deviations.

This information should enable a better understanding of the context in which we are working. A solid knowledge of the basic facts about anatomy and neurophysiology will help us to improve our diagnoses and especially to develop the 'sixth-sense' which alerts the diagnostician when an unusual situation is encountered. In discussions with colleagues about the – rare – occasions when they found severe problems while examining children, almost all of them admitted that before they actually identified the diagnostic problem they had had a hunch that something was not quite as it should be. The information contained in the following pages should help to alert one to these unusual cases.

Or to put it another way, the chapters in Section 1 can be seen as an antidote against too much confidence of the style 'I am so successful that I don't bother about the details'. If we keep reminding ourselves how much there is to know about the incredibly complex web of dependencies we will maintain a healthy fear of overlooking something. This is even more important in MTC than in other specialties as there are times when one 'simple' case seems to follow another, and lulled into a false sense of security with our 'diagnostic auto pilot' we might overlook the small sign that should warn us.

Last but not least, these chapters (and Hori's in particular) remind us about the differential diagnosis of all the phenomena that may comprise KISS – but may be a sign of quite another underlying pathology, too.

References

Cattaneo A, Davanzo R, Bergman N et al 1998 Kangaroo mother care in low-income countries. International Network in Kangaroo Mother Care. Journal of Tropical Pediatrics 44(5):279–282

Cleary G M, Spinner S S, Gibson E et al 1997 Skin-to-skin parental contact with fragile preterm infants. Journal of the American Osteopathic Association 97(8):457–460

Feldman R, Weller A, Sirota L et al 2002 Skin-to-skin contact (Kangaroo care) promotes self-regulation in premature infants: sleep-wake cyclicity, arousal modulation, and sustained exploration. Developmental Psychology 38(2):194–207

Fohe K, Kropf S, Avenarius S 2000 Skin-to-skin contact improves gas exchange in premature infants. Journal of Perinatology 20(5):311–315

Ludington-Hoe S M, Hadeed A J, Anderson G C 1991 Physiologic responses to skin-to-skin contact in hospitalized premature infants. Journal of Perinatology 11(1):19–24

Simkiss D E 1999 Kangaroo mother care. Journal of Tropical Pediatrics 45(4):192–194

Tessier R, Cristo M, Velez S et al 1998 Kangaroo mother care and the bonding hypothesis. Pediatrics 102(2):e17

Wilkinson R G 1996 Unhealthy societies: the afflictions of inequality. Routledge, London

Wolf S, Bruhn J G 1997 The power of clan: the influence of human relationships on heart disease. Transaction, London

Chapter 3

Development and topographical anatomy of the cervical spine

R. Huang, B. Christ

'The neck, *cervix (collum)*, is a mobile connecting structure between head and trunk. The supporting element of the neck is the cervical spine (cervical spinal column), the most cranial part of the vertebral column. The vertebral column and parts of the cranium represent the axial structures of the human body. The vertebral column comprises 33 vertebral segments, *vertebrae*, connected to each other by fibrocartilaginous intervertebral disks, ligaments and muscles. Its function is to support the trunk and protect the spinal cord. The cervical spine provides a morphological basis for an extensive freedom of head movement. In addition, the cervical vertebral column serves as a bridge for numerous blood and lymphatic vessels and nerves, linking head, trunk and upper limb.

Developmental abnormalities of the cervical vertebral column can affect these functions. For example, the Klippel–Feil syndrome, in which a short cervical vertebral column develops, is characterized by a reduction of head mobility, migraine headache and paresthesia of the arm and hand. Further examples of vertebral abnormalities are cervical ribs and spina bifida, atlas assimilation and fused vertebrae.

In the thoracic vertebral column, the costal processes grow laterally to form a series of ribs. The costal processes normally do not extend distally in the cervical vertebral column, but occasionally they do so in the case of the seventh cervical vertebra, even developing costovertebral joints. Such cervical ribs may even reach the sternum. Neural arches and their ligaments form a protective roof over the vertebral canal for the spinal cord. Occasionally the coalescence of vertebral laminae is incomplete, a cleft of variable width being left through which dura and arachnoid mater may protrude. Part of the spinal cord with its pia mater also commonly projects, a condition known as spina bifida.

The malformation is more common in the lumbosacral regions, but may also occur at thoracic or cervical levels. Fusion of two or more vertebrae may occasionally be observed in the developing vertebral column. The atlas, normally forming an articulation between the cranial end of the vertebral column and the head, may fuse with the occipital bone, so-called atlas assimilation or occipitalization of the first cervical vertebra. An understanding of normal development and topography of the cervical vertebral column could help in understanding the basis for such vertebral abnormalities and their symptoms.

PRENATAL DEVELOPMENT

The most specialized part of the cervical vertebral column is the cervico-occipital transitional region. Striking features of this region are already apparent during development. Although the posterior part of the cranium and the vertebral column derive from the same primordium, a boundary develops between the head and the neck. The primordium located cranially to this boundary is included in the development of the head. The cervico-occipital transitional region represents a very special body part that not only provides the material for the formation of the axial skeleton but also participates in the development of essential organs such as heart, gastrointestinal tract, and kidney.

The vertebral column develops from somites, the first visible segmental units of the embryo. In older papers the somites have been called 'protovertebrae' and therefore have been related to the

'vertebrae', the definitive structures of the vertebral column. The development of the vertebral column reveals a primary segmentation (the somite formation) and secondary segmentation (resegmentation of the vertebral column). The specification of the vertebrae is controlled by a genetic program, namely the *Hox* genes. The primary and secondary segmentation and the segmental specification will be discussed in the next section.

Primary segmentation and somite formation

The occipital bone, the vertebral column and their skeletal musculature develop commonly from a compartment of the intermediate layer (mesoderm) (Fig. 3.1). This can be divided into paraxial mesoderm, intermediate mesoderm and the lateral plate mesoderm. The paraxial mesoderm flanks the axial organs (neural tube and notochord). It consists of a preotical part, located cranially to the ear placode, and a postotical part, extending caudally from the ear placode into the neck and the trunk. The postotical paraxial mesoderm becomes segmented, while the preotical part does not. Segmentation of the paraxial mesoderm is characterized by somite formation. The somites are the first clearly delineated segmental units. They are formed in pairs by epithelialization from the paraxial mesoderm. The first somite pair arises directly behind the ear placode and the further somites develop one by one in a craniocaudal direction. New mesenchymal cells enter the paraxial mesoderm at its caudal end as a consequence of gastrulation. The newly formed paraxial mesoderm is not immediately segmented. The part of the paraxial mesoderm prior to somite formation is called the segmental plate or presomitic mesoderm.

The fundamental prerequisite for somite formation is the growth of the paraxial mesoderm. This growth is controlled by gastrulation genes and the fibroblast growth factor 8 (FGF-8) that is produced in the caudal part of the segmental plate. The

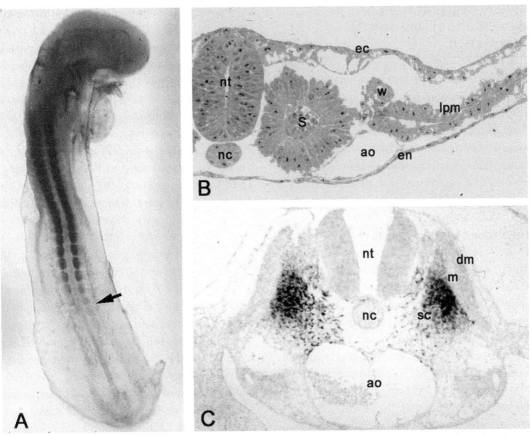

Figure 3.1   A: *Pax-1* expression in the somites of a 2-day-old chick embryo. The arrow marks the boundary between the newly formed somite and the segmental plate. B: Transverse section through a cervical somite. C: Transverse section through a 3-day-old chick embryo. Division of the somite in a dermomyotome (dm) and a sclerotome (sc). Expression of *Pax-1* in sclerotome. ao, aorta; ec, ectoderm; en, endoderm; nc, notochord; nt, neural tube; S, somite; w, Wolff's duct; lpm, lateral plate mesoderm.

quantity of FGF-8 secretion determines the size of the developing somite (Dubrulle et al 2001).

Segmentation was found to be controlled by a molecular mechanism called the 'segmentation clock' (Pourquie 2000). This clock contains molecular oscillators that are characterized by the rhythmic production of mRNAs. The 'hairy, lunatic fringe' gene and genes of the Delta-Notch signaling pathway belong to these segmentation genes. The expression pattern of these genes appears as waves that roll through the segmental plate from its caudal to its cranial end, and each wave is initiated once during formation of one somite. This means that these genes are expressed 12 times in each segmental plate cell before it becomes integrated in a somite at its cranial end.

The gene oscillation leads to a maturation of the segmental plate. Morphologically, this maturation is characterized by a cell condensation and a mesenchymal-to-epithelial transition of the cells in the cranial part of the segmental plate. The epithelialization requires the expression of the bHLH gene *paraxis* (Burgess et al 1996). Epithelialization of the segmental plate mesoderm and somite formation are severely affected in *paraxis* null mutant mice. As a consequence, these mice develop a vertebral column that is not regularly segmented.

Secondary segmentation (resegmentation) and somite differentiation

Remak (1850), who was studying whole mount chick embryos, made the observation that the boundaries of the definitive vertebrae are shifted one half segment as compared to those of the 'protovertebrae' (somites). This so-called 'Neugliederung' (resegmentation) was observed in various species and was thought to be achieved by a new combination of somite halves. A secondary segmentation appears within each somite: an intrasegmental fissure divides its ventral compartment, the sclerotome, into a cranial and caudal half and marks the boundary of the definitive vertebra. This means that the fusion of the caudal half of one sclerotome with the cranial half of the next one forms one vertebra. Two neighboring vertebrae are thereafter articulated by an intervertebral disk whose primordium is situated caudally to an intrasegmental fissure, the so-called von Ebner fissure (von Ebner 1889). Muscle cells develop from the dorsal compartment of the somite, the dermomyotome, and are not affected by this craniocaudal subdivision. Muscles derived from one somite are therefore attached to two adjacent vertebrae. This means that resegmentation is required for appropriate movement of the vertebral column.

To form a functional vertebral column, somites undergo a dorsoventral and a craniocaudal compartmentalization. Newly formed somites are masses of mesodermal cells with a small cavity in the middle, the somitocoel (Fig. 3.1). The cells are arranged epithelially and radially arround the somitocoel, which is occupied by mesenchymal cells. Extracellular matrix connects the somite to adjacent structures (neural tube, notochord, ectoderm, endoderm, aorta, Wolffian duct). A continuous cell layer connects the lateral portion of the somite to the intermediate mesoderm and thus indirectly to the lateral plate mesoderm. Under the influence of ventralizing signals such as Sonic hedgehog (Shh) from the notochord and the floor plate of the neural tube, *Pax-1* and *Pax-9* become

expressed in the somitocoel cells and the ventral somite half (Fig. 3.1). This leads to an epithelio-mesenchymal transition of this somite part. Their cells form the mesenchymal sclerotome which gives rise to basioccipital bone, vertebrae, intervertebral disks and ribs. Dorsal signals are derived from both the surface ectoderm and the dorsal neural tube, which belongs to the *Wnt* family of genes. *Wnt-1* and *Wnt-3a* are expressed in the dorsal neural tube and *Wnt-6* in the ectoderm. These signals promote the development of the dorsal compartment which keeps its epithelial structure and forms the dermomyotome. *Pax-3* and *Pax-7* are expressed by their cells. Cells located in the four edges of the dermomyotome de-epithelialize and elongate in a longitudinal direction. These cells differentiate into myogenic cells and form a cell layer, the myotome, between dermomyotome and sclerotome. Both ventral (Shh) and dorsal signals (Wnt proteins) are required for the specification of myogenic cells in the epaxial domain of the somite.

The sclerotome divides into a cranial and a caudal half along the longitudinal axis (Fig. 3.2). Determination of this craniocaudal polarization is acquired prior to somite formation in the cranial portion of the segmental plate and depends on the Delta/Notch signaling pathway. The prospective

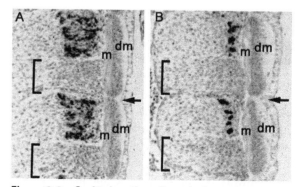

Figure 3.2 Sagittal sections through the metameric primordium of the spinal ganglia (A) and the spinal nerves (B). The nerve placode is visualized with antibody. dm, dermomyotome; m, myotome; the brackets mark the caudal sclerotome halves and the arrows the boundary between two adjacent somites.

somitic halves can be identified by the expression domains of various genes. *Delta 1, Mesp1,2* are expressed in the caudal half and *EphA4* in the cranial half of the prospective somites in the cranial part of the segmental plate. The craniocaudal compartmentalization is indispensable for the development of the metameric vertebral column and for the secondary metamerism of the peripheral nervous system. Different genes are activated in the cranial and caudal sclerotome halves. The transmembrane protein ephrin and the Eph receptors are important molecules of these compartments. Eph receptor is situated in the cell membrane of the migrating neural crest cells, while ephrin is expressed exclusively in the caudal sclerotome half. The interaction between ephrin and its receptor stops the migration of neural crest cells. So the axons of motor nerves and the neural crest cells forming the dorsal root ganglia invade the cranial half-segment whereas the caudal half-segment acts as a barrier to axon and neural crest cell invasion.

Uncx4.1 is expressed in the caudal sclerotome half and is essential for the formation of the neural arch. When *Uncx4.1* function is lost experimentally, the neural arch cannot be formed and the dorsal root ganglia fuse together to form an unsegmented cell mass next to the spinal cord.

As discussed above, the sclerotome is the derivative of the ventral half of the somite epithelium and the mesenchymal somitocoel cells. Ventral signals are able to induce the expression of *Pax-1* and *Pax-9* in the sclerotome. However, it has to be kept in mind that only the ventromedial part of the sclerotome continues to express *Pax-1* and *Pax-9*. Sclerotome cells that do not express these *Pax*-genes are situated at the ventrolateral and the dorsomedial angles of the sclerotome. *Pax-1*-positive cells of the ventromedial sclerotome migrate into the initially cell-free perinotochordal space to form the mesenchymal perinotochordal tube, which develops into the vertebral bodies and intervertebral disks.

The fate of the cells in the dorsomedial angle is not quite clear. Grafting experiments indicate that these cells migrate in a dorsomedial direction to form the dorsal mesenchyme which contributes to the dorsal part of the neural arch and the spinous process. *Msx1* and *Msx2* have been found to be expressed in this mesenchyme and to be controlled by the roof plate of the neural tube and possibly the surface ectoderm via BMP4 signaling. Interruption of this cross-talk could be one of the reasons for the malformations of the dorsal vertebral column, such as spina bifida. *Pax-3* is expressed in the dorsal neural tube and in *Splotch* mice in which the homeobox domain of the *Pax-3* gene is mutated, the development of the dorsal neural tube is affected, resulting in the formation of a spina bifida.

The fate of the cells in the ventrolateral angle of the sclerotome remains to be studied. These cells are located in the transitional region of the paraxial to the intermediate mesoderm and might contribute to kidney formation. In addition, these cells could represent a cell population that participates in the development of the ribs. Recent studies have suggested a two-stage model of rib development. In the first instance, Shh emanating from the axial structures induces the development of the sclerotome and also the expression of *Fgf-8* in the myotome. Secondly, the ventrolateral domain of the sclerotome becomes expanded, controlled by FGFs secreted by myotome cells.

The vertebral disks located between adjacent surfaces of vertebral bodies from C_2 (axis) to the sacrum are the main junction between the vertebral bodies. Each disk consists of an outer laminated *annulus fibrosus* and an inner *nucleus pulposus*. The intervertebral disk is derived from somitocoel cells (Huang et al 1994, 1996). The cells of the intervertebral disk still express *Pax-1* when it is already downregulated in the vertebral body anlagen. *Pax-1* expression is most likely to promote proliferation of disk cells (Wilting et al 1995). An early downregulation of *Pax*-expression is observed in the basioccipital germ, in which the disk primodia degenerate leading to a fusion of the chondrogenic vertebral anlagen. Pathologically fused vertebrae can occasionally arise after an early downregulation of *Pax-1* expression. In the late development, the notochord disappears from the vertebral bodies and expands into the condensed mesenchymal primordia of the intervertebral disks. In the adult, the notochord persists as nucleus pulposus, while somitocoel-derived mesodermal cells form the annulus fibrosus of the intervertebral disk.

The morphogenesis of the vertebral column reflects the development of the vertebral motion segment. The vertebral motion segment is a functional entity consisting of two adjacent vertebrae, the intervertebral disk, ligaments, and muscles that act on the segment (Schmorl and Junghanns 1968). Therefore, one vertebra is part of two adjacent motion segments. The motion segment also includes spinal nerves and blood vessels. The relationship between the somite and the motion segment has been investigated by using the biological cell tracing method of quail-chick chimeras (Huang et al 1996, 2000a, 2000b). Skeletal elements, ligaments, muscle, and connective tissue of a motion segment originate from one somite. Somitocoel cells give rise to primordial material of the intervertebral disks and are positioned in the articulation part of the motion segment. The intersegmental muscle is made up of myogenic cells from one somite, whereas the superficial segment-overlapping muscle consists of myogenic cells from several somites.

Segmental identity

The vertebral column consists of 7 cervical, 12 thoracic, 5 lumbar, 5 sacral and 4 coccygeal vertebrae. The cervical vertebrae show very special characteristics. For example, the seven cervical vertebrae are typified by a foramen in each transverse process. The vertebral artery and its vein run through the foramina. Furthermore, the cervical pedicles and laminae enclose a large, roughly triangular vertebral foramen, forming a channel for the spinal cord.

Comparing the seven cervical vertebrae with each other, one can find conspicuous differences in size and shape. In particular, the first (atlas) and second (axis) have special features and differ greatly from the other cervical vertebrae. The atlas consists of two lateral masses connected by a short anterior and a longer posterior arch. The transverse ligament retains the dens against the anterior arch. The transverse processes are longer than those of all cervical vertebrae except the seventh vertebra. They act as strong levers for the short neck muscles, making fine adjustments for keeping the head balanced. The axis is an axle for rotation of the atlas and head around the dens, which projects cranially from the axis body. The third to sixth cervical vertebrae have small, relatively broad vertebral bodies, and short and bifid spinous processes. The seventh cervical vertebra has a long spinous process.

As described above, each cervical vertebra has its own identity, so-called segmental identity. The segmental individualization of sclerotomal derivatives along the craniocaudal axis is already determined in the segmental plate. When cervical somites are grafted into the thoracic region, ribs and scapula do not develop in this thoracic region (Kieny et al 1972).

Each newly formed somite is identical to every other somite, in so far as it gives rise to the same cell types (muscle, bone, dermis, endothelial cells). The developmental fate of somites at different axial levels has been found to be determined by the *Hox* genes, which include at least 38 members representing 13 paralogous groups aligned in four clusters (a–d). Expression of the *Hox* genes begins dynamically in the prospective somites and persists stably in the somite until the beginning of chondrification in the primordia of the vertebrae. *Hox* genes show a cranial-to-caudal expression pattern with a sequence of cranial expression boundaries that corresponds to their alignment on the chromosomes (Duboule and Dolle 1989). The identity of the vertebrae may be specified by a unique combination of *Hox* genes, called the *Hox* code (Kessel and Gruss 1991).

For example, in the mouse the atlas is characterized by the expression of *Hoxb-1, Hoxa-1, Hoxa-3* and *Hoxd-4*. The axis is specified by these four, plus *Hoxa-4* and *Hoxb-4*. Changes in *Hox* gene expression lead to a homeotic transformation of the vertebrae. When *Hox-1.1* transgene was introduced into the germline of mice, the cranial part of the vertebral column was posteriorized. The base of the occipital bone was transformed into a vertebra (proatlas), and the atlas was fused with its centrum, resulting in an axis that did not possess an odontoid process.

The question of how *Hox* genes are regulated and how they act on the behavior of sclerotome cells remains to be studied. It has been shown that retinoic acid controls the activity of *Hox* genes. Application of retinoic acid can cause cranial or caudal level shifts in the overall segmental organization of the vertebrae. It has been suggested that *Hox* genes regulate downstream genes that control the level-specific identity. These genes determine the proliferation, apoptosis, migration and differentiation of sclerotome cells.

As discussed above, the basioccipital bone and spine generally develop from the somites. The boundary between these two axial structures is located in the middle of somite 5. Thus, sclerotome of the first 4.5 somites lose their segmental characteristic and fuse to form a skeletal mass, the basioccipital bone. This process coincides with a downregulation of *Pax-1* in the intervertebral disks (Wilting et al 1995). The atlas and the axis differ not only in their morphology but also in their development from the typical vertebra. The typical vertebra is formed by two adjacent somite halves. However, the atlas is formed only by the caudal half of somite 5, while the axis arises from three somites: the caudal half of somite 5, the whole of somite 6 and the cranial half of somite 7. So the axis can be considered as the result of the fusion of two vertebrae. The cranial part of the axis derives from the caudal half of somite 5 and the cranial half of somite 6, while the caudal part originates from the caudal half of somite 6 and the cranial half of somite 7. The fusion of these two vertebrae is due to the degeneration of the original intervertebral disk between them during development (Huang et al 2000a, Wilting et al 1995). The

notochord between the basioccipital and the dens axis forms a ligament, the apical ligament of dens. The third, fourth, fifth, sixth and seven cervical vertebrae derive from sclerotome halves of two adjacent cervical somites, respectively.

POSTNATAL DEVELOPMENT

The structure of the vertebral column undergoes progressive change in the postnatal period, affecting its growth and morphology. This process continues in adulthood. Vertebral column morphology is influenced externally by mechanical as well as environmental factors and internally by genetic, metabolic and hormonal factors. These all affect its ability to react to dynamic forces, such as compression, traction and shear. The postnatal development of the cervical spine will be discussed here from different aspects, such as ossification, uncovertebral articulation and curvatures.

Ossification of the cervical vertebrae

A typical cervical vertebra consists of hyaline cartilage with three separate primary ossification centers, which appear in the ninth to tenth week after birth. One is located in each half of the vertebral arch and the other one in the body. Centers in the arches appear at the roots of the transverse processes and from there the ossification spreads backwards, forwards, upwards, downwards and laterally into the adjacent parts of the vertebra. The major part of the body, the centrum, ossifies from a primary center located dorsally to the notochord.

The atlas is normally ossified from three centers. Each lateral mass has one ossification center at about the seventh week. Both centers extend gradually into the posterior arch and fuse together between the third and fourth year. The third center appears in the anterior arch at the end of the first year and fuses with the lateral masses between the sixth and eighth year. Ossification of the axis is more complex (Ogden 1984).

It has five primary and two secondary centers. Each vertebral arch and the body is ossified from one center, as in a typical vertebra. The two centers in the vertebral arch appear about the seventh or eighth week, and the one in the body about the fourth or fifth month. The dens is ossified from two primary and two secondary bilateral centers. The primary centers of the dens appear about the sixth month and are separated from the center in the vertebral body by a cartilaginous region. The primary centers of the dens and the body most often fuse between the fifth and eighth years, but sometimes even later, at about the twelfth year. Before fusion of these three centers, the synchondrosis between them is situated below the level of the atlantoaxial joints. It must be distinguished from a fracture, which usually spreads along this structure in infants and children. Two secondary ossification centers, so-called ossiculum terminale, appear in the apex of the dens at 8–10 years. Fusion of the ossiculum terminale with the rest of the dens occurs between the tenth and thirteenth years.

Development of the uncovertebral joint

At birth the intervertebral disks are composed mainly of the nucleus pulposus. It is a large, soft, gelatinous structure of mucoid material with a few multinucleated notochord cells, invaded also by cells and fibers from the inner zone of the adjacent annulus fibrosus. Notochordal cells disappear in the first decade, followed by gradual replacement of mucoid material by fibrocartilage, mainly derived from the annulus fibrosus and the hyaline cartilaginous plate adjoining vertebral bodies. The nucleus pulposus becomes much reduced in the adult as the annulus fibrosus develops. A further characteristic feature of the developing cervical vertebral column is a gradual appearance of a cross-fissure in the intervertebral disk (Töndury 1958). After examination of over 150 cervical vertebral columns, Töndury made the observation that this so-called uncovertebral

fissure begins to form first at the age of 9 years. The annulus fibrosus is torn in its lateral part under the influence of gliding by vertebral rotation. This tearing occurs in normal tissue and cannot be considered a degeneration phenomenon of the intervertebral disk. It seems to be a prerequisite for the extensive cervical vertebral rotation. The tear extends from the peripheral to central region. Finally the cells of the nucleus pulposus come out of the disk through the fissure. While at the age of 18–20 years, one can still find intact intervertebral disks in the cervical vertebral column, after the age of 20 years, each cervical intervertebral disk reveals a fissure.

The uncinate process develops almost synchronously with the uncovertebral fissure. At the age of 9 years the bone tissue of the neural arch rises up adjacent to the lateral lip of the upper surface of the vertebral body. At the end of the proliferation period, the uncinate process has a shovel-shaped bony ridge and fuses with the vertebral body. Thus the superior surface of the vertebral body is saddle-shaped, while the inferior surface is flat or minimally concave. The intervertebral disk, which is split into cranial and caudal halves by the uncovertebral fissure, forms a gliding surface on the two adjacent vertebral bodies. So an uncovertebral joint forms between two adjacent vertebral bodies. This articulation makes the extensive mobility of the cervical spine easier.

Development of curvatures of the cervical spine

In the normal vertebral column, there are no lateral curvatures, but S-shaped curvatures are seen in the sagittal plane. Curvatures appear as a response to fetal movements as early as 7 weeks in utero. Primary thoracic and pelvic curves are due to the bending posture of the embryo. Muscle development leads to the early appearance of secondary cervical and lumbar spinal curvatures. However, the vertebral column has no fixed curvatures in the neonate. It is so flexible that when dissected free from the body it can easily be bent into a perfect half circle. The cervical curvature develops when the head can be held erect from 3 months of age onwards and the lumbar curvature when walking starts from 1 year of age onwards. In adults, the cervical curve is bent forwards forming a lordosis. It extends from the atlas to the second thoracic vertebra, with its apex between the fourth and the fifth cervical vertebrae.

TOPOGRAPHY

The neck is the bridge between head and trunk. Great vessels and nerves as well as the visceral structures run through the neck. The vertebral arteries, the important arteries of the brain, are topographically the closest vessels to the cervical spine. The vertebral artery arises from the subclavian artery, ascends caudocranially, and finally enters the foramen transversarium of vertebra C_6. The artery passes through the foramina of the cervical transverse processes of C_6–C_1, curves medially behind the lateral mass of the atlas and then enters the cranium via the foramen magnum. Occasionally, it may enter the bone at the fourth, fifth or seventh cervical transverse foramen. Its vein passes through the same pathway as the artery.

The cervical spinal nerves are also topographically very closely related to the cervical spine. Their dorsal rami originate just beyond the spinal ganglion and pass backward on the side of the superior articular process. They supply the skin and the deep (intrinsic) muscles of the back. Deep muscles of the back developed from the epaxial myotome (see above in the section on secondary segmentation and somite differentiation) are found dorsally to the cervical vertebral column. The topography of these muscles is shown in a dissection of a fetus (Fig. 3.3). The splenius muscle (Fig. 3.3A) wraps around the other deep muscles in the neck, as its name implies (Latin: splenius = a bandage). It arises from the lower half of the ligamentum nuchae and from the upper thoracic spinous processes. The muscle separates into two

parts: splenius cervicis and splenius capitis. The splenius cervicis muscle joins the levator scapulae muscle to share its attachments to the transverse processes C_1–C_4. The splenius capitis shares the attachments of the sternocleidomastoid muscle to the superior nuchal line and the mastoid process. The semispinalis capitis muscle is located beneath the splenius muscle. The semispinalis capitis muscle passes from the upper thoracic and lower cervical transverse processes (C_4 to T_5) to the occipital bone between the superior and inferior nuchal lines.

The semispinalis cervicis and the suboccipital muscles are located beneath the semispinalis capitis muscle (Fig. 3.3B). The semispinalis cervicis muscle arises from the transverse process of T_6–C_7 and inserts into the cervical spinous processes (C_6–C_2).

The suboccipital muscles are shown in Figure 3.3B and C. The rectus capitis posterior minor muscle arises from the posterior tubercle of the atlas, the rectus capitis posterior major muscle from the spinous process of the axis. These two muscles are attached side by side to the occipital bone between the inferior nuchal line and the foramen magnum. The obliquus capitis inferior muscle passes from the spinous process of the axis obliquely upward and forward to the tip of the transverse process of the atlas. The obliquus capitis superior muscle passes from the tip of the transverse process of the atlas obliquely upward and backward to be inserted between the two nuchal lines of the occipital bone.

The four suboccipital muscles are very well innervated (Voss 1958). They have many more muscle spindles than other neck muscles and are able to precisely inform the position of the head in relation to the neck. These muscles are innervated by the suboccipital nerve, the dorsal ramus of the first cervical spinal nerve. It emerges between the occipital bone and the atlas, and then reaches its target muscles.

The great occipital nerve, the dorsal ramus of the second cervical spinal nerve, emerges between the posterior arch of the atlas and the lamina of the axis (Fig. 3.3D), below the inferior oblique muscle (Fig. 3.3C). It then ascends between the inferior oblique and semispinalis capitis muscles, and pierces the occipital attachments of the semispinalis capitis and the trapezius muscles. It supplies the skin of the scalp as far as the vertex.

The trapezius and the sternocleidomastoid muscles are superficial cervical muscles of the neck. Both of them are split from one sheet of embryonic muscle that originates from the higher cervical somites. Both muscles are innervated by the accessory nerve. Cranially, these two muscles have a continuous attachment extending from the mastoid process to the protuberantia occipitalis externa. Caudally they have a discontinuous attachment to the clavicle. Both of them are enveloped in the superficial lamina of the cervical fascia.

The ventral rami of the upper four cervical spinal nerves form the cervical plexus. It supplies some neck muscles, the diaphragm and areas of the skin in the head, neck and chest. The superficial branches of the cervical plexus perforate the cervical fascia behind the sternocleidomastoid muscle to supply the skin of the occipital and cervical region, while the deep branches (ansa cervicalis and phrenicus nerve) supply infrahyoid and diaphragm muscles. The superficial branches are

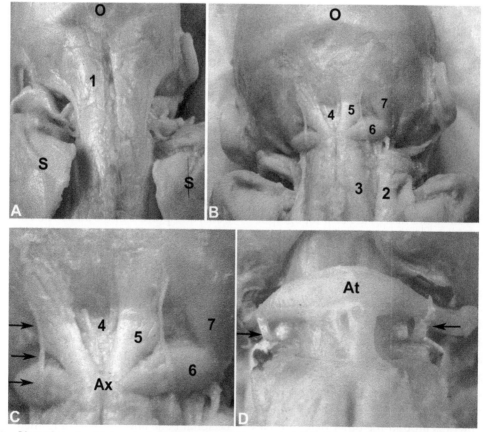

Figure 3.3 Dissection of a fetal neck. A: Semispinalis capitis muscle (1). B: Suboccipital muscles (4–7). C, D: Topography of the great occipital nerve (arrows). 2, caudal part of transversely cut semispinalis capitis muscle; 3, semispinalis cervicis muscle; 4, rectus capitis posterior minor muscle; 5, rectus capitis posterior major muscle; 6, obliquus capitis inferior muscle; 7, obliquus capitis superior muscle; Ax, the spinous process of the axis; At, the posterior arch of the atlas; O, occipital bone; S, scapula.

lesser occipital (C_2), greater auricular (C_2, C_3), transverse cutaneous nerve of the neck (C_2, C_3) and supraclavicular nerves (C_3, C_4).

The ventral rami of the lower four cervical and the first thoracic spinal nerves tie into the brachial plexus, which supplies the shoulder girdle and upper limb muscles. The brachial plexus emerges between the scaleni anterior and medius that arise from the upper cervical transverse processes and descend to the first rib. Inferior to the brachial plexus, the subclavian artery also passes through the gap between the scaleni anterior and medius. In the case of a cervical rib the scaleni gap could become narrow, leading to a compression of the brachial plexus.

While the dorsal neck musculature is relatively compact, the ventral one is divided into several layers and enveloped by three lamina of the cervical fascia. The superficial lamina of the cervical fascia is continuous with the ligamentum nuchae. It forms a thin covering for the trapezius muscle, covers the posterior triangle of the neck, encloses the sternocleidomastoid muscle, covers the anterior triangle of the neck and reaches forwards to the midline. Here it meets the corresponding lamina from the opposite side.

The pretracheal lamina of the cervical fascia is very thin, and provides a fine fascial sheath for the infrahyoid muscles. The four paired infrahyoid muscles are depressors of the larynx and hyoid bone. The sternohyoid and omohyoid muscles attach side by side to the hyoid body. The sternohyoid runs down to the posterior aspect of the capsule of the sternoclavicular joint and adjacent bone. The omohyoid muscle leaves the sternohyoid muscle abruptly below the level of the cricoid cartilage, passes beneath the sternocleidomastoid muscle, and crosses the posterior triangle to the upper border of the scapula. The thyrohyoid muscle extends upward to the greater horn and the body of the hyoid bone. The sternothyroid muscle converges on its fellow as it descends, until their medial borders meet at the center of the posterior surface of the manubrium. The pretracheal cervical fascia envelops these muscles and attaches to the prevertebral cervical fascia laterally to the omohyoid muscle. Our study of the development of avian tongue muscles showed that the infrahyoid muscles are formed by the myogenic cells migrating from the occipital and higher cervical somites, like the intrinsic tongue muscles (Huang et al 1999). Thus they are innervated by the hypoglossal nerve and the ansa cervicalis.

The carotid sheath is a condensation of the pretracheal lamina of the cervical fascia around the common and internal carotid arteries, the internal jugular vein, and the vagus nerve. The common carotid arteries originate from the brachiocephalic trunk (right carotid artery) and directly from the aortic arch (left carotid artery). The carotid arteries ascend to the thyroid cartilage's upper border, where they divide into external and internal carotid arteries. The internal jugular vein collects blood from the skull, brain, face and neck. It begins at the cranial base in the jugular foramen and descends in the carotid sheath, joining with the subclavian vein. The vagus nerve descends vertically in the neck in the carotid sheath. After emerging from the jugular foramen the vagus has two enlargements, the superior and inferior ganglion.

The prevertebral lamina of the cervical fascia covers the deep anterior vertebral muscles and extends laterally on the scalenus anterior, scalenus medius and levator scapulae muscles. Deep anterior cervical muscles are the longus colli (cervicis) and longus capitis muscles. The longus colli muscle extends from the body of the third thoracic vertebra to the anterior tubercle of the atlas, and it is attached to the bodies of the vertebrae in between. The longus capitis muscle arises from the third, fourth, fifth and sixth anterior tubercles and ascends to the basioccipital bone to be attached behind the plane of the pharyngeal tubercle.

The cervical sympathetic trunk is an upward extension of the thoracic sympathetic nerves. It ascends through the neck between the longus colli muscle and the prevertebral lamina of the cervical fascia. It has three interconnected ganglia. The superior cervical ganglion is located at the level of the second and third cervical vertebrae. The middle one is usually found at the sixth cervical vertebra level. The third one is the cervico-thoracic ganglion, which lies between the seventh cervical transverse process and the neck of the first rib.

The viscera cord, consisting of the pharynx, esophagus, larynx and trachea as well as the thyroid gland, runs through the space between the pretracheal and prevertebral lamina. The whole larynx is located at the axial level between the hyoid bone and the cricoid cartilage in adult men. These three structures extend over three cervical vertebrae (Fig. 3.4). The hyoid bone is at the level of the intervertebral disk between the fourth and the fifth vertebral bodies. The upper border of the larynx is about one vertebral body deeper than the hyoid bone and thus located at the level of the intervertebral disk between the fifth and the sixth vertebral bodies. The lower border of the cricoid cartilage is nearly at the level of the boundary between the cervical and thoracic vertebral column.

The larynx of adult women is placed a bit higher than in men. The lower border of the cricoid cartilage corresponds to the level of the intervertebral disk between the sixth and seventh vertebrae. In childhood, the larynx is considerably higher than in the adult. Before birth the cricoid cartilage corresponds to the level of the fourth cervical vertebra bottom. Owing to the growth of visceral cranium and descent of the thoracic and cervical organs, the larynx descends during postnatal development. The descent of the larynx is schematically illustrated in Figure 3.4. In puberty the larynx reaches the adult position.

CONCLUSION

In summary, our review shows that the morphological and topographical complexity of the cervical spine arises from its regional specific and genetically well-coordinated development. This leads to the ability for wide and precise movements and, on the other hand, guarantees the function of the structures situated in it.

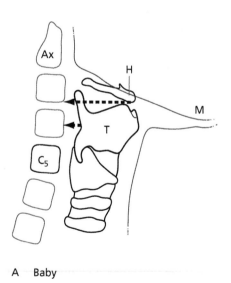
A   Baby

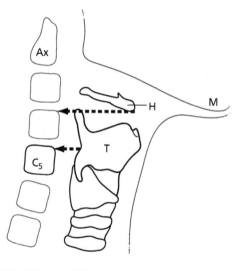
B   6–7 years old

Figure 3.4 Position of the larynx at different ages (adapted from von Lanz and Wachsmuth 1955). Ax, axis; C_5, the fifth cervical vertebra; h, hyoid bone; T, thyroid cartilage; m, mandible.

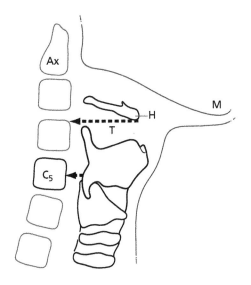

C   10–12 years old

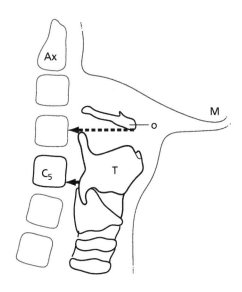

D   15–17 years old

Figure 3.4   *Continued*

References

Burgess R, Rawls A, Brown Dl 1996 Requirement of the paraxis gene for somite formation and musculoskeletal patterning. Nature 384(6609):570–573

Duboule D, Dolle P 1989 The structural and functional organization of the murine HOX gene family resembles that of *Drosophila* homeotic genes. EMBO Journal 8(5):1497–1505

Dubrulle J, McGrew M J, Pourquie O 2001 FGF signaling controls somite boundary position and regulates segmentation clock control of spatiotemporal *Hox* gene activation. Cell 106(2):219–222

Huang R, Zhi Q, Wilting J, Christ B 1994 The fate of somitocoele cells in avian embryos. Anatomy and Embryology (Berlin) 190(3):243–250

Huang R, Zhi Q, Neubuser A et al 1996 Function of somite and somitocoele cells in the formation of the vertebral motion segment in avian embryos. Acta Anatomica 155:231–241

Huang R, Zhi Q, Izpisua-Belmonte J-C et al 1999 Origin and development of the avian tongue muscles. Anatomy and Embryology (Berlin) 200(2):137–152

Huang R, Brand-Saberi B, Christ B et al 2000a New experimental evidence for somite resegmentation. Anatomy and Embryology (Berlin) 202(3):195–200

Huang R, Zhi Q, Patel K et al 2000b Contribution of single somites to the skeleton and muscles of the occipital and cervical regions in avian embryos. Anatomy and Embryology (Berlin) 202(5):375–383

Kessel M, Gruss P 1991 Homeotic transformations of murine vertebrae and concomitant alteration of Hox codes induced by retinoic acid. Cell 67(1): 89–104

Kieny M, Manger A, Sengel P 1972 Early regionalization of the somite mesodermas studied by the development of the axial skeleton of the chick embryo. Developmental Biology 28:142–161

Ogden J A 1984 Radiology of postnatal skeletal development. XII. The second cervical vertebra. Skeletal Radiology 12(3):169–177

Pourquie O 2000 Segmentation of the paraxial mesoderm and vertebrate somitogenesis. Current Topics in Developmental Biology 47:81–105

Remak R 1850 Untersuchungen über die Entwicklung der Wirbeltiere. Reimer, Berlin

Schmorl G, Junghanns H 1968 Die gesunde und die kranke Wirbelsäule im Röntgenbild und Klinik. Thieme, Stuttgart

Töndury G 1958 Entwicklungsgeschichte und Fehlbildungen der Wirbelsäule. In: Unghanns H (ed) Wirbelsäule in Forschung und Praxis. Hippokrates, Stuttgart

von Ebner V 1889 Urwirbel und Neugliederung der Wirbelsäule. Sitzungeberatungen Akademischen Wissenschaften, Wien 97: 194–206

von Lanz T, Wachsmuth W 1955 Praktische Anatomie. In: Der Hals. Springer, Berlin

Voss H 1958 Zahl und Anordnung der Muskelspindeln in den unteren Zungenbeinmuskeln, dem M.sternocleidomastoideus und den Bauch-und tiefen Nackenmuskeln. Anatomischer Anzeiger 105:265–275

Wilting J, Ebensberger C, Müller TS et al 1995 *Pax-1* in the development of the cervico-occipital transitional zone. Anatomy and Embryology (Berlin) 192:221–227

Chapter 4

Development of the central nervous system

A. Hori

INTRODUCTION

It is usually possible to specify the critical time period of the onset of malformations of the central nervous system (CNS) by morphological examination. These anomalies can be induced by either intrinsic or exogenous factors, or both.

The specificity of exogenous factors does not usually determine the type of CNS malformation but rather it is the time and/or period of the influence of these factors that is decisive. This principle is termed the teratogenetic determination period (the time span during which pathogens can influence the development of a certain malformation) or teratogenetic termination time (the time point after which the effect of the pathogens can no longer result in a certain malformation). The experimental administration of ethanol at different stages of pregnancy produced different types of brain malformations in fetuses of rats (Sakata-Haga et al 2002). While the teratogenetic determination time is relatively easy to estimate, the pathogenic factors are, on the other hand, not always identifiable with modern diagnostic tools such as in situ hybridization or immunohistochemistry due to the complexity of both the intrauterine and postnatal environment. In addition, the mother often did not notice anything unusual or had not felt ill at the teratogenetically suspicious period.

Endogenous disorders such as chromosomal anomalies usually affect the brain heterochronously and result in typical, though not specific, morphological changes which do not provide any clues to the teratogenetic determination period. Recent advances in molecular genetics have shown that normal and pathological neuroembryonal developmental mechanisms at molecular levels are closely related to genes and their product proteins. In this chapter, however, clinical neuropathological aspects will be emphasized and the molecular genetic embryology will only be dealt with briefly.

Malformations are easily understood by comparison with the features of normal CNS development. Therefore, several malformations will be described after brief review of each embryofetal developmental stage. The most frequent malformations are neural tube defects, disturbance of lateral differentiation of the brain, and migration disorders, which we will review here. Further CNS anomalies, largely caused by environmental factors, will be described separately for the various developmental stages. Maternal factors or disorders which influence the environs of the embryo/fetus such as alcohol consumption, drug intake, state of nutrition, hormonal imbalance, diabetes mellitus, etc., may result in unspecific malformations since the influence of these exogenous factors is not limited to a certain period but usually continues throughout embryonal/fetal development.

EARLY DEVELOPMENT OF THE CNS

Neural tube formation

The central nervous system (CNS) is the first organ that appears in the embryonal stage. The nervous system begins to develop from the neural plate that forms the neural groove, which is present until the eighteenth gestational day, on the dorsal side of the embryo.

A scheme of neural tube formation during ontogenesis of CNS is provided in Figure 4.1.

The primary neural tube is formed from the neural plate via the neural groove between the twenty-second and the twenty-eighth gestational day (*neurulation*). Fusion of the dorsal raphe of the neural groove, beginning at the level of the mesencephalon, does not occur in a zipper fashion uniformly along the entire spinal cord, but rather at different points simultaneously. This explains the individually different sites of the spina bifida. Clinically well-known neural tube defects such as spina bifida or anencephaly may occur as early as in the fourth week of gestation.

The dorsoventral differentiation of the neural tube is an essential development of the CNS since the motor neurons arise from the ventral and the sensory neurons from the dorsal part of the neural tube. Both areas are sharply divided by the limiting sulcus at the lateral wall of the central canal. The development of the ventral part of the neural tube is inducted by sonic hedgehog protein (Shh), which is produced by the notochord, and later by the floor plate. Sensory motor differentiation is also regulated by several genes such as dorsalin-1 (*drs-1*).

Neural tube defect: dysraphism

Dysraphism varies greatly in intensity. The most common locations of dysraphism are the lumbar and lumbosacral areas at the spinal level, and the occipital area at the cranial level (Hori 1993). Different manifestations of the dysraphism in the cranial and spinal areas are summarized in Table 4.1.

The morphogenesis of the dysraphism is considered to be a disturbance of the closure of the neural tube as proposed for the first time by von Recklinghausen in 1886. This disturbance may also be induced by a local amnion adhesion. The classic observations by Marin-Padilla (1970) on the reduction of the number of neuroblasts at the rim of the neural groove in normal human embryos as well as by Patten (1952) on the 'overgrowth of neuroectodermal tissue' (i.e. overproduction of neuroblasts) causing disturbance of the neural tube closure, may be an anomaly of developmentally programed cell death (apoptosis). Another hypothesis on the morphogenesis of dysraphism is the secondary reopening of the dorsal neural tube after its closing by embryonal 'hydromelia' (Ikenouchi et al 2002), which has also been induced experimentally by cyclophosphamide, resulting in necrosis of the dorsal neural tube (Padmanabhan 1988).

Although the causes of neural tube defects are still not clear, folic acid deficiency is considered to be one of the most important factors in neural tube defect formation. Prophylactic evidence has been shown by giving folic acid to a group of women at risk (see later section on maternal diabetes, hyperthermia and epilepsy, p. 41).

Anencephaly and encephalocele: dysraphism in the brain

If the dysraphism occurs in the cranium (Fig. 4.2B), the brain is exposed to the amniotic fluid, an 'exencephaly'. Such a brain is also more or less dysraphic and the basicranium (chondrocranium) is usually dysmorphic. An exencephalic brain will be destroyed during intrauterine life. Destroyed tissue fragments are occasionally swallowed by

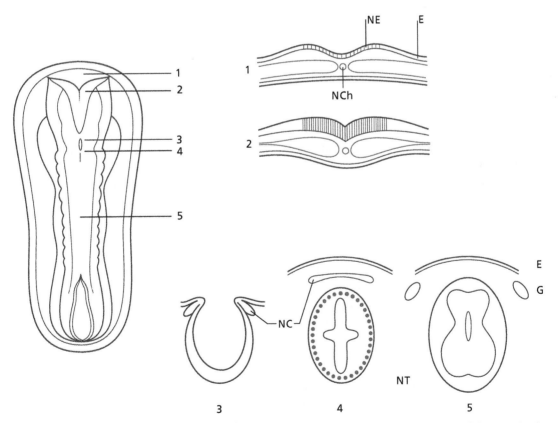

Figure 4.1   Schema of an embryo at the later phase of neural tube formation. Different stages of the neural tube formation are observed on the cut surfaces. 1, Neural plate structure; 2 and 3, neural groove structure (neural groove does not close like a zip-fastener, but closes multilocularly); 4 and 5, complete neural tube structure. E, Ectoderm; G, ganglion; NE, neuroectoderm; NCh, notochord; NC, neural crest; NT, neural tube.

Table 4.1 Neural tube defects in the cranial and spinal region

CNS	Neural tube defect/dysraphism
Brain	Anencephaly
	Exencephaly
	Encephalocele
	Meningocele
Brainstem	Encephalocele
	Meningocele
	Chiari anomaly type 2
	Tectocerebellar dysraphy
	Dandy–Walker anomaly
Spinal cord	Myeloschisis
	Myelocele
	Chiari anomaly type 3
	Myelocystocele
	Meningocele
	Diastematomyelia
	Dermal sinus
	Spina bifida
	Cyst of the terminal ventricle
	Tethered cord

the fetus together with amniotic fluid, in some rare cases resulting in a heterotopic brain mass in the buccal cavity, lung or gastrointestinal tract (Okeda 1978). Exencephaly is most likely a pre-stage of anencephaly, although anencephaly can manifest without exencephalic stages.

The destruction of the dysraphic brain is followed by tissue repair with intensive proliferation of the connective tissue, especially by vascularization, resulting in the meshwork of proliferated vessels and remaining dysplastic brain tissues, called 'area cerebrovasculosa', which was earlier incorrectly believed to be an angiomatous malformation. In about 50% of anencephalic babies the pituitary gland is lacking, with corresponding adrenocortical hypoplasia and endocrinological anomalies. The absence of the pituitary was also incorrectly believed to be due to agenesis of the pituitary. However, the pituitary is in fact also destroyed during the intrauterine period in anencephaly and replaced by connective tissue. Agenesis of the pituitary in anencephaly is excluded by

the continuing existence of the pharyngeal pituitary (Hori et al 1999).

Encephalocele is a partial dysraphism in the cranium, appearing as a protruding sac, usually seen on the midline in the occipital or frontal areas. The contents of the sac may be a part of the brain tissue (encephalocele), or merely leptomeningeal tissue without protrusion of the brain (meningocele). Encephalocele may occur in the frontal base area, resulting in the protrusion of the cerebral tissue into the nasopharyngeal cavity. This condition is often diagnosed as nasal glioma, not meaning a neoplasm, but a malformation.

Spinal dysraphism

The listed dysraphisms of the spinal regions differ only in the severity of the defects (Table 4.1 and Fig. 4.2A). Myelocystocele is a type of myelocele in which the contents of the cele sac include the dilated central canal of the spinal cord. If the sac does not contain the spinal cord tissue but only the leptomeninges and/or dura, this is termed a meningocele, analogous to that of the cranial region. The dysraphism may be limited within the spinal column without protrusion of the spinal cord tissue, which remains inside the dura in the spinal canal. This condition is known as a spina bifida occulta.

Patients with spina bifida occulta may occasionally complain of lumbago, motor disturbance and other symptoms, but this condition can be clinically silent. The author knows personally an athlete who has an asymptomatic spina bifida occulta. A focal trichosis or skin pigmentation on the lumbosacral midline may indicate an occult dysraphism.

CEREBRAL LATERAL DIFFERENTIATION

Normal development of the forebrain

After neural tube formation, the brain vesicles at the oral end of the neural tube develop further,

Figure 4.2   Examples of different CNS diseases. A: Neural tube defect at the spine: spina bifida aperta lumbosacralis. B: Neural tube defect in the cranium: anencephaly. C: Multicystic encephalopathy with hydrocephalus (frontal cut slices). D, E: Fetal brain disruption sequences with microcephaly and posthemorrhagic hydranencephaly in a newborn resulting from a severe maternal trauma in the later fetal phase. F, Porencephaly (from Hori 1999, with permission of Igaku–Shoin Ltd). G: Microcephaly and cyclopia (holoprosencephaly) in swine littermates due to intrauterine mercury poisoning at the gold mine region in Brazil (courtesy of Dr S. U. Dani, Sao Paulo).

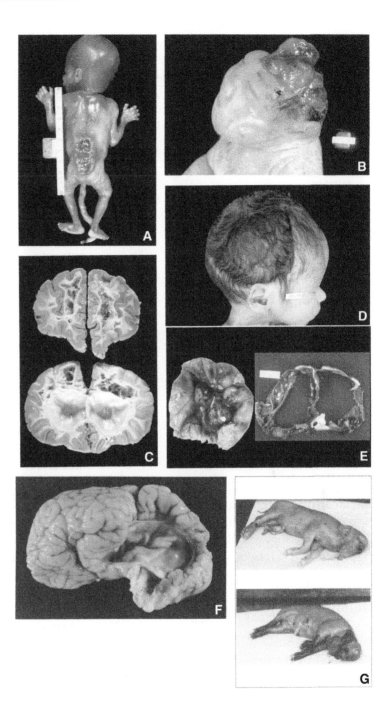

rendering telencephalic hemispheres (cerebrum), diencephalon, mesencephalon (midbrain), rhombencephalon (hind brain = cerebellum and brainstem), and myelencephalon (spinal cord). It is during this period that brain malformation such as holoprosencephaly, rhombencephalosynapsis, agenesis of the corpus callosum or cerebellar vermis develop, namely anomaly of the brain organogenesis. The correlation of normal organogenesis and its malformations in this phase is shown in Table 4.2. The

Table 4.2   Brain organogenesis and possible malformation

Normal brain development	Anomalies	Subtypes of anomalies
Lateral differentiation of the forebrain (eighth week of gestation)	Holoprosencephaly	Alobar holoprosencephaly Semilobar holoprosencephaly Lobar holoprosencephaly (according to the severity)
Lateral differentiation of the metencephalon (fifth week of gestation)	Fusion of thalami (unithalamus)	
Lateral differentiation of the rhombencephalon (fifth week of gestation)	Rhombencephalosynapsis	Typical and incomplete forms of rhombencephalosynapsis
Commissural fiber formation (beginning at the fifth week of gestation, completed in the sixth month)	Agenesis of the corpus callosum	Total and partial agenesis with anomaly of the gyral pattern of the medial surface of the cerebral hemispheres
Differentiation of cerebellum	Agenesis of the cerebellum Agenesis of a part of the cerebellum	Agenesis and hypoplasia of the cerebellum Agenesis of the cerebellar vermis
Twin	Duplication as an incomplete form of duplicitas	Craniopagus, including Janus anomaly
		Duplication of a part of the brain, e.g. pituitary, cerebellum, brainstem and spinal cord
Sulcus and gyral formation	Lissencephaly (agyria)	Lissencephaly Partial agyria

formation of the cerebral sulci and gyri also belongs to organogenesis, but occurs much later (from the fourteenth week of gestation, intensively after the twenty-first week). In this section, only holoprosencephaly is reviewed.

Holoprosencephaly

Holoprosencephaly is a relatively common malformation of the brain which is due to disturbance of its lateral differentiation, occurring around the eighth week of gestation. The brains of typical cases display no divided hemispheres and a single ventricular system. The metencephalon (thalamus) is also not divided but is singular. The eye is also single, being termed cyclopia. The olfactory bulbs and tracts are lacking. This was why holoprosencephaly was synonymously – and incorrectly – termed arhinencephaly.

Different craniofacial anomalies are frequently accompanied by holoprosencephaly. A typical manifestation is a spectrum of hypotelorism, including cyclopia or proboscis instead of a nose (Table 4.3). Since a typical holoprosencephaly displayed typical facial anomalies, the principle 'face predicts brain anomaly' was proposed earlier. However, because of the broad morphological spectrum of the intensity of the malformations in craniofacial as well as brain anomalies, this principle is no longer of use. In our own archives there are two cases of (lobar or semilobar) holoprosencephaly without craniofacial anomalies. In holoprosencephaly, some non-obligatory facial anomalies may be complicated such as different intensity of cheilopalatoschisis.

Table 4.3 Morphological spectrum of the intensity of brain and craniofacial anomalies in holoprosencephaly

Slight anomaly	$\rightarrow$	$\rightarrow$	Severe anomaly
Normal eyes	Hypotelorism	Synopia	Cyclopia
Normal nose	Only one opening of the nose		No nose but nostril (proboscis) above
Lobar holoprosencephaly	Semilobar holoprosencephaly		Alobar holoprosencephaly

Corresponding to the clinically broad spectrum of the intensity of holoprosencephaly (Table 4.3), many different genes play a complex role in constructing this abnormal morphology. Some of the genes of familial holoprosencephaly ('HPE' 1~5) are identified and located on the chromosomes. For example, sonic hedgehog (*Shh* = HPE3), which was found to produce double formation in an individual, is located on chromosome 7q36. Haploinsufficiency for *Shh* was considered to be one of the causes of holoprosencephaly (Roessler et al 1996, 1997). A component of the *Shh* pathway, the receptor PTCH (Patched-1), was recently identified, a mutation of which can cause holoprosencephaly (Ming et al 2002).

On the other hand, extrinsic factors may also cause holoprosencephaly as described in the literature, for example antiepileptics taken by the mother (Homes and Harvey 1994, Kotzot et al 1993, Rosa 1995), maternal alcohol abuse (Bonnemann and Meinecke 1990b) or intrauterine cytomegalovirus infection (Byrne et al 1987). In a gold mining district in Brazil, holoprosencephaly occurs frequently in cattle, probably due to the mercury pollution (Fig. 4.2G), although intrauterine mercury intoxication does not cause holoprosencephaly in humans but developmental anomalies of motoric nerve bundles and commissural bundles (e.g. fetal Minamata disease due to industrial pollution in Japan).

Clinically, patients are severely or very severely handicapped due to the prosencephalic malformations. In less severe cases, it is possible to survive to adulthood.

MIGRATION AND CELLULAR DIFFERENTIATION IN THE BRAIN AND ITS PATHOLOGY

Migration of neuroblasts is an essential part of the histogenesis of CNS. In principle, organogenesis is followed by histogenesis, although both phases overlap. In the early phase of neurulation, a stem cell wall attaches to the central canal side with one end and reaches the mantle side with the other end. The nuclei of these stem cells shuttle inside the elongated cytoplasm between the central canal side and the mantle side ('elevator movement') in accordance with the cell cycle: the nuclei display mitosis and division while they are situated in the central canal side (M phase) and DNA synthesis is active while they are located in the outer surface side of the neural tube (S phase).

Migration

During and after their production in the periventricular zone, the neuroblasts migrate along the radial glia towards the brain mantle in the phase of brain vesicle formation. The speed of the neuroblast migration is estimated at a maximum of 70 µm/h in the region of the olfactory bulb (Tamamaki et al 1999). In the mantle zone, the cortical cell layers are formed where neuroblasts differentiate to the nerve cells. The neuroblasts migrate along the radiating glia from the subependymal zone in the direction of the marginal mantle zone where Cajal–Retzius cells are found. Cajal–Retzius cells, the first differentiated cells containing neurofibrils, recognizable as early as the forty-third gestational day (Marin-Padilla and Marin-Padilla 1981) and constantly observed from the fiftieth day on, produce the extracellular protein 'reelin' that inactivates the migration of the neuroblasts. The next migrating neuroblasts pass over the neuroblasts that have already arrived at the cortex and ceased to migrate, until they come in contact with reelin. In this manner the outer cortical layer is formed by newcomer neuroblasts: 'inside-out law'.

The Cajal–Retzius cells reduce in number by apoptosis in the peri- and postnatal period. Excessive residual Cajal–Retzius cells were previously discussed as one of the possible causes of seizures in epileptic patients.

Disturbed migration results in heterotopically located nerve cell groups; heterotopia refers to a nerve cell group that is found in anatomically incorrect regions such as the subependyma or the subcortical white matter and have either nodular or band form. These anomalies may be caused by genetic defects as well as by many kinds of extrinsic factors such as intrauterine exposure to radiation (see section on intrauterine radiation exposure, p. 42), fetal circulatory disturbance (see section on micropolygyria below).

Cortical differentiation, heterotopia, double cortex, and agyria (lissencephaly)

The neuroblasts that arrived in the cortex then differentiate to the cortical nerve cells with a topographically typical laminar structure, usually consisting of six layers.

A migration anomaly results in nodular heterotopia (periventricular heterotopia), subcortical laminar (band) heterotopia (double cortex syndrome), and agyria/pachygyria (lissencephaly) (Schull et al 1992). Nodular heterotopia is a focal arrest of migration, usually identified in the periventricular areas as single or multiple nodules of nerve cell accumulation, and clinically may be a focus of epileptic discharge. In our experience, there is silent single heterotopia in 0.7% of routine necropsy series. In X-linked dominant periventric-

ular nodular heterotopia, filamin 1 (FLN1) mutation was identified as a genetic defect causing the hereditary nodular heterotopia (Fox et al 1998). Familial nodular heterotopia is linked to the gene located in chromosome Xq28 in females. In males, the same Xq28 gene is considered to be responsible for bilateral nodular heterotopia combined with frontonasal malformation (Guerrini and Dobyns 1998). Pathomechanisms of the migration disturbance can be explained by the disruption of the radial glia along which the neuroblasts migrate from the subependymal to cortical zone (Santi and Golden 2001). This condition may explain a non-hereditary occurrence of nodular heterotopia.

Laminar (band) heterotopia is a diffuse arrest of migration and is found in the (subcortical) white matter as an additional nerve cell layer (hence, double cortex syndrome). The gene DCX is located on the X chromosome and produces the protein named doublecortin. The mutation of this single gene is the cause of two different types of migration disturbances: double cortex syndrome in females and lissencephaly in males. In females (karyotype XX), mutant X disturbs the neuronal migration; however, non-mutant X forwards the migration, i.e., some of the neurons migrate regularly but the migration of others is disturbed and they therefore make up the subcortical heterotopia in a laminar form. This condition is termed 'double cortex syndrome'. In males (karyotype XY), the migration is completely disturbed by mutant X so that a severe form of lissencephaly occurs, but no double cortex. Another lissencephaly, morphologically identical to the hereditary ones, is caused by the LIS1 gene, located on chromosome 17.

Clinically, lissencephaly and laminar heterotopia (double cortex syndrome) form a morphological substrate for severe psychomotor retardation.

Micropolygyria

Micropolygyria (or polymicrogyria) is not a precise description although the term is generally accepted since the cortical surface of this anomaly does not consist of small gyri.

The gyri themselves are rather pachygyric and the surface has the appearance of a cobble stone pavement. Histologically, the cortical surface is, corresponding to its gross appearance, very irregularly configured and the surface neurons invade randomly into the leptomeninges through the broken subpial limiting glial membrane. The cortical architecture is also abnormal, with small islets of neuronal mass, and the virtual molecular layers are irregularly confluent. Another typical cortical feature is a four-layer pattern due to an intermediate nerve fiber layer between the neuronal layer (1, molecular layer; 2, external nerve cell layer; 3, myelinated nerve fiber layer; 4, internal nerve cell layer). The abnormal cortical layer may show an abrupt boundary to the intact six-layered cortex. This suggests focal injury and thus an exogenous cause in micropolygyria, although endogenous micropolygyria may also be focally limited. The lesions are, in the majority of cases, not diffusely distributed but localized or coexistent with other lesions such as porencephaly (see later section on porencephaly, p. 39). A representative case is that of a 27-week-old fetus in which micropolygyria was limited to the disturbed supplying area of the middle cerebral artery (Richman et al 1974). Further reports of intrauterine CO intoxication at the fifth gestational month or at the twenty-fourth week (Bankl and Jellinger 1967) confirm an exogenous cause of micropolygyria. Intrauterine infection with cytomegalovirus (CMV) is known to cause a brain malformation (micropolygyria, micrencephaly). However, there is other evidence that micropolygyria in congenital CMV infection is a result of circulatory disturbance (Marques Dias et al 1984). Small focal micropolygyria may also be observed in endogenous CNS anomalies such as thanatophoric dysplasia (Hori et al 1983). The teratogenic determination period is thought to be between 17 and 26 weeks of gestation (Golden 2001).

Micropolygyria accompanied by widespread pachygyria (pachygyric micropolygyria) is termed lissencephaly type 2. This type 2 is typical in the group of muscle–eye–brain diseases, Walker–Warburg syndrome (linked mostly to chromosome 17q) or the Fukuyama type of muscle dystrophy (linked to chromosome 9q31–33), known as autosomal recessive hereditary diseases, and is not exogenous.

Clinical manifestations of micropolygyria generally consist of psychomotor retardation and typically seizures.

BRAIN ANOMALIES IDENTIFIABLE IN THE NEONATAL AND INFANTILE PERIOD

Brain anomalies recognizable in the postnatal period may have occurred either during intrauterine life or in the perinatal as well as postnatal period. The majority of these anomalies are due to an encephaloclastic process of extrinsic causes, for example birth trauma, perinatal hypoxia, infection, etc. Complications in twin conception (such as fetofetal transfusion syndrome) may also be included in this group although they are not exogenous in the strict sense of the word. The disorders described in this section include different syndromes and diseases which are not grouped systematically and which exclude brain malformations.

Fetal brain disruption sequences and hydranencephaly

This clinical concept includes all encephaloclastic processes which involve a collapse of the skull or microcephaly with organic brain damage in mentally and physically handicapped babies (Fig. 4.2D).

Etiopathogenetically, these disorders may occur in every embryofetal stage from very different causes, such as viral or parasitic infection or circulatory disturbances in later fetal stages, analogous to hydranencephaly. The majority of the reported cases are sporadic. However, Alexander reported an occurrence in sisters, suggesting some genetic component (Alexander et al 1995). In this context, a recessively inherited vasculopathy resulting in hydranencephaly-hydrocephaly disorder (Harding et al 1995) should also be included in this group of disorders.

Microcephaly or overlapping sutures is a typical clinical manifestation (Fig. 4.2D). The baby has a normal craniofacial appearance. Hydrocephalus may also occur but is not obligatory. Sonographic and radiological examination as well as transillumination of the head confirm the diagnosis. Neurological symptoms include seizures, spasticity, myoclonus, cortical blindness and optical atrophy. Prognosis is very poor and most patients die shortly after birth. Surviving babies are severely handicapped.

The brain changes largely include hydranencephaly (Fig. 4.2E) and/or cerebrocortical damage. Hydranencephaly is essentially not a type of malformation but a residual state of the encephaloclas-

tic processes. The brain shows only a contour of the cerebral mantle and is filled with cerebrospinal fluid since the majority of the telencephalic structures are destroyed and replaced by fluid (Fig. 4.2E). In extreme cases, only the molecular layer and residual parts of the cerebral cortex are preserved, but there is practically no white matter or internal structures. The brain substance is destroyed by colliquation necrosis. If the brainstem is preserved, the fetus usually survives for a short time.

Hydranencephaly can occur after the fourth gestational month, though usually after the seventh month (gestational week 28) when the brain is formally 'completed' (though immature), since cortical dysgenesis such as micropolygyria or migration disturbances and other kinds of brain malformations are usually lacking in hydranen-

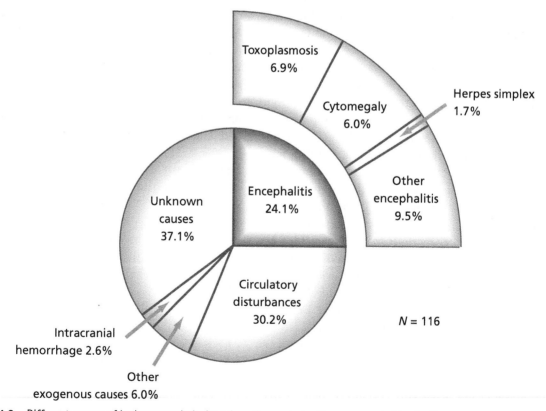

Figure 4.3 Different causes of hydranencephaly, based on the analysis of cases reported in the literature as well as from the author's own archives. Note that a quarter of all cases of hydranencephaly are caused by intrauterine encephalitis.

cephaly. The cortical gyral structures are normally recognizable although the subcortical structures are totally or subtotally destroyed. Normal configuration of the ventricular system is therefore radiologically or sonographically often not detectable.

The causes of hydranencephaly vary greatly; for a majority of the cases, intrauterine encephalitis and trauma are responsible (Fig. 4.3). No matter what the initial cause is, an additional circulatory disturbance of the brain followed by diffuse necrosis plays a major role in establishing hydranencephaly. A recessively inherited vasculopathy is another cause of hydranencephaly, as already cited (Harding et al 1995). In a few cases, hydranencephaly may occur after birth as a result of cerebral infarction complicated by widespread meningitis and/or intracerebral hemorrhage (Lindenberg and Swanson 1967).

Neonatal (including perinatal) meningitis is often complicated by focal or multiple infarction, followed by hydrocephalus due to absorption disturbance of the cerebrospinal fluid if the patients survive the acute phase of the infection. Intrauterine meningitis is extremely rare. We observed one such case with evidence of the transplacental infection (Hori and Fischer 1982).

Multicystic encephalopathy

Multicystic encephalopathy is one of the severest cerebral disorders with multiple cavity formation in the cerebral hemispheres due to encephaloclastic processes (Fig. 4.2C). This condition is usually accompanied by hydrocephalus and lack of septum pellucidum. The remaining cortical ribbon is very thin. Basal ganglia, thalamus or even brainstem may also show microcystic changes and there is severe nerve cell depopulation or calcification of dead nerve cells. As a result of the parenchymal destruction, glial scar formation (including ulegyria) is usually observed.

Severe circulatory disturbance during the late intrauterine and/or neonatal phase is the main pathogenesis of this condition, for example stenosis of the carotid arteries. However, the causes of the cerebral circulatory disturbance resulting in multicystic encephalopathy are very different – birth trauma, intrauterine viral infection, etc. Several twins with this condition have been recorded in the literature. The majority of patients are neonates with different neurological manifestations since the brain changes occur usually in the perinatal phase. Rarely, surviving 'shaken baby syndrome' patients also manifest multicystic encephalopathy together with other typical signs of the syndrome.

Porencephaly

In contrast to hydranencephaly and fetal brain disruption sequences, porencephaly displays congenital, partial cerebral destruction (Fig. 4.2F). Porencephaly is defined as a communication between the internal and external cerebrospinal spaces due to partial destruction of the brain, occurring in the middle and later fetal stages. Postnatal porencephaly is an exception (Cross et al 1992). The lesions are usually seen bilaterally and often in the central to parietal regions. The tissue of the lesion shows glial scar formation and sometimes micropolygyric changes in the cortex at the margin of the destructive lesion (Tominaga et al 1996). Rarely heterotopic neurons are observed near the lesion. However, the micropolygyric or heterotopic changes are interpreted as secondary, since the encephaloclastic damage is thought to be a result of extrinsic causes at the time of migration. In some cases of porencephaly, however, this condition is observed in successive generations or in twins and a genetically defined etiopathogenesis has also been considered (Brewer et al 1996, Jung et al 1984).

Pathological myelination: status marmoratus (marbled state) of the basal ganglia

Normal myelination begins in the second fetal trimester in the brainstem. In the spinal cord, the sensory fascicles show earlier myelination than the motor fascicles, but the motor spinal roots are myelinated earlier than the sensory spinal roots. The cerebral white matter myelination is completed by 1 postnatal year. The complete myelination of the reticular formation may be as late as puberty.

Status marmoratus (marbled state) of the basal ganglia, occasionally also of the thalamus, represents glial scars with irregular hypermyelination associated with neuronal loss. This indicates that the disorder is not a congenital malformation but an acquired condition. Since the myelination in the basal ganglia commences at the sixth month of postnatal life, the status marmoratus is thought to occur around this period at the sites of the scars that may have occurred earlier than 6 months of age. The clinical features of patients prior to this critical period include birth complications such as asphyxia as well as cyanosis, resuscitation and convulsions. These complications result in damage to the basal ganglia and thalamic regions. In older infants, rigidity or choreoathetosis is a common clinical manifestation. Mental retardation or movement disturbances such as spastic paraplegia may also manifest. The average life expectancy of children with status marmoratus is approximately 12 years of age.

Nuclear jaundice (kernicterus)

Severe neonatal hyperbilirubinemia may result in 'nuclear jaundice'. One of the major causes of this disorder is megakaryocytosis due to Rh incompatibility. However, the nuclear jaundice is merely an unspecific 'bilirubin encephalopathy', regardless of the cause of hyperbilirubinemia. Since the blood–brain barrier is still immature in neonates, bilirubin reaches brain parenchyma so that the caudate nucleus, putamen, globus pallidus, subthalamic nucleus, hippocampus, cerebellar dentate nucleus and olivary nucleus are selectively and bilaterally yellowish colored and nerve cells undergo degeneration. The different distribution of the changes in patients of different ages may be related to differences in the topographical development of the blood–brain barrier. Choreoathetotic movement disorders and psychomotor retardation are major clinical manifestations of this 'nuclear' jaundice.

EMBRYOFETOPATHY DUE TO MATERNAL DISEASE OR MEDICATION

Fetal alcohol syndrome

Maternal chronic or excessive alcohol consumption, in particular in the first trimester after the conception, can lead to the unspecific congenital anomaly of the baby, an (embryo)-fetal alcohol syndrome. Not only ethanol itself, but also its intermediate metabolite acetaldehyde is considered to be embryotoxic.

The newborn baby is small for dates, which may be recognized during in utero examination, and shows craniofacial dysmorphism. Some authors describe the craniofacial anomalies in fetal alcohol syndrome as typical: short eyelids, broad nasal root, flat and long philtrum, thin upper lip, occasionally blepharophimosis and anti-Down eyelids. Generalized malformations in these patients are usually not remarkable. Slight craniofacial dysmorphism may partly regress by the time of adolescence; the body weight may also normalize while the lower IQ remains unchanged. However, a long-term prognostic study showed that adequate education may improve learning ability since the postnatal development of these patients varies (Streissguth et al 1991). Recorded brain anomalies are various and unspecific in contrast to the relatively uniform craniofacial anomalies: hydrocephalus, cerebral heterotopia, agenesis of the corpus callosum, dysraphism, or porencephaly; even holoprosencephaly has been recorded (Bonnemann and Meinecke 1990a).

Experimentally, reduction in the number of pyramidal nerve cells (Barnes and Walker 1981), depression of glutamate release and decrease in glutamate binding (Farr et al 1988), and changes in neurotrophic activity (Heaton et al 1995) of the hippocampus are demonstrated, the latter being an important area for memory function. In animal experiments, different brain malformations were produced in both the cerebrum (including leptomeningeal heterotopia) and cerebellum by intrauterine exposure to ethanol. Scheduled alcohol consumption at different times in the pregnancy induced different types of cerebral malformation in fetuses (Sakata-Haga et al 2002).

Maternal diabetes, hyperthermia and epilepsy

Maternal diabetes mellitus possibly influences the morphology of embryos/fetuses. Babies born to diabetic mothers are usually large for dates. A high incidence of anomalies such as Down syndrome (Narchi and Kulaylat 1997), preaxial polydactyly (Slee and Goldblatt 1997) or caudal regression syndrome (Passarge and Lenz 1966, Williamson 1970) have been recorded in the literature. Other malformations have also been sporadically reported. Early intellectual development in children of diabetic mothers is poorer than in those of non-diabetic mothers (Yamashita et al 1996). The teratogenic mechanism of maternal diabetes mellitus is not known; however, not only diabetes mellitus, but also the effect of medical control of diabetes should be discussed.

Maternal hyperthermia is shown to result in embryofetal malformations experimentally (Shiota 1988, Shiota et al 1988). Several case reports describe dysraphism or facial dysmorphism in humans.

Epileptic mothers have a risk of giving birth to malformed children with or without CNS anomalies. According to the study by Canger et al (1999), the overall incidence of malformations (not only CNS malformations) in siblings born to epileptic mothers was 9.7%. The majority of the mothers were treated with antiepileptic drugs.

The incidence of malformation among infants of epileptic mothers who were not taking antiepileptic drugs was 4.8%. Intrauterine head growth was correlated to the number of antiepileptic drugs taken by mothers (Battino et al 1992). Serum and cerebrospinal fluid levels of folate were reduced in a high percentage of epileptic patients treated with antiepileptic drugs (Raynolds 1973). Folate is known to be an important factor in preventing the risk of neural tube defect, so that mothers who already have dysraphic babies are advised to take folic acid as a prophylaxis, even prior to the planned conception. Therefore, it is likely that antiepileptic-drug-related factors predominate over genetic predisposition as the cause of malformation in cases of maternal epilepsy. However, the mother's convulsion itself should also be regarded as a possible teratogenic factor (Leppert and Wieser 1993) in addition to the genetic factors.

Maternal infection and trauma

In cases of maternal infection, virus or bacteria may be transported via the placenta to the fetus and fetal CNS. Cytomegalovirus is known to cause micropolygyria with microcephaly; however, the teratogenic determination period is limited to the later migration phase (till the end of the fourth gestational month; see section on micropolygyria, p. 36). Other viral infections in the later fetal period, e.g. herpes virus, are known to cause severe encephaloclastic processes such as hydranencephaly (see section on fetal brain disruption sequences and hydranencephaly, p. 37). However, other factors such as circulatory disturbances are assumed to play a much more important role in the pathological morphogenesis than the virus itself.

Severe maternal trauma with uterine injury and/or bleeding may also cause fetal anomaly. Hydranencephaly is documented (in the literature as well as in our archives) as one of the results of accidental severe trauma to the mother.

Intrauterine radiation exposure

Therapeutic or accidental exposure to irradiation as well as nuclear bomb exposure during embryo-fetal life may also cause CNS anomalies.

Much tragedy was seen in children born to surviving pregnant victims of the atomic bombs (ionizing radiation) in Hiroshima and Nagasaki. Significantly, frequent mental retardation and microcephaly was observed in such children (Otake et al 1989) exposed to atomic bomb irradiation before the twenty-sixth gestational week, and mostly between the eighth and fifteenth week. The children who were exposed in the eighth and ninth weeks of gestation showed mental retardation as a result of bilateral periventricular heterotopia which was ascertained by magnetic resonance imaging. The fetuses that were exposed to the atomic bomb during the twelfth/thirteenth week of gestation showed no heterotopia but pachygyria. Even low-dose ionizing irradiation in utero resulted experimentally in migration anomalies (Fushiki et al 1994, 1996). Intrauterine X-irradiation was experimentally ascertained as the cause of a deceleration in the migration of neuroblasts (including cortical derangement) (Fushiki et al 1997).

Therapeutic or prophylactic X-ray irradiation to the head in leukemic children is known eventually to result in meningiomas (or gliomas and other brain tumors) about 10 years later as a delayed side effect.

CONCLUSION

Knowledge of the process of normal neuroembryonal development helps in interpreting the malformations of the central nervous system, especially in cases of neural tube defects (including anencephaly), holoprosencephaly and migration anomalies such as lissencephaly or heterotopia. These anomalies can be induced endogenously by genetic errors and also by environmental (exogenous) factors. Exogenous factors, such as infection, trauma, intoxication and other maternal conditions, may induce different malformations, mostly independent of the factors but dependent on the pathogenically effective time period. Chronic effects of exogenous factors or chromosomal anomalies may produce unspecific though typical anomalies due to their heterochronous pathomechanism. Clinically severe brain disorders may be produced by encephaloclastic processes due to hypoxia, circulatory disturbance, trauma, and many other causes mostly during the perinatal phase as well as in the latest fetal stage. Despite having the same etiopathogenetic factors, phenotypically different brain anomalies may be produced depending on the time of onset of the causes, for example a series of hydranencephaly, porencephaly and polycystic encephalopathy due to brain circulatory disturbances. The search for possible causes of CNS anomalies should lead to the prevention of the disorders.

References

Alexander I E, Tauro G P, Bankier A 1995 Fetal brain disruption sequence in sisters. European Journal of Pediatrics 154(8):654–657

Bankl H, Jellinger K 1967 Zentralnervöses Schäden nach fetaler Kohlenoxydvergiftung [Central nervous system injuries following fetal carbon monoxide poisoning]. Beitrage zur pathologischen Anatomie 135(3):350–376

Barnes D E, Walker D W 1981 Prenatal ethanol exposure permanently reduces the number of pyramidal neurons in rat hippocampus. Brain Research 227(3):333–340

Battino D, Granata T, Binelli S et al 1992 Intrauterine growth in the offspring of epileptic mothers. Acta Neurologica Scandinavica 86(6):555–557

Bonnemann C, Meinecke P 1990a Holoprosencephaly as a possible embryonic alcohol effect: another observation. American Journal of Medical Genetics 37(3):431–432

Bonnemann C G, Meinecke P 1990b Fetal brain disruption sequence: a milder variant. Journal of Medical Genetics 27(4):273–274

Brewer C M, Fredericks B J, Pont J M et al 1996 X-linked hydrocephalus masquerading as spina bifida and destructive porencephaly in successive generations in one family. Developmental Medicine and Child Neurology 38(7):632–636

Byrne P J, Silver M M, Gilbert J M et al 1987 Cyclopia and congenital cytomegalovirus infection. American Journal of Medical Genetics 28(1):61–65

Canger R, Battino D, Canevini M P et al 1999 Malformations in offspring of women with epilepsy: a prospective study. Epilepsia 40(9):1231–1236

Chiari H 1891 Über Veränderungen des Kleinhirns infolge Hydrocephalus des Großhirnes. Deutsche Medizinische Wochenschrift 17:1172–1175

Chiari H 1895 Über Veränderungen des Kleinhirns, des Pons und der Medulla oblongata infolge von kongenitaler Hydrocephalie des Großhirns. Denkschrift für Akademischen Wissenschaften, Wien 63:71–116

Cross J H, Harrison C J, Preston P R et al 1992 Postnatal encephaloclastic porencephaly – a new lesion? Archives of Disease in Childhood 67(3):307–311

DeJonge M, Poulik J 1997 Pathological case of the month. Fetal brain disruption sequence. Archives of Pediatrics and Adolescent Medicine 151(12):1267–1268

Farr K L, Montano C Y, Paxton L L et al 1988 Prenatal ethanol exposure decreases hippocampal 3H-glutamate binding in 45-day-old rats. Alcohol 5(2):125–133

Fox J W, Lamperti E D, Eksioglu Y Z et al 1998 Mutations in filamin 1 prevent migration of cerebral cortical neurons in human periventricular heterotopia. Neuron 21(6):1315–1325

Fushiki S, Hyodo-Taguchi Y, Kinoshita C et al 1997 Short- and long-term effects of low-dose prenatal X-irradiation in mouse cerebral cortex, with special reference to neuronal migration. Acta Neuropathologica (Berlin) 93(5):443–449

Fushiki S, Matsushita K, Yoshioka H et al 1994 Effects of low doses of ionizing radiation on the developing brain – experimental studies in vivo and in vitro. In: Seki T (ed) Brain damage associated with prenatal environmental factors. Sanyo Kogyo, Tokyo, p 31–39

Fushiki S, Matsushita K, Yoshioka H et al 1996 In utero exposure to low-doses of ionizing radiation decelerates neuronal migration in the developing rat brain. International Journal of Radiation Biology 70(1):53–60

Golden J A 2001 Cell migration and cerebral cortical development. Neuropathology and Applied Neurobiology 27(1):22–28

Guerrini R, Dobyns W B 1998 Bilateral periventricular nodular heterotopia with mental retardation and frontonasal malformation. Neurology 51(2):499–503

Harding B N, Ramani P, Thurley P 1995 The familial syndrome of proliferative vasculopathy and hydranencephaly-hydrocephaly: immunocytochemical and ultrastructural evidence for endothelial proliferation. Neuropathology and Applied Neurobiology 21(1):61–67

Heaton M B, Paiva M, Swanson D J et al 1995 Prenatal ethanol exposure alters neurotrophic activity in the developing rat hippocampus. Neuroscience Letters 188(2):132–136

Holmes L B, Harvey E A 1994 Holoprosencephaly and the teratogenicity of anticonvulsants. Teratology 49(2):82

Hori A 1993 A review of the morphology of spinal cord malformations and their relation to neuro-embryology. Neurosurgical Review 16(4):259–266

Hori A 1999 Morphology of brain malformation: beyond the classification, towards the integration. No Shinkei Geka (Neurol Surg Tokyo) 27:969–985

Hori A, Fischer G 1982 Intrauterine purulent leptomeningitis. Acta Neuropathologica 58(1):78–80

Hori A, Friede R L, Fischer G 1983 Ventricular diverticula with localized dysgenesis of the temporal lobe in cloverleaf skull anomaly. Acta Neuropathologica 60(1–2):132–136

Hori A, Schmidt D, Rickels E 1999 Pharyngeal pituitary: development, malformation, and tumorigenesis. Acta Neuropathologica (Berlin), 98(3):262–272

Ikenouchi J, Uwabe C, Nakatsu T et al 2002 Embryonic hydromyelia: cystic dilatation of the lumbosacral neural tube in human embryos. Acta Neuropathologica (Berlin) 103(3):248–254

Jung J H, Graham J M Jr, Schultz N et al 1984 Congenital hydranencephaly/porencephaly due to vascular disruption in monozygotic twins. Pediatrics 73(4):467–469

Karagöz F, Izgi N, Sencer S 2002 Morphometric measurements of the cranium in patients with Chiari type I malformation and comparison with the normal population. Acta Neurochirurgica (Wien) 144:165–171

Kotzot D, Weigl J, Huk W et al 1993 Hydantoin syndrome with holoprosencephaly: a possible rare teratogenic effect. Teratology 48(1):15–19

Leppert D, Wieser H G 1993 Schwangerschaft, Antikonzeption und Epilepsie [Pregnancy, contraception and epilepsy]. Nervenarzt 64(8):494–503

Lindenberg R, Swanson P D 1967 'Infantile hydranencephaly' – a report of five cases of infarction of both cerebral hemispheres in infancy. Brain 90(4):839–850

Marin-Padilla M 1970 Morphogenesis of anencephaly and related malformations. Current Topics in Pathology 51:145–174

Marin-Padilla M, Marin-Padilla T M 1981 Morphogenesis of experimentally induced Arnold–Chiari malformation. Journal of the Neurological Sciences 50(1):29–55

Marques Dias M, Harmant-van Rijkevorsel G, Landrieu P et al 1984 Prenatal cytomegalovirus disease and cerebral microgyria: evidence for perfusion failure, not disturbance of histogenesis, as the major cause of fetal cytomegalovirus encephalopathy. Neuropediatrics 15:18–24

Ming J E, Kaupas M E, Roessler E et al 2002 Mutations in PATCHED-1, the receptor for SONIC HEDGEHOG, are associated with holoprosencephaly. Human Genetics 111(4–5):464

Narchi H, Kulaylat N 1997 High incidence of Down's syndrome in infants of diabetic mothers. Archives of Disease in Childhood 77(3):242–244

Okeda R 1978 Heterotopic brain tissue in the submandibular region and lung. Acta Neuropathologica 43:217–220

Otake M, Yoshimaru H, Schull W 1989 Prenatal exposure to atomic radiation and brain damage. Congenital Anomaly 29:309–320

Padmanabhan R 1988 Light microscopic studies on the pathogenesis of exencephaly and cranioschisis induced in the rat after neural tube closure. Teratology 37(1):29–36

Passarge E, Lenz W 1966 Syndrome of caudal regression in infants of diabetic mothers: observations of further cases. Pediatrics 37(4):672–675

Patten B 1952 Overgrowth of the neural tube in young human embryos. Anatomical Record 113:381–393

Raynolds E 1973 Anticonvulsants, folic acid and epilepsy. Lancet i:1376–1378

Richman D P, Stewart R M, Caviness V S Jr 1974 Cerebral microgyria in a 27-week fetus: an architectonic and topographic analysis. Journal of Neuropathology and Experimental Neurology 33(3):374–384

Roessler E, Belloni E, Gaudenz K et al 1996 Mutations in the human Sonic Hedgehog gene cause holoprosencephaly. Nature Genetics 14(3):357–360

Roessler E, Belloni E, Gaudenz K et al 1997 Mutations in the C-terminal domain of Sonic Hedgehog cause holoprosencephaly. Human Molecular Genetics 6(11):1847–1853

Rosa F 1995 Holoprosencephaly and antiepileptic exposures. Teratology 51:230

Roth M 1986 Cranio-cervical growth collision: another explanation of the Arnold–Chiari malformation and of basilar impression. Neuroradiology 28(3):187–194

Sakata-Haga H, Sawada K, Hisano S et al 2002 Administration schedule for ethanol containing diet in pregnancy affects types of offspring brain malformation. Acta Neuropathologica 104:305–312

Santi M R, Golden J A 2001 Periventricular heterotopia may result from radial glial fiber disruption. Journal of Neuropathology and Experimental Neurology 60(9):856–862

Schull W, Nishitani H, Hasuo K et al 1992 Brain abnormalities among the mentally retarded prenatally exposed atomic bomb survivors. RERF Technicak Report Series 1–16

Shiota K 1988 Induction of neural tube defects and skeletal malformations in mice following brief hyperthermia in utero. Biology of the Neonate 53(2):86–97

Shiota K, Shionoya Y, Ide M et al 1988 Teratogenic interaction of ethanol and hyperthermia in mice. Proceedings of the Society for Experimental Biology and Medicine 187(2):142–148

Slee J, Goldblatt J 1997 Further evidence for preaxial hallucal polydactyly as a marker of diabetic embryopathy. Journal of Medical Genetics 34(3):261–263

Streissguth A P, Aase J M, Clarren S K et al 1991 Fetal alcohol syndrome in adolescents and adults. Journal of the American Medical Association 265(15):1961–1967

Tamamaki N, Sugimoto Y, Tanaka K et al 1999 Cell migration from the ganglionic eminence to the neocortex investigated by labeling nuclei with UV irradiation via a fiber-optic cable. Neuroscience Research 35(3):241–251

Tominaga I, Kaihou M, Kimura Y et al 1996 [Cytomegalovirus fetal infection. Porencephaly with polymicrogyria in a 15-year-old boy]. Revue Neurologique (Paris) 152(6–7):479–482

von Recklinghausen F 1886 Untersuchungen über die Spina bifida. Virchows Archiv 105:243–330

Williamson D A 1970 A syndrome of congenital malformations possibly due to maternal diabetes. Developmental Medicine and Child Neurology 12(2):145–152

Yamashita Y, Kawano Y, Kuriya N et al 1996 Intellectual development of offspring of diabetic mothers. Acta Paediatrica 85(10):1192–1196

Chapter 5

Adaptive properties of motor behavior

J.-M. Ramirez

INTRODUCTION

The ability to walk and to maintain posture depends on a complex integration of many intrinsic and extrinsic factors. The basic walking rhythm is generated by a neuronal network, which is located within the spinal cord (Kiehn and Kjaerulff 1998). This network is capable of generating reciprocal neural activity, which is sent via motor neurons to the periphery where it activates muscles that produce alternating limb movements. Each of these limb movements is the result of a complex activation of numerous antagonistic and agonistic muscles that lead to the generation of a step, which consists of a swing and stance phase. The exact timing and also the shape of activation of each of these muscles is highly influenced by the properties of the muscles and the activation of sense organs located within the muscles and tendons of each limb, the so-called proprioceptors. The activation of proprioceptors feeds back to the neuronal network located within the central nervous system, which adjusts the intrinsically generated motor activity in a cycle-by-cycle manner to the constantly changing extrinsic conditions, such as the surface of the ground (McCrea 2001, Pearson and Ramirez 1997).

Besides these rapidly occurring adaptive processes, long-term changes are also very characteristic and essential for normal locomotor behavior. The timing of proprioceptive feedback has to be adjusted to long-term changes in body size. In the developing child, new locomotor movements are learned, or existing movements are refined as the child is growing. This motor learning will be associated with a complex change in the activation pattern of individual muscles (Okamoto et al 2001), in neuronal networks located within the spinal cord (Nakayama et al 2002), as well as complex changes in the afferent feedback (Roncesvalles and Woollacott 2000). Adaptive processes are not only critical during development, but also important in the adult as body weight may change drastically over weeks and months (Barbeau and Fung 2001, Pearson 2000). Injury will also change the gain of proprioceptive reflexes over several months, which will affect not only locomotion, but also posture (Barbeau et al 2002, Bouyer et al 2001, De Leon et al 2001, Rossignol 2000, Whelan and Pearson 1997). Vice versa, changes in posture may affect step size and timing during locomotion. Many of these long-term changes may be explained by changes in the response of the central nervous system to afferent inputs from proprioceptors or by changes in the excitatory drive to proprioceptors that derives from gamma motor neurons, which can change the gain of reflexes in a state-dependent manner (Lam and Pearson 2002, Pearson 2000, 2001, Prochazka 1989). An important role in these adaptive changes can be attributed to neuromodulators, which are substances that alter membrane properties of neurons involved in the generation of rhythmic motor activity. In injury, for example, endorphins are released. These peptides can potentially alter not only reflexes, but also membrane and synaptic properties of neurons within the central nervous system, thus resulting in long-term changes in walking behavior.

This chapter will review concepts and principles that have been established in various animal models in order to explain how the nervous system produces a locomotor behavior. Many of the principles that are directly relevant for human locomotion have been established in a variety of animal models, which were used to study not only locomotion, but also other rhythmic behaviors. Here I will summarize these general principles of rhythm generation, which are applicable not only to how the nervous system produces walking in particular, but rhythmic activity in general.

THE GENERATION OF RHYTHMIC ACTIVITY: THE CONCEPT OF A CENTRAL PATTERN GENERATOR (CPG)

As mentioned above, the nervous system generates not only walking, but many forms of rhythmic activity, which dominate our daily life. When we become tired in the evening, this is not only because we are physically exhausted. More likely, it is because our 'internal clock' tells us that it is time to sleep (Kuller 2002, Zisapel 2001). In the morning we wake up, because our internal clock 'reminds' us, that it is time to get up. We do not necessarily wake up because we regained our physical strength during the sleep, as everybody knows, who cannot go back to sleep in the morning, even if the preceding night was highly disturbed. A similarly common experience is the jet-lag that affects people who travel overseas (Boulos et al 1995, Brown 1994, Zisapel 2001), or the problems associated with shift work (Rajaratnam and Arendt 2001). The internal clock that is responsible for these phenomena has been identified as a small neuronal network, located in the so-called supra-chiasmatic nucleus (SCN, Cheng et al 2002, Reppert and Weaver 2002). This network is both sufficient and necessary for generating the circadian rhythm. Isolated from the remaining central nervous system, the SCN maintains a 24-hour rhythm even in a Petri dish (Gillette and Tischkau 1999, Weaver 1998). This experiment indicates that the SCN is sufficient to generate a 24-hour rhythm and that this rhythmic activity is generated endogenously by the central nervous system, and does not depend on the presence or absence of light. The SCN controls various circadian rhythms and is responsible, for example, for the generation of circadian fluctuations in hormone levels (e.g. the growth hormone) or for rhythmic changes in body temperature. Lesions of the SCN abolish these circadian rhythms in otherwise intact animals (Weaver 1998), indicating that this network is necessary for generating circadian rhythms. Neural networks that are capable of generating rhythmic activity in the absence of a sensory input (e.g. a visual input, light) are called *central pattern generators* or CPGs (Marder and Calabrese 1996).

The SCN is only one of many central pattern generators in the central nervous system. The thalamus generates rhythmic activity, which highly influences our cortical activity. The thalamic rhythmicity is state-dependent, and associated with well-known changes in neuronal properties of thalamic neurons (McCormick 2002). The transition from being rhythmic to non-rhythmic is controlled by inputs from the brainstem and cortex, which play important functions in regulating the role of the thalamus as a relay nucleus in sensory processing. As described for the SCN, isolated slices from the thalamus are still capable of generating rhythmic activity (McCormick and Bal 1997). Knowing how the thalamus generates rhythmic activity is not only important for understanding the transitions from wakefulness to sleep, but this understanding is also clinically relevant. Rhythmic activity generated by the thalamus can be pathophysiological and thalamic oscillations have been associated with the generation of absence seizures (McCormick and Contreras 2001).

The cortex also exhibits various forms of rhythms, which can be used to characterize different states of sleeps and wakefulness (McCormick 2002, Steriade 2001, Steriade and Amzica 1998, Steriade et al 1994). The generation of rhythmic cortical activity has been associated with consciousness, as well as psychiatric disorders (Llinas et al 1999). As already mentioned for the thalamic oscillations, pathophysiological forms of cortical rhythms underlie various forms of epileptic seizures (McCormick 2002). Understanding how these rhythms are generated by the nervous system is therefore essential to the development of rational therapies for treating epilepsy and mental disorders.

Various rhythm-generating networks also exist in the brainstem. Rhythms controlled by the brainstem include chewing, licking, swallowing, vomiting, sneezing, coughing and breathing. Best understood is the neural network which controls breathing. Respiratory neurons are distributed in a neuronal column within the ventrolateral medulla, which is called the 'ventral respiratory group', VRG (McCrimmon et al 2000). One area within the VRG that is of particular importance for the generation of the respiratory rhythm is the so-called pre-Bötzinger complex (Smith et al 1991). As in the case of the SCN, this nucleus is both sufficient and necessary for generating respiratory rhythmic activity. Lesions of the pre-Bötzinger complex in an intact animal abolish respiration, indicating its necessity for breathing (Ramirez et al 1998). Isolation of the pre-Bötzinger complex in a brainstem slice preparation retains respiratory rhythmic activity (Ramirez et al 1996, Smith et al 1991), thus indicating that this nucleus is sufficient for generating a respiratory rhythm (Fig. 5.1).

More recently it has been demonstrated that the pre-Bötzinger complex is important for the generation of different forms of breathing including 'eupnea', gasping and sighing (Lieske et al 2000). The transition from eupnea to gasping and the generation of the sigh are generated by the same neuronal network, which is, however, reconfigured in a state-dependent manner (Lieske et al 2000).

As already mentioned in the introduction, the generation of the walking rhythm depends also on a neural network, which is located in the spinal cord (Kiehn and Kiaerulff 1998). The same principles as established for other rhythm-generating neural networks also apply for the central pattern generator for walking. The rhythm-generating network responsible for the generation of walking can be isolated in a spinal cord preparation from neonatal rats. Even after isolation, this network is still capable of generating a 'fictive' locomotor rhythm (i.e. neuronal activity that represents a locomotor rhythm in the absence of actual

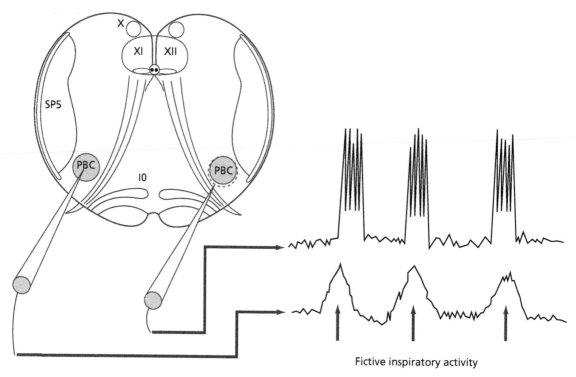

Figure 5.1 Medullary slice generates fictive respiration. PBC, pre-Bötzinger complex.

locomotor movements), indicating that the circuitry located within the spinal cord is sufficient for generating a locomotor rhythm (Fig. 5.2).

Studying fictive locomotor activity in these spinal cord preparations has led to important new insights into the mechanisms that underlie the generation of walking. For further details see various reviews (Hamm et al 1999, Jordan et al 1992, Kiehn and Kiaerulff 1998, Kiehn and Tresch 2002, Kiehn et al 2000, Schmidt and Jordan 2000). One important take-home message is that these 'in vitro' experiments indicate that the isolated spinal cord is capable of generating locomotor activity in the absence of sensory (proprioceptive) input.

THE ROLE OF PROPRIOCEPTIVE INPUT IN THE GENERATION OF RHYTHMIC ACTIVITY

Although central pattern generators can generate rhythmic activity in the absence of sensory input,

it must be emphasized that this is only the case under artificial conditions, for example following deafferentation, or following the isolation of a network under in vitro conditions. In the presence of actual movements, this is certainly not the case, and sensory feedback will highly influence the generation of rhythmic activity. In the example of the circadian clock, daylight constantly resets the circadian rhythm so we wake up in the morning, when daylight shines into our bedroom. Intense light exposure helps to overcome jet-lag and it has been used therapeutically in shift-workers to help them overcome problems associated with constant changes in the sleep–wake cycle. The lack of sensory stimulation is a major problem for blind people, in whom daylight does not constantly reset the circadian clock. These individuals have major problems with their 'free-running' circadian clocks. Circadian changes in body temperature and in hormone levels are non-synchronized, which greatly affects the daily life of blind people.

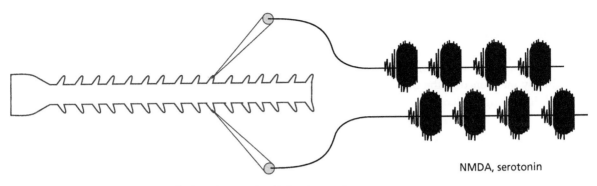

NMDA, serotonin

Figure 5.2 Isolated brainstem spinal cord generates fictive locomotion.

Sensory inputs also play a very important role in the generation of walking (Rossignol 2000, Pearson and Ramirez 1997). It is now well established that sensory inputs contribute to the generation and maintenance of the rhythmic activity. Phasic sensory input initiates major phase transitions from swing to stance and from stance to swing phase. Sensory inputs are important in regulating the magnitude of the ongoing motor activity. The concept that proprioceptive input can regulate the transitions from one phase to another has been demonstrated in various studies (Andersson and Grillner 1983, Grillner and Rossignol 1978, Kriellaars et al 1994). The proprioceptors responsible for these phase transitions seem to be muscle spindle afferents that are located in hip flexor muscles (Hiebert and Pearson 1999, Hiebert et al 1996). However, Golgi tendon organs are also important for regulating phase transitions. Located in extensor muscles, input from these so-called Ib afferents has, during locomotion, an excitatory effect on extensor motor neurons (Pearson and Collins 1993, Pearson et al 1998). Interestingly, stimulation of the same tendon organs has an opposite effect in the standing animal, indicating that reflexes are state-dependent, a phenomenon that is also known as

'reflex-reversal' (Hess and Buschges 1999, Knop et al 2001, Pearson et al 1998). This has important implications as it indicates that different regulatory mechanisms contribute to the neural control of posture and walking.

In walking, the regulation of phase transitions and the duration of a step are directly correlated. For example, electrical stimulation of group I afferents from knee and ankle extensor muscles during the extensor phase, prolongs the stance phase in walking, decerebrate cats (Pearson and Ramirez 1997). The unloading of extensor muscles is therefore thought to be a necessary condition for the initiation of the swing phase during normal walking. This sensory signal is produced by a decreased activity in the tendon organs of extensor muscles.

The role of proprioceptors in regulating the timing of phase transitions is functionally very adaptive. This regulatory mechanism guarantees that phase transitions are precisely timed according to the specific internal and environmental conditions. Proprioceptors are ideal for assuming this role as they synthesize information from the state of the moving body and from the state of the environment.

STATE-DEPENDENT MODULATION OF REFLEX PATHWAYS

The state-dependency of proprioceptive integration was already mentioned in the context of the reflex reversal. Increasing evidence indicates that reflexes are not as simple as initially thought. Reflexes can drastically change due to a direct modulation by efferent gamma-innervation, which is highly state-dependent (Prochazka 1989). However, reflex pathways are also chemically modulated within the central nervous system. For the respiratory system it has been demonstrated that pulmonary reflexes are transmitted to the central respiratory network via the nucleus tractus solitarius (NTS), an area that contains numerous neuromodulatory substances (Bonham 1995, Maley 1996, Moss and Laferriere 2002) known to play an important role in modulating breathing. These modulatory substances (serotonin, substance P, acetylcholine, endorphins, thyrotropin-releasing hormone (TRH)) are known to affect membrane properties of respiratory neurons (Dekin et al 1985, Telgkamp et al 2002) and hence transmission of reflex pathways. When released during hypoxia, the modulators may contribute to an increased ventilatory drive by altering transmission in reflex pathways from afferents of the carotid body (Wickstrom et al 1999).

NEUROMODULATION AND RECONFIGURATION OF RHYTHM-GENERATING NETWORKS WITHIN THE CENTRAL NERVOUS SYSTEM

Neuromodulatory processes also play important roles in controlling the rhythm-generating network within the central nervous system. Although, the spinal cord is capable of generating fictive locomotion in the absence of higher brain centers, they are not capable of generating locomotion spontaneously. To initiate fictive locomotor activity it is necessary to apply serotonin and NMDA exogenously, presumably in order to compensate for the missing descending aminergic input from the

brainstem (Kiehn et al 2000). There are reasons to believe that these findings also apply to the neural control of walking in humans (Calancie et al 1994, Dimitrijevic et al 1998, Duysens and van de Crommert 1998, Lamb and Yang 2000). If this is the case, these findings have important implications for various forms of spinal cord injuries. In spinal cord injured people, the inability to walk is often due to the interruption of descending inputs from higher brain centers, which are necessary to initiate and maintain locomotion. If the absence of these descending inputs is indeed responsible for the loss of locomotion, an important consequence is that the spinal network responsible for generating the walking rhythm should still be 'intact'. Therefore, it should theoretically be possible to replace these missing descending inputs pharmacologically in order to activate the dormant walking rhythm-generating network. Important chemical messengers released from descending neurons include serotonin, dopamine and noradrenaline (norepinephrine) and, in theory, exogenous application of these amines should activate locomotion. It is well established that exogenous application of either of these substances can evoke forms of locomotion in cats following spinal cord transection. And in fact it was possible to initiate stepping movements in paraplegic patients using aminergic substances (Remy-Neris et al 1999, Rossignol et al 1996, Wainberg et al 1990).

Why is the rhythm generator for walking inactive in the absence of descending inputs and how can amines activate a rhythm-generating neuronal network? One possible explanation is that descending inputs provide a tonic excitation, which is necessary to activate the neural network for walking. If this were the case, any excitatory stimulus that depolarizes the membranes of locomotor neurons should initiate locomotion. This is, however, not the case. For example, raising the potassium concentration in an isolated spinal cord would depolarize locomotor neurons, but this treatment will not initiate locomotion. It is necessary to apply aminergic substances in order to activate the rhythm-generating neural network. How could amines such as serotonin or also dopamine lead to the activation of a rhythm-generating network? There is a huge body of literature indicating that amines act as neuromodulators in neuronal network, leading to the modulation of membrane properties and synaptic transmission (Nusbaum et al 2001). Some of these properties are known to play important roles in the generation of rhythmic activity.

Membrane properties that are very important for the generation of most rhythmic activities are the so-called plateau potentials or pacemaker properties. Pacemaker properties have been demonstrated in neurons of the thalamus (Luthi and McCormick 1999), SCN (Nitabach et al 2002, Wang et al 2002), cortex (Brumberg et al 2002), and pre-Bötzinger complex (Thoby-Brisson and Ramirez 2001; Thoby-Brisson et al 2000). In many cases, it has been demonstrated that these pacemaker properties are dependent on the presence or absence of neuromodulators, such as serotonin (Pena and Ramirez 2002). This is very well documented for rhythmic activity in thalamic relay neurons, which can be induced or suppressed depending on the presence of serotonin or adrenaline (epinephrine) (McCormick and Pape 1990). Pacemaker properties can also be induced by NMDA. This has been demonstrated in spinal cord neurons, thus explaining the ability to induce fictive walking in isolated spinal cord preparations (Parker and Grillner 1999).

In many motor systems, it has also been demonstrated that amines can induce long-lasting constant discharges, which are due to the activation of so-called plateau-potentials. The induction of plateau-potentials by serotonin has been demonstrated in spinal motor neurons (Hounsgaard and Kiehn 1993) and there is good evidence that these plateau-potentials are important for the control of posture (Kiehn and Eken 1997).

Presumably the most important synaptic mechanism for the generation of rhythmic activity is reciprocal inhibition. The so-called half-center model predicts that two groups of neurons, which are connected via synaptic inhibition and which receive a tonic excitatory drive, become bi-stable and are capable of generating reciprocal rhythmic activity. Indeed, computational models have demonstrated that two groups of neurons can generate rhythmic activity if the neurons contain certain membrane properties, such as for example the so-called Ih current (Sharp et al 1996). The concept of a half-center network has been very influential and has been adopted to explain the generation of rhythmic motor activities in many motor systems, such as the swimming movements in lamprey (Grillner et al 2000), locomotion in *Xenopus* (Tunstall et al 2002), and the breathing movements in mammals (Richter and Spyer 2001). Similarly, reciprocal inhibition seems to play a role in establishing the different phases of locomotion in spinal cord preparation of neonatal rats. Synaptic interactions, such as those necessary for establishing rhythmic motor activity, are known to be targets of neuromodulators like serotonin and dopamine (Ayali et al 1998). Thus, it can be assumed that descending aminergic drive may influence the generation of walking by modulating synaptic interaction between rhythm-generating neurons in the spinal cord.

An important concept derives from these and many other findings obtained in rhythm-generating neuronal networks (e.g. Pearson and Ramirez 1997): a rhythm generating neural network is not 'hard-wired', but flexible. In the presence of neuromodulators, pacemaker properties and synaptic transmission can be modulated, changing the characteristics and connectivity of rhythm-generating networks. This is highly relevant as we have to envision that a rhythm-generating network is embedded in a 'soup of neuromodulators' which are released in a state-dependent manner from descending as well as local neurons and which constantly change the properties of the network and the proprioceptive pathways as discussed in the previous paragraph. The exact composition of this 'soup of neuromodulators' will not only be state-dependent, but it will be highly variable in different individuals and will also change dramatically during ontogenetic development. This characteristic may at least partly explain why the details of locomotion, and also the details of posture, will not be the same in any two individuals.

THE DEVELOPMENT OF MOTOR NEURAL NETWORKS

There is increasing evidence that synaptic and membrane properties change dramatically during postnatal development. For example, the composition of the glycine receptor changes postnatally (Laube et al 2002). These changes are associated with physiological changes in the properties of synaptic transmission. As the glycine receptor is abundant in the spinal cord, these changes may play an important role in establishing reciprocal activity during walking. However, the changes in the glycine receptor are only one example, and similar ontogenetic changes have been described for most other transmitter receptors and ion channels, indicating that presumably most neural networks undergo dramatic, ontogenetic changes. This will presumably result in strikingly different adaptive properties of most behaviors. However, we are far from understanding the details of how these postnatal changes at the molecular level translate into changes in behavior. This lack of understanding is partly due to the complexity of developmental changes. For example, the time course of any of the known postnatal changes differs in different regions of the brain. Postnatal changes described in one cortical layer may be different from postnatal changes that occur in another layer of the cortex. The same presumably applies to all other parts of the central nervous system.

Despite this complexity, and despite the lack of a concrete understanding of how these molecular and cellular changes translate into changes at the behavioral levels, these findings emphasize that the central nervous system has to be considered as a very plastic entity, which undergoes dramatic short-term and long-term changes. These changes will result in dramatic changes in behavior, which for the most part will be adaptive, adjusting the organism to changes in postnatal development, in the external environment, in body size and in body weight. However, these changes may not only be adaptive and one might speculate that a behavior may become maladaptive if any of these changes is disturbed, either in its time course or in its magnitude. Such ontogenetic changes at the molecular level may explain why many diseases are very characteristic for a certain stage of ontogenetic development. There are numerous examples, such as sudden infant death syndrome (SIDS), schizophrenia, manic disorders or Alzheimer's disease, which occur or begin typically in very specific age groups. Understanding which molecular factors are maladaptive will be one of the important challenges in future medical research.

CONCLUSIONS

In this chapter, principles were summarized that are relevant not only for the generation of walking, but for the generation of rhythmic activity in general. One of the most important messages is that these networks are highly flexible. In the case of the motor behavior, locomotor circuits and reflex pathways can rapidly adapt a motor behavior to changes in the external environment. As important, however, are long-term changes that alter network properties and reflex pathways to adjust a motor behavior to changes in body size and weight. In particular, during ontogenetic development, these adjustments are essential to guarantee a well-adapted motor behavior. Long-term changes occur also in association with motor learning, a form of plasticity that is particularly relevant for a developing child. This chapter has summarized possible neural mechanisms that could contribute to long-term and short-term changes and emphasized the potential role of chemical modulators in regulating membrane properties and synaptic transmission. These modulatory changes can result in varying degrees of changes in the network configuration, which can lead to a complete reconfiguration of a neural network, such as in the case of the respiratory network where it can generate significantly different forms of breathing, such as gasping or sighing. Network reconfigurations, however, occur not only in response to the release of neuromodulators. Dramatic changes can also occur as part of a genetic program during ontogenetic development. It is well established that all molecular components of a neural network undergo dramatic changes and reorganizations that translate into developmental changes of a motor behavior.

Thus, an important lesson learned from these studies is that neuronal networks are amazingly plastic and continuously changing depending on the developmental, internal and external conditions. It is therefore not surprising that the posture and walking behavior of any individual will differ from that of another individual. Given the complexity and plasticity of these neural networks it is indeed surprising that most individuals manage to produce a well-adapted 'normal' locomotor behavior and posture. This indicates that strong self-regulating mechanisms must exist that constantly adjust neuronal network properties in order to avoid major deviations from a 'normal' behavior.

References

Andersson O, Grillner S 1983 Peripheral control of the cat's step cycle. II. Entrainment of the central pattern generators for locomotion by sinusoidal hip movements during 'fictive locomotion'. Acta Physiologica Scandinavica 118(3):229–239

Ayali A, Johnson B R, Harris-Warrick R M 1998 Dopamine modulates graded and spike-evoked synaptic inhibition independently at single synapses in pyloric network of lobster. Journal of Neurophysiology 79(4):2063–2069

Barbeau H, Fung J 2001 The role of rehabilitation in the recovery of walking in the neurological population. Current Opinion in Neurology 14(6):735–740

Barbeau H, Fung J, Leroux A, Ladouceur M 2002 A review of the adaptability and recovery of locomotion after spinal cord injury. Progress in Brain Research 137:9–25

Bonham A C 1995 Neurotransmitters in the CNS control of breathing. Respiration Physiology 101(3):219–230

Boulos Z, Campbell S S, Lewy A J et al 1995 Light treatment for sleep disorders: consensus report. VII. Jet lag. Journal of Biological Rhythms 10(2):167–176

Bouyer L J, Whelan P J, Pearson K G, Rossignol S 2001 Adaptive locomotor plasticity in chronic spinal cats after ankle extensors neurectomy. Journal of Neuroscience 21(10):3531–341

Brown G M 1994 Light, melatonin and the sleep-wake cycle.Journal of Psychiatry and Neuroscience 19(5): 345–353

Brumberg J C, Nowak L G, McCormick D A 2002 Ionic mechanisms underlying repetitive high-frequency burst firing in supragranular cortical neurons. Journal of Neuroscience 20(13):4829–4843

Calancie B, Needham-Shropshire B, Jacobs P et al 1994 Involuntary stepping after chronic spinal cord injury. Evidence for a central rhythm generator for locomotion in man. Brain 117 (Pt 5):1143–1159

Cheng M Y, Bullock C M, Li C et al 2002 Prokineticin 2 transmits the behavioural circadian rhythm of the suprachiasmatic nucleus. Nature 417(6887):405–410

De Leon R D, Roy R R, Edgerton V R 2001 Is the recovery of stepping following spinal cord injury mediated by modifying existing neural pathways or by generating new pathways? A perspective. Physical Therapy 81(12):1904–1911

Dekin M S, Richerson G B, Getting P A 1985 Thyrotropin-releasing hormone induces rhythmic bursting in neurons of the nucleus tractus solitarius. Science 229(4708):67–69

Dimitrijevic M R, Gerasimenko Y, Pinter M M 1998 Evidence for a spinal central pattern generator in humans. Annals of the New York Academy of Science 860:360–376

Duysens J, Van de Crommert H W 1998 Neural control of locomotion; the central pattern generator from cats to humans. Gait and Posture 7(2):131–141

Gillette M U, Tischkau S A 1999 Suprachiasmatic nucleus: the brain's circadian clock. Recent Progress in Hormone Research 54:33–58

Grillner S, Rossignol S 1978 On the initiation of the swing phase of locomotion in chronic spinal cats. Brain Research 146(2):269–277

Grillner S, Cangiano L, Hu G et al 2000 The intrinsic function of a motor system – from ion channels to networks and behavior. Brain Research 886(1–2):224–236

Hamm T M, Trank T V, Turkin V V 1999 Correlations between neurograms and locomotor drive potentials in motoneurons during fictive locomotion: implications for the organization of locomotor commands. Progress in Brain Research 123:331–339

Hess D, Buschges A 1999 Role of proprioceptive signals from an insect femur-tibia joint in patterning motoneuronal activity of an adjacent leg joint. Journal of Neurophysiology 81(4):1856–1865

Hiebert G W, Pearson K G 1999 Contribution of sensory feedback to the generation of extensor activity during walking in the decerebrate cat. Journal of Neurophysiology 81(2):758–770

Hiebert G W, Whelan P J, Prochazka A, Pearson K G 1996 Contribution of hind limb flexor muscle afferents to the timing of phase transitions in the cat step cycle. Journal of Neurophysiology 75(3):1126–1137

Hounsgaard J, Kiehn O 1993 Calcium spikes and calcium plateaux evoked by differential polarization in dendrites of turtle motoneurones in vitro. Journal of Physiology 468:245–259

Jordan L M, Brownstone R M, Noga B R 1992 Control of functional systems in the brainstem and spinal cord. Current Opinion in Neurobiology 2(6):794–801

Kiehn O, Eken T 1997 Prolonged firing in motor units: evidence of plateau potentials in human motoneurons? Journal of Neurophysiology 78(6):3061–3068

Kiehn O, Kjaerulff O 1998 Distribution of central pattern generators for rhythmic motor outputs in the spinal cord of limbed vertebrates. Annals of the New York Academy of Sciences 16; 860:110–129

Kiehn O, Tresch M C 2002 Gap junctions and motor behavior. Trends in Neurosciences 25(2):108–115

Kiehn O, Kjaerulff O, Tresch M C, Harris-Warrick R M 2000 Contributions of intrinsic motor neuron properties to the production of rhythmic motor output in the mammalian spinal cord. Brain Research Bulletin 53(5):649–659

Knop G, Denzer L, Buschges A 2001 A central pattern-generating network contributes to 'reflex-reversal'-like leg motoneuron activity in the locust. Journal of Neurophysiology 86(6):3065–3068

Kriellaars D J, Brownstone R M, Noga B R, Jordan L M 1994 Mechanical entrainment of fictive locomotion in the decerebrate cat. Journal of Neurophysiology 71(6):2074–2086

Kuller R 2002 The influence of light on circarhythms in humans. Journal of Physiological Anthropology Applied Human Sciences 21(2):87–91

Lam T, Pearson K G 2002 The role of proprioceptive feedback in the regulation and adaptation of locomotor activity. Advances in Experimental Medicine and Biology 508:343–355

Lamb T, Yang J F 2000 Could different directions of infant stepping be controlled by the same locomotor central pattern generator? Journal of Neurophysiology 83(5):2814–2824

Laube B, Maksay G, Schemm R, Betz H 2002 Modulation of glycine receptor function: a novel approach for therapeutic intervention at inhibitory synapses? Trends in Pharmacological Science 23(11):519–527

Lieske S P, Thoby-Brisson M, Telgkamp P, Ramirez J M 2000 Reconfiguration of the neural network controlling multiple breathing patterns: eupnea, sighs and gasps. Nature Neuroscience 3(6):600–607

Llinas R R, Ribary U, Jeanmonod D, Kronberg E, Mitra P P 1999 Thalamocortical dysrhythmia: A neurological and neuropsychiatric syndrome characterized by magnetoencephalography. Proceedings of the National Academy of Sciences, U S A 96(26):15222–15227

Luthi A, McCormick D A 1999 Modulation of a pacemaker current through Ca(2+)-induced stimulation of cAMP production. Nature Neuroscience 2(7):634–641

Maley B E 1996 Immunohistochemical localization of neuropeptides and neurotransmitters in the nucleus solitarius. Chemical Senses 21(3):367–376

Marder E, Calabrese R L 1996 Principles of rhythmic motor pattern generation. Physiological Reviews 76(3):687–717

McCormick D A 2002 Cortical and subcortical generators of normal and abnormal rhythmicity. International Review of Neurobiology 49:99–114

McCormick D A, Bal T 1997 Sleep and arousal: thalamocortical mechanisms. Annual Review of Neuroscience 20:185–215

McCormick D A, Contreras D 2001 On the cellular and network bases of epileptic seizures. Annual Review of Physiology 63:815–846

McCormick D A, Pape H C 1990 Noradrenergic and serotonergic modulation of a hyperpolarization-activated cation current in thalamic relay neurones. Journal of Physiology 431:319–342

McCrea D A 2001 Spinal circuitry of sensorimotor control of locomotion. Journal of Physiology 533(Pt 1):41–50

McCrimmon D R, Ramirez J M, Alford S, Zuperku E J 2000 Unraveling the mechanism for respiratory rhythm generation. Bioessays 22(1):6–9

Mignot E, Taheri S, Nishino S 2002 Sleeping with the hypothalamus: emerging therapeutic targets for sleep disorders. Nature Neuroscience 5 Suppl:1071–1075

Moss I R, Laferriere A 2002 Central neuropeptide systems and respiratory control during development. Respiratory Physiology and Neurobiology 131(1–2):15–27.

Nakayama K, Nishimaru H, Kudo N 2002 Basis of changes in left-right coordination of rhythmic motor activity during development in the rat spinal cord. Journal of Neuroscience 22(23):10388–10398

Nitabach M N, Blau J, Holmes T C 2002 Electrical silencing of *Drosophila* pacemaker neurons stops the free-running circadian clock. Cell 109(4):485–495

Nusbaum M P, Blitz D M, Swensen A M, Wood D, Marder E 2001 The roles of co-transmission in neural network modulation. Trends in Neuroscience 24(3):146–154

Okamoto T, Okamoto K, Andrew P D 2001 Electromyographic study of newborn stepping in neonates and young infants. Electromyography and Clinical Neurophysiology 41(5):289–296

Parker D, Grillner S 1999 Long-lasting substance-P-mediated modulation of NMDA-induced rhythmic activity in the lamprey locomotor network involves separate RNA- and protein-synthesis-dependent stages. European Journal of Neuroscience 11(5):1515–1522

Pearson K G 2000 Plasticity of neuronal networks in the spinal cord: modifications in response to altered sensory input. Progress in Brain Research 128:61–70

Pearson K G 2001 Could enhanced reflex function contribute to improving locomotion after spinal cord repair? Journal of Physiology 533(Pt 1):75–81

Pearson K G, Collins D F 1993 Reversal of the influence of group Ib afferents from plantaris on activity in medial gastrocnemius muscle during locomotor activity. Journal of Neurophysiology 70(3):1009–1017

Pearson K G, Ramirez J M 1997 Sensory modulation of pattern-generating circuits. In: Stein P S G, Grillner S, Selverston A, Stuart D (eds) Neurons, networks and motor behaviour. MIT Press, Cambridge, MA, p 225–237

Pearson K G, Misiaszek J E, Fouad K 1998 Enhancement and resetting of locomotor activity by muscle afferents. Annals of the New York Academy of Sciences 16;860:203–215

Pena F, Ramirez J M 2002 Endogenous activation of serotonin-2a receptors is required for respiratory rhythm generation in vitro. Journal of Neuroscience 22:11055–11064

Prochazka A 1989 Sensorimotor gain control: a basic strategy of motor systems? Progress in Neurobiology 33(4):281–307

Rajaratnam S M, Arendt J 2001 Health in a 24-h society. Lancet 358(9286):999–1005

Ramirez J M, Quellmalz U J, Richter D W 1996 Postnatal changes in the mammalian respiratory network as revealed by the transverse brainstem slice of mice. Journal of Physiology 491:799–812

Ramirez J M, Schwarzacher S W, Pierrefiche O, Olivera B M, Richter D W 1998 Selective lesioning of the cat pre-Botzinger complex in vivo eliminates breathing but not gasping. Journal of Physiology 507(Pt 3):895–907

Remy-Neris O, Barbeau H, Daniel O, Boiteau F, Bussel B 1999 Effects of intrathecal clonidine injection on spinal reflexes and human locomotion in incomplete paraplegic subjects. Experimental Brain Research 129(3):433–440

Reppert S M, Weaver D R 2002 Coordination of circadian timing in mammals. Nature 418(6901):935–941

Richter D W, Spyer K M 2001 Studying rhythmogenesis of breathing: comparison of in vivo and in vitro models. Trends in Neuroscience 24(8):464–472

Roncesvalles M N, Woollacott M H 2000 The development of compensatory stepping skills in children. Journal of Motor Behavior 32(1):100–111

Rossignol S 2000 Locomotion and its recovery after spinal injury. Current Opinion in Neurobiology 10(6):708–716

Rossignol S, Chau C, Brustein E et al 1996 Locomotor capacities after complete and partial lesions of the spinal cord. Acta Neurobiologiae Experimentalis (Warsz) 56(1):449–463

Schmidt B J, Jordan L M 2000 The role of serotonin in reflex modulation and locomotor rhythm production in the mammalian spinal cord. Brain Research Bulletin 53(5):689–710

Sharp A A, Skinner F K, Marder E 1996 Mechanisms of oscillation in dynamic clamp constructed two-cell half-center circuits. Journal of Neurophysiology 76(2):867–883

Smith J C, Ellenberger H H, Ballanyi K, Richter D W, Feldman J L 1991 Pre-Botzinger complex: a brainstem region that may generate respiratory rhythm in mammals. Science 254(5032):726–729

Steriade M 2001 Impact of network activities on neuronal properties in corticothalamic systems. Journal of Neurophysiology 86(1):1–39

Steriade M, Amzica F 1998 Coalescence of sleep rhythms and their chronology in corticothalamic networks. Sleep Research Online 1(1):1–10

Steriade M, Contreras D, Amzica F 1994 Synchronized sleep oscillations and their paroxysmal developments. Trends in Neuroscience 17(5):199–208

Telgkamp P, Cao Y Q, Basbaum A I, Ramirez J M 2002 Long-term deprivation of substance P in PPT-A mutant mice alters the anoxic response of the isolated respiratory network. Journal of Neurophysiology 88(1):206–213

Thoby-Brisson M, Ramirez J M 2001 Identification of two types of inspiratory pacemaker neurons in the isolated respiratory neural network of mice. Journal of Neurophysiology 86(1):104–112

Thoby-Brisson M, Telgkamp P, Ramirez J M 2000 The role of the hyperpolarization-activated current in modulating rhythmic activity in the isolated respiratory network of mice. Journal of Neuroscience 20(8):2994–3005

Tunstall M J, Roberts A, Soffe S R 2002 Modelling inter-segmental coordination of neuronal oscillators: synaptic mechanisms for uni-directional coupling during swimming in Xenopus tadpoles. Journal of Computational Neuroscience 13(2):143–158

Wainberg M, Barbeau H, Gauthier S 1990 The effects of cyproheptadine on locomotion and on spasticity in patients with spinal cord injuries. Journal of Neurology, Neurosurgery and Psychiatry 53(9):754–763

Wang J, Chen S, Nolan M F, Siegelbaum S A 2002 Activity-dependent regulation of HCN pacemaker channels by cyclic AMP: signaling through dynamic allosteric coupling. Neuron 36(3):451–461

Weaver D R 1998 The suprachiasmatic nucleus: a 25-year retrospective. Journal of Biological Rhythms 13(2):100–112

Whelan P J, Pearson K G 1997 Plasticity in reflex pathways controlling stepping in the cat. Journal of Neurophysiology 78(3):1643–1650

Wickstrom H R, Holgert H, Hokfelt T, Lagercrantz H 1999 Birth-related expression of c-fos, c-jun and substance P mRNAs in the rat brainstem and pia mater: possible relationship to changes in central chemosensitivity. Brain Research. Developmental Brain Research 112(2):255–266

Zisapel N 2001 Circadian rhythm sleep disorders: pathophysiology and potential approaches to management. CNS Drugs 15(4):311–328

Chapter 6

Neuromotor development in infancy and early childhood

S. Huber

INTRODUCTION

Learning complex motor skills up to their virtuoso performance is a very long and protracted process which normally extends over several years. If we compare motor control in children and adults, young adolescents still show substantial differences in efficiency and accuracy of performance in motor tasks. Even elementary motion sequences like smiling, grasping of an object, sitting, walking and speaking take months to years to be performed efficiently. The movement of newborns, in contrast, appears very uncontrolled and variable.

For a long time, it was considered as fact that brain maturation alone is responsible for the development of motor skills. The theory of maturation, which was predominant during the 1920s to 1940s, was mainly developed and pushed forward in the domain of motor development by Gesell (1933, 1946) and McGraw (1945, 1946). They assumed that the regularities that can be observed in the process of motor development reflect the development of brain maturation, i.e. the unfolding of a genetic program that was supposed to be the same in all infants. The underlying idea of their theory was that the maturation of motor skills reflects the hierarchy of the central nervous system: When an infant matures, higher brain areas of the motor cortex take over the tasks of the subcortex and inhibit the subcortex. Reflexive and immature motion patterns are replaced by coordinated and directed movements controlled by the cortex. The theory of maturation also assumed that there is a fixed sequence of motor development in which practice and the environment play only a subordinate role.

Phenomenological experiments have been conducted to support this view. Catalogues were developed with lists of stages (Gesell 1933, McGraw 1945, Shirley 1931) detailing age-specific behavior as well as how children gain control over their movements. For throwing objects, for instance, 58 stages were specified, for rattling 53 stages, etc. One of the studies cited repeatedly as evidence for the maturation theory was a culture study, dating back to 1940, on the development of walking in infants of Hopi Indians (Dennis and Dennis 1940). Infants from the Hopi community spend most of their first year of life wrapped up tightly in a cradle and carried around on their mothers' backs. According to this study, although these babies can hardly move, they learn to walk only slightly later than infants from Western traditions. The fact that these infants were only slightly delayed in learning to walk despite an apparent lack of constant practice was cited as evidence that behavioral changes in motor control are directly linked to changes in the brain.

This view of a direct causal link between maturation of the brain and behavioral changes is highly plausible and is still held today to some extent. Until the mid 1980s, this view of motor development was actually predominant. It was only when Bernstein's new way of looking at motor coordination became known that a paradigm shift occurred (Bernstein 1967) (for review see Sporns and Edelman 1993).

Bernstein (1967) challenged the view of a 1 : 1 mapping of neural code, firing of motor neurons and actual movement, which had been postulated by brain maturation theories. He took a fresh look at the problem of motor development, suggesting that a movement can be caused by a variety of different motion patterns, and the pattern of how movement is executed can, in turn, be executed in a variety of ways. This implies that movement has to be planned on a much more abstract level, as it would be far too complex for the central nervous system to program all the local and context-dependent, dynamic variables in advance.

Bernstein thus described movement as a problem of coordination, i.e. as the coordination of a cooperative interaction of many partners to gain a uniform result. The problem, according to Bernstein, is how the organism with its almost indeterminable number of combinations of body segments and positions finds a solution to enable all parts to work together harmoniously and efficiently, without every step being programed in advance. This new way of thinking about movement control has led to a rethinking of the principles of motor development, resulting in theories that put forward a multicausal view of motor development (Newell 1986, Thelen 2000). These theories assume a dynamic system where the environment, the development of the perceptual system, biomechanics and muscle power complement the maturation of the brain as principal components.

These more recent theories (e.g. *dynamic systems theory* – Thelen 1995, 2000) assume that due to only few movement restrictions at the beginning of life, the infant can draw upon a large variety of motion patterns to execute spontaneous movements. This variety of motion patterns implies that all possibilities of motor control can be explored. At the same time it makes these patterns suitable for a changing environment. The infant learns to restrict this variability as more functional motor programs develop.

Practice, as gained by the increasing experience of the motor system as well as the sensory system, plays a crucial role in the development of specific motor skills. Visual, vestibular and proprioceptive information allows the infant to fine-tune balance, head and body control as well as grasping movements on the basis of visual, tactile and kinesthetic information. This integration of new motor strategies is brought about by a process of neural selection. At the beginning, the infant executes spontaneous movements which are subject to high variability. Motion patterns can be evaluated via sensory feedback and connections can be selected which fulfill current needs or which seem to lead to an important skill for the future. Finally, neural connections that are related to the most efficient motor patterns are strengthened and others are inhibited.

But why does motor development take so long? One reason is that motor control is only possible based on a highly complex nervous system with a huge number of connections. These connections send out motor signals, but provide a continuous feedback about the current state of the system, too, during the movement being executed (Fig. 6.1).

Eliot (1999) illustrates the problem of movement control with a simple example: When a straightforward arm movement is executed, the biceps bends and the triceps is stretched at the same time. The command of such a voluntary movement is generated in the motor area of the cerebral cortex. There are three motor areas which are all located in the back part of the frontal lobe: the primary motor cortex, the supplementary motor area and the pre-motor cortex. The primary motor cortex triggers voluntary movement, while the other two operate on a higher level and control more complex sequences of motion. The motor cortex – like the somatosensory cortex – contains a distorted upside-down map of the body, the homunculus: the lateral regions of this area control the muscles of the head and the face, the middle regions control the arms and hands, and the medial regions are in control of the legs and feet (Penfield and Rasmussen 1950). This distorted map allocates bigger areas for those body parts – such as hands and the face – that possess more muscles, since they have to execute more complex movements than for example the trunk or the legs.

If a voluntary movement of the arm is executed, the neurons of the arm region of the left motor cortex send action potentials to the spinal cord, which is connected via the corticospinal tract. In the spinal cord, the neurons of the corticospinal tract excite motor neurons, which send out their axons via peripheral nerves to reach the muscle fibers in the arm. The electrical excitation leads to a contraction of the relevant muscles. At the beginning

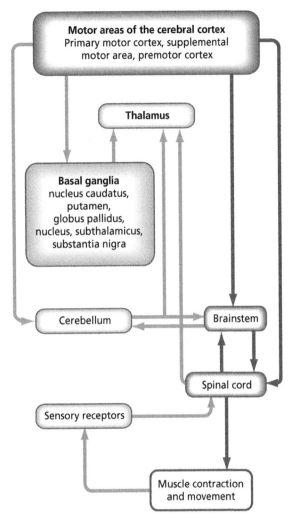

Figure 6.1   Motor circuits involved in the execution of voluntary movements (Ghez 1991).

of the movement, the muscle undergoes changes in tension and length, which again are perceived by special sensory neurons, the proprioceptors. Proprioceptive information feeds back to the spinal cord, where the firing of muscle motor neurons is modified, and on to the cerebral cortex where the arm position is perceived. Proprioceptive information allows the movement of the arm to be felt and to be fine-tuned millisecond by millisecond. All this is most likely to happen parallel to hand and finger movements. In addition, information is integrated from the visual system, which provides information about the arm position to the motor cortex in order to control muscle contraction and relaxation. Highly elaborate tasks, such as walking or postural balance of the whole body, where dozens of muscles are involved, are even more complex tasks for the motor control system.

The cerebellum is mainly responsible for the precise coordination and timing of all these movements. It receives input from the motor cortex (i.e. information about the kind of movement that is to be executed) as well as from different sensory systems, such as vision, hearing, balance and proprioception (i.e. information about the actual movement). The cerebellum controls and times the movements by comparing the incoming information, and modifies the motor commands to achieve the best possible result for the execution of the movements. The basal ganglia play a central part in movement control, too. Here motor actions and inhibiting involuntary movements are selected. Patients with Parkinson's disease or Huntington's disease, for instance (who show disorders in the basal ganglia), have great problems initiating voluntary movements. They often have difficulty talking or walking, or their movements are very slow. In contrast to patients suffering from paralysis, however, they move quite a lot, though most of their movements are involuntary. The basal ganglia also have a strong connection to the thalamus, which receives sensory as well as motor information (from the cerebellum, the spinal cord and the basal ganglia) and sends it on to the cortex.

BRAIN MATURATION AND MYELINATION

It cannot be denied that maturation of the central nervous system plays a crucial role in the development of motor skills, although it is clear today that there is no exact mapping between the two because of the environmental influences that have just been described. The motor cortex undergoes a great deal of modification during the first year. The most important neuromotor changes, which lead to a predictable sequence of development of motor skills, are described below.

The higher areas of the brain are hardly developed at birth. Maturation of the brain areas develops from caudal to cranial areas and from dorsal to ventral areas (Grodd 1993, Staudt et al 2000): motor connections in the spinal cord mature first, long before birth, followed by the neurons of the brainstem and the connections in the primary motor cortex. Finally, the higher brain areas located in the frontal lobe attain maturation. The motor neurons which leave the spinal cord are among the first fibers in the brain to myelinate (by mid-gestation). Myelination of the motor areas in the brainstem starts in the last trimester of pregnancy. The fibers and connections of the primary motor cortex begin to myelinate around birth. Myelination in this area takes about 2 years. The myelination in the frontal lobe progresses very slowly. The fibers of the premotor cortex and the supplementary motor area, for instance, do not begin to myelinate until about the age of 6 months and then continue to do so for several years.

With the brainstem maturing early, the order of motor development is from central to peripheral body parts, since the muscles of the trunk and the head are mainly controlled by the motor connections in the brainstem, whereas the muscles of the peripheral body segments are controlled by the motor cortex. In fact, infants are able to control their trunk and their head muscles before they can control their arms and legs or their hands and fingers. The maturation of the primary motor cortex also influences the sequence of motor development. Myelination and maturation start in the lower areas of the primary motor cortex and progress upwards, i.e. control over the muscles of the face is gained before that over hands or feet. Infants, therefore, can turn their head and smile before they learn to grasp, crawl and walk.

DEVELOPMENT OF MOTOR SKILLS

Neuromotor development is a long-lasting process. It sets in some weeks after fertilization and then continues several years after birth until reaching completion during puberty. Thanks to the advanced use of ultrasonic imaging, there is now a fairly clear and comprehensive understanding of the prenatal development of motor skills.

The fetus is active from the 8th to 10th week of gestation, showing spontaneous activity as well as structured activity patterns from the very beginning (Prechtl 1985, 1993). Initially these are movements of the whole fetus, spontaneous arches and curls, but very soon the limbs themselves move and initiate entire body movements. Isolated arm and leg movements start at about the 10th week, finger movements set in 2 weeks later. From the 11th week onwards, the fetus starts to bring a hand to its head, but it only starts to suck its thumbs after approximately 5 months.

Other astonishing motor skills which develop in the first 3 months are hiccups, stretching, yawning, swallowing and grasping. These movements are already highly coordinated right from the start. In the second half of pregnancy, the fetus commences with continuous breathing movements. The lungs, at this point still filled with liquid, start to expand and compress together with the diaphragm and thorax in a rhythmic and coordinated fashion. Sucking and swallowing become more coordinated from the 28th week onwards. From week 33 onwards both swallowing and sucking are coordinated with breathing movements. These processes seem to be at least in part an expression of the launch of activity of the developing neural system. In addition, some of these behavioral patterns also fulfill functions of adaptation, provide behavioral patterns for later use (such as breathing and sucking) or constitute precursors of later movement patterns (Hall and Oppenheim 1987).

BIOMECHANICS, PRACTICE AND ENVIRONMENT

Recently, a number of studies have been conducted to show which other factors besides the maturation of the brain have an impact on motor development. The organism, biomechanics, and muscle power are said to play an important role at every step of motor development. Already in 1931, Shirley documented that differences in infants' physical growth, muscle tone, and energy levels were related to differences in the onset of various motor skills.

Physical dimensions, biomechanics and movement styles are still seen as an important part of motor development (Thelen 2000). The influence of biomechanics has been studied by Thelen and her colleagues in a series of experiments testing walking skills. If newborns are lifted up so that their feet touch the ground while being supported under their arms, they will readily show step-like movements which have a close resemblance to the walking pattern of older infants. It is astonishing how coordinated these movements are already in newborns, who can hardly control their head. After a few weeks, this reflex disappears, only reappearing later in the year when the infant is ready to learn to walk.

Traditionally, the disappearance of the step-like movements, the so-called walking reflex, in newborns after just a few weeks was explained by the fact that the first subcortically driven reflex is inhibited by the developing motor cortex (McGraw 1945). This inhibition is only suspended if the motor cortex is mature enough to take over control of the subcortically driven processes in a coordinated way.

Investigations of the rhythmic kicking behavior of infants who are just a few months old and lying on their back show, however, that the walking reflex does not disappear at all. The kicking movements directly match the rhythmic step-like movements of newborns. The only difference is the position in which the infant's body experiences the effect of gravity: infants lying on their back can lift up their legs more easily than those in an upright position.

Thelen and her colleagues showed that infants that seem to have lost their walking reflex also start to show the pattern spontaneously when their legs are under water (Thelen et al 1984). Underwater gravitation has less effect due to buoyancy. They also demonstrated that younger infants do not show this walking pattern if their legs are made heavier with little weights (Adolph and Avolio 2000, Thelen et al 1987). Infants, thus, seem to stop showing the stepping reflex because their weight gain during the first months of life is not matched by an increase in muscle mass or force, therefore depriving the infants of sufficient power to lift the legs in an upright position. This interaction between intrinsic and environmental constraints has also been studied in the domain of reaching by Savelsbergh and van der Kamp (1994). They showed that body orientation with respect to gravity has an effect on the quantity and quality of infants' reaching behavior.

Besides the influence of biomechanics and body layout, important factors are the possibilities to practice motor control, and perceptual stimulation from the environment. New insights in motor development strongly emphasize the role of exploration and selection in the acquisition of new motor skills. The infants' first step is to discover configurations that enable them to perform a certain motor task; these must then be fine-tuned to the required smoothness and efficiency. Thelen (1994) demonstrated that by the age of 3 months infants can, given an appropriate and novel task, already transform their seemingly spontaneous kicking movements into new and efficient motor patterns.

Thelen and her colleagues investigated the kicking movements of 3-month-old infants who were allowed to control the movement of an overhead mobile by means of a string attached to their legs. In one group, the infants additionally had their two legs tied loosely together at the ankles. The soft elastic allowed the infants to move their legs in any coordinated pattern of alternating, single, or simultaneous kicks, but simultaneous kicks provided the strongest activation of the mobile. All infants kicked more often as well as faster when their kicks activated the mobile as compared to when their kicks did not have any effect.

However, only the infants with loosely tied legs moved their legs in an increasingly simultaneous pattern.

The study suggests that infants at the age of 3 months can discover and learn a match between inter-limb coordination patterns and a specific task. Acquisition of new motor skills, thus, seems to depend on learning processes such as these, rather than autonomous brain 'maturation' (Thelen 1994). At the age of 3 months infants are already able to quickly solve new tasks in which, for instance, certain knee positions (such as bending and stretching of the knee) have gained positive feedback (Angulo-Kinzler et al 2002). Another example comes from a study by Goldfield et al (1993). They investigated how infants learn to use a Jolly Jumper (a baby seat attached to elastic ropes): infants started with only a few bounces, which had irregular amplitudes and periods. As the weeks passed, infants increased the number of bounces and at the same time decreased their period and amplitude variability, settling in on a frequency which was consistent with the predicted resonant frequency of the infant-bouncer-spring system.

PERCEPTION AND MOTOR DEVELOPMENT

Recent advances in the understanding of human movement control have enabled developmental psychologists to discover unique patterns of organization and control in infant motor behavior and development, and triggered new interest in this topic. The tuning of movement patterns shown in several examples above is most probably established through repeated cycles of perception and action as well as through the consequences of the action in relation to the goal. We will come back to this in the next section where we consider the development of eye–hand coordination in detail. Besides perception influencing the development of action, some researchers postulate not only that motor development is supported by perceptual development but also that motor development may play a predominant role in determining developmental sequences or 'timetables' in the domain of perception (Bushnell and Boudreau 1993). Specifically, they argue that particular motor achievements may be integral to the development in the domains of haptic and depth perception. In both cases, there is a high degree of fit between the developmental sequence in which certain perceptual sensitivities unfold and the age of onset of corresponding motor abilities (Fig. 6.2).

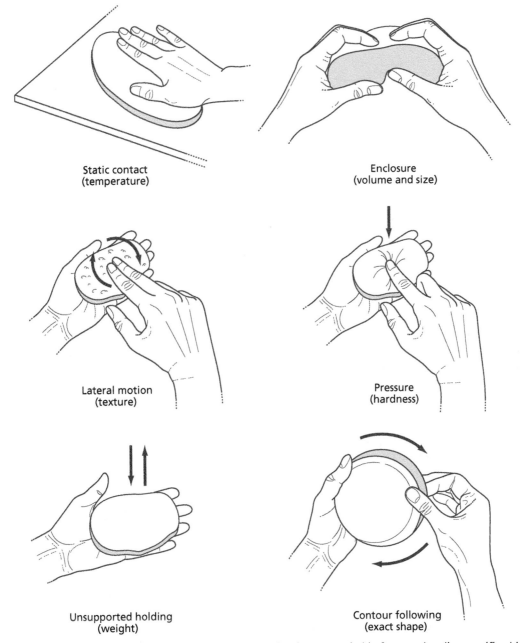

Static contact
(temperature)

Enclosure
(volume and size)

Lateral motion
(texture)

Pressure
(hardness)

Unsupported holding
(weight)

Contour following
(exact shape)

Figure 6.2 Hand movement patterns which have been found to be most suitable for apprehending specific object properties (from Lederman and Klatzky 1987, with permission of Elsevier Science).

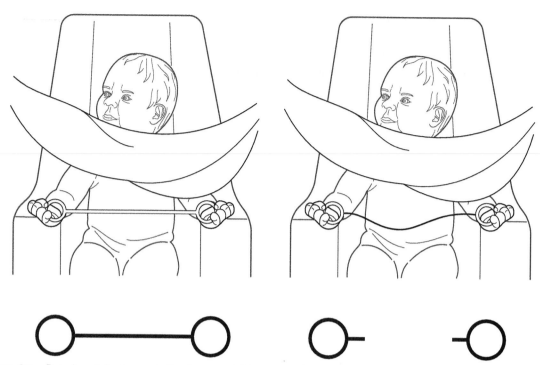

Figure 6.3 Experimental setup and stimulus material in an experiment on haptic perception (from Streri and Spelke 1988, with permission of Elsevier Science).

Evidence for these connections is found, for instance, in experiments conducted by Streri and Spelke (1988; Streri et al 1993). They investigated 4.5-month-old infants' perception of the unity and boundaries of haptically presented objects (Fig. 6.3). When infants actively explored the two handles of an unseen object assembly, perception of the unity of the assembly depended on the handles' motion. Infants perceived a single, connected object if the handles moved rigidly together, and they perceived two distinct objects if the handles underwent vertical or horizontal motion.

EYE–HAND COORDINATION IN THE FIRST YEAR OF LIFE

In this section we take a closer look at the development of a special skill, eye–hand coordination, which is probably the most intensively investigated field in motor development (for an overview see also Wilkening and Krist 1998). Eye–hand coordination undergoes profound development throughout the first year of life, when children learn how to grasp for objects and how to manipulate them. Besides the development of efficient motor programs, the development of object perception as well as proprioceptive and visual perception of the hand play important roles in developing skilled motor control of the arm, hand and fingers.

For newborns, arm and hand movements are closely linked. The bending and stretching of the arm is often accompanied by the bending and stretching of the hand. Only at about the age of 2 months does this coupling disappear. At this age, the hand is mostly formed to a fist when the arm is stretched. Especially at this age (2 to 4 months), the hand possesses an important function for perception, i.e. in the haptic experience of objects.

Hand and eye work more or less independently from each other at this age. Infants often fixate one object with their eyes and investigate another one with their hands (Hatwell 1987). At the age of 3 months, infants resume opening their hand while stretching the arm, when they fixate an object. But infants younger than 4 months are generally not able to target and grasp a seen object. Infants, on the other hand, who are about to start grasping are not interested anymore in just haptically exploring the target object (Hatwell 1987).

Because of this developmental sequence, the belief was widely shared for a long time that initially eye and hand are controlled independently from another. Only at about the age of 3 or 4 months, when infants begin to grasp, does the coordination of eyes and hands start. However, recent studies show this view not to be correct. Although the spontaneous arm movements of newborns seem to be aimless under supporting conditions – one of which is support of the body of the infant – studies show that the movements depend on the direction of the visual goal. Von Hofsten (1982) was able to demonstrate that 5–9-day-old infants already show a rudimentary eye–hand coordination. As the arm movements of newborns typically consist of several uncoordinated sub-movements, von Hofsten chose only the sub-movements that brought the hand nearest to the aimed target. He compared the direction of movements where the infants fixated the target with their eyes with direction of movements where they did not fixate the target. The results showed that infants miss the target with fixation by on average 32° and without fixating the target by about 52°. Thus, eye and hand do not work independently of each other in newborns.

Eye–hand coordination is, however, only rudimentary in newborn infants. Newborns direct the arm approximately by fixing the goal. This *ballistic movement* is triggered by the visual input. Infants at the age of 5 months, on the other hand, start to move their hand under constant visual control and systematically move their hand nearer to the target. The movement is visually guided (Bushnell 1985). Before infants start to guide their movements visually, it can be observed that they show an increased tendency to fixate their hand and fol-

low the hand with their gaze (Piaget 1973, 1975b, White et al 1964).

Only from the age of 5 months onwards do infants, when reaching for an object, show a better result if they can see not only the target but also the grasping hand (Lasky 1977, McDonnell 1975). This is not to mean, however, that coordinated grasping attempts are executed solely under the visual guidance of the hand. Important empirical evidence comes from a number of studies on grasping in the dark and grasping for moving objects. Infants aged 4 to 7 months can grasp for objects in the dark even if they can only be located by sound, if they glow in the dark or if they were located before it got dark (Clifton et al 1973). Nevertheless, if continuous sight of the object is available, infants use vision during the reach. However, they can still reach for an illuminated object even if it is darkened during the reach (McCarty and Ashmead 1999). These results are astonishing in light of the fact that infants from this age until the age of 8–9 months do not reach for an object if it disappears behind another object in front of their eyes (Piaget 1975b). Diamond showed that it seems to be important that the object can be reached on a direct path without having to plan detours (Diamond 1990). Taken together these results indicate that infants do not necessarily have to guide their hand visually when reaching for an object.

Experiments on reaching for moving objects have been conducted mainly by von Hofsten and co-workers (von Hofsten 1980, 1983, 2002). Von Hofsten and Lindhagen (1979) examined infants between 12 and 30 weeks of age once every 3 weeks as to their development in reaching for moving objects. An object was moved back and forth in front of the infant such that it got into reaching distance for a certain amount of time. At the same time as infants learned to reach for static objects, they successfully reached for moving objects. At the age of 18 weeks, they successfully grasped for objects that moved at about 30 cm/s. At this speed, they had to start the reaching movement before the object was in reaching distance. Thus, the infants at this early age anticipated the intersection point and planned the movement accordingly. The visually triggered movement that is observable in adults when they grasp accurately for all kinds of objects is, therefore, already present in infants and does not develop from visually guided reaching. Von Hofsten (1983) also showed that at 34 to 36 weeks of age, infants can already catch an object, even if it moves at 120 cm/s.

Recent studies investigated which critical variables guide the extrapolation of object movement (von Hofsten et al 1998). Six-month-old children were sitting in front of a screen when objects were presented to them which came into grasping distance on four different paths (Fig. 6.4): two were linear and crossed each other in the middle of the screen and two contained an abrupt change in the direction of the crossing. The reaching movements and gaze direction of the children showed that the infants extrapolated the object motion along a linear path, according to the laws of inertia. This behavior was still present when confronting the infants several times with the non-linear object movement. Further studies show that infants from the age of 5 to 7.5 months reach for moving objects that glow in the dark. Thus, even in such a complex reaching task the proprioceptive information and the sight of the object are sufficient for an infant to successfully reach for the object. Again the reaching movement is directed towards an anticipated intersection point (Robin et al 1996).

In follow-up studies, von Hofsten et al investigated what happens if the target is occluded at the point of crossing in the brief period before it comes within reach (von Hofsten et al 1994). Infants now either tended to reach for the object only rarely or they interrupted the grasping movement very often. When presented with the same movement several times in a row (in a linear or non-linear fashion), 6-month-old infants showed a predictive gaze behavior after just a few trials for

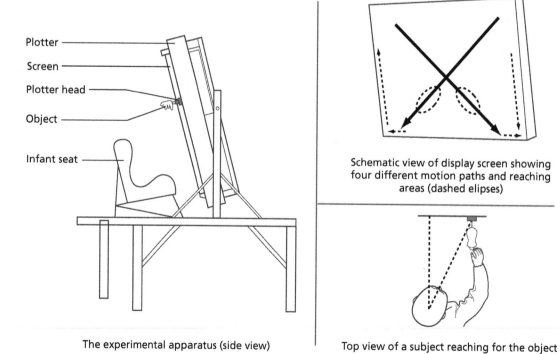

Plotter
Screen
Plotter head
Object
Infant seat

The experimental apparatus (side view)

Schematic view of display screen showing four different motion paths and reaching areas (dashed elipses)

Top view of a subject reaching for the object

Figure 6.4 Experimental setup in a grasping experiment (from von Hofsten et al 1998, with permission of Elsevier Science).

linear object motion (von Hofsten et al 2000), whereas the ability to predict non-linear object motion is only learnt slowly.

Further studies have shown that reaching behavior did not improve if the occluder was transparent such that the object could be seen behind the occluder. Thus, reaching behavior was not reduced due to perceiving the occluder as a barrier for reaching (Spelke and von Hofsten 2001). The influence of the visual control of the hand wanes during the second half of the first year in favor of pre-programed movements, but it does not disappear completely. During this phase, infants, just like adults, use the visually perceived relation between hand and target to reach for the target precisely in the final phase of the movement and to compensate for unexpected replacements of the target (Ashmead et al 1993). The more precisely the reach can be pre-programed by the infants the less dependent they are on other correction mechanisms. In fact, after already a few months of reaching practice, the infant is able to reach for objects with one quick arm movement.

Nevertheless, difficulties may still arise if increasing demands are made on the motor skill. It has been confirmed time and again that infants of 5 to 6 months can reach and grasp for a freestanding object, but fail to retrieve the same object if it is mounted on top of a larger object. Studies by Diamond and Lee (2000) suggest that the findings can be explained by the lack of fully developed motor skills. If infants reached for the upper object but – due to an imprecise movement – touched the lower object, they could not inhibit the reflex of grasping the lower object instead of continuing to reach for the upper object. If the demands on the motor skill, however, were reduced by decreasing the possibility of the infant accidentally touching the base object (by just using smaller base objects), infants successfully retrieved the upper object. These new results replaced the long accepted view according to which infants do not understand conceptually that the object continues to exist when placed on another object and, therefore, stop grasping for it.

Apart from the tendency to grasp for an object that is accidentally touched, systemic one- or two-handed motor tendencies in the reaching behavior of infants seem to be in conflict with the development of efficient grasping skills. Corbetta et al (2000) addressed this issue by investigating 5- to 9-month-old infants' reaching and grasping behavior for objects of different sizes and textures. Only infants older than 8 months were able to scale their actions according to the visual and haptic information available to them about the object. Younger infants seemed to be locked into one motor pattern: they could not select and switch between one- and two-handed reaching behavior.

A number of studies show that the ability to pre-program anticipatory hand and finger movements develops mainly in the second half of the year. At that time infants not only learn to open and close their hand at the right moment but they also start to consider the orientation of the hand with respect to the object and other spatio-temporal aspects of the movement (Lockman 1990, von Hofsten 1989, von Hofsten and Rönquist 1988). For example, they start to use a two-finger grip at about the age of 9 to 10 months. Infants at this point in time are able to coordinate thumb and index finger such that a small object can be grasped and lifted between the finger tips.

The role of postural adjustment during spontaneous and goal-directed reaching behavior has been investigated for example by van der Fits et al (1999). They investigated particularly whether the immature postural control of newborns and young infants is responsible for the relatively poor quality of pre-reaching movements.

Parallel to the development of the reaching and grasping behavior, changes in postural control can be observed. Newborns are already able to adapt their posture to the current position, 3-month-old infants can stabilize head and trunk and by the age of 6 to 7 months, infants can sit upright with the help of arm support. At the age of 9 months, infants sit upright even without support. In lying and sitting adults, voluntary arm movements are accompanied, in particular, by activity in the neck and trunk muscles. The neck and upper trunk muscles seem to be responsible for opposing reaction forces which are generated by the reaching movements and the lower trunk muscles serve to stabilize the center of mass. Fits et al found that in pre-reaching infants the spontaneous arm movements are accompanied by postural muscle activity which is highly variable (van der Fits et al 1999).

As the infants get older, successful reaching and adult-like temporal characteristics of the postural adjustment seem to emerge in parallel. These results suggest a fundamental coupling between arm movements and postural control.

MOTOR DEVELOPMENT BEYOND THE FIRST YEAR OF LIFE

The ability to pre-program and execute the movement efficiently increases up to young adolescence continuously (see also Wilkening and Krist 1998). Firstly, this is due to increased speed of planning, preparing and performing movements. Secondly, this is closely connected to the ability to plan the movement accurately. The more accurate the pre-programming, the fewer and less significant are the corrections that have to be made dur-

ing the movement's execution. Both spatial and temporal accuracy as well as speed of the movement seem to improve with age. However, there are some notable exceptions for certain tasks which are related to qualitative changes in the way of controlling the movement, as these qualitative changes seem to be correlated to strategic changes in movement control (Connolly 1968, Hay 1984). Hay tested 5-, 7-, 9- and 11-year-old children in a pointing task (Hay 1984). Children had to point to one of several target points which lit up randomly on a horizontal line, the view of hand and arm being occluded by a screen. Children, thus, had to pre-program the arm movement or use proprioceptive information to adjust arm and hand position with respect to the target.

Mean accuracy was high for 5- and 11-year-old children but low for 7- and 9-year-old children. However, 5-year-olds produced a high intra-individual variability, which decreased considerably with age. Taking movement time into account as well, it can be seen that the movement pattern produced by the different age groups differs considerably (Fig. 6.5). Five-year-olds produced a ballistic-like pattern with very sudden acceleration and deceleration phases. At the age of 7 and still at the age of 9 years, the pointing movement consists

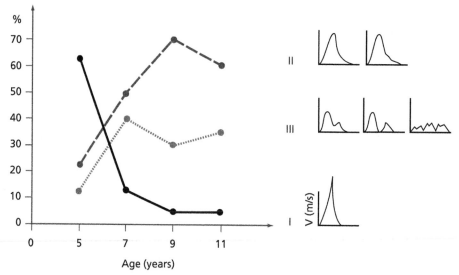

Figure 6.5 Percentage of each type of velocity pattern per age (from Hay 1984, with permission of Springer-Verlag, © Springer-Verlag).

of several sub-movements with braking activity and processing of (proprioceptive) feedback, whereas some 9-year-olds and especially the 11-year-olds again produce a ballistic movement in which feedback control is now concentrated at the end of the movement sequence and all parts of the movement are better coordinated.

Another experiment with 6- to 10-year-old children and adults on sequential pointing revealed a similar non-linear development (Badan et al 2000). Badan et al manipulated the task difficulty by changing the number, size and spacing of the targets in the sequences. Children's temporal and spatial parameters of the motor sequences showed large age-dependent trends, but did not reach the adult values. This is consistent with the view that the neurophysiological mechanisms mediating perceptual and motor functions are well developed at the age of 6 and improvements are due to a continuing process of fine-tuning the system. However, the authors also found that increasing the difficulty of the task did not affect behavior in a similarly uniform fashion. The performance of the 7-year-olds, in particular, showed that the motor planning strategy characteristic of older children seems to emerge at this age, though it has not yet superseded the less effective planning mode adopted at earlier stages of development. Thus, it seems that motor development is not a uniform fine-tuning of stable strategies. Instead, each stage of development is best characterized by a set of strategic components potentially available at that stage, and by the age-dependent rules for the selection of components in a given context.

Pellizzer and Hauert (1996) conducted a study to gain information about the origin of the temporary decrease in visuo-manual performance occurring around the age of 7 and 8 years. They assumed that changes occurring on a behavioral level are consequences of those taking place on the neuronal level. They tested children between the age of 6 and 10 years in a visuo-manual aiming task. Results showed non-monotonic changes, which were linked to age, spatial accuracy, reaction time and movement time. Spatial accuracy in the right

visual field decreased between 6 and 8 years and increased afterwards. Reaction time and movement time decreased with age, except at the age of 8 years when both tended to increase.

The same children participated in two control tasks which showed that the non-monotonic trend is not present if reaction time is tested where no spatial processing is required and vice versa if spatial processing is tested but reaction time is not a constraint. The authors concluded that this asymmetry in the data seems to be due to different processes involved in each task and that these processes undergo a qualitative change at the age of 8 years. Moreover their results seem to suggest that the prevailing processes that are transformed are located in the left cerebral hemisphere (Pellizzer and Hauert 1996). In fact, this observed asymmetry is compatible with studies indicating that homologous regions of both cerebral hemispheres develop asynchronously (Rabinowicz et al 1977, Thatcher et al 1987).

COGNITION AND PERCEPTION

For many years, motor skills and cognition were believed to be unrelated, since many studies have shown only a modest correlation between motor and intellectual development (Piaget 1975a, Shirley 1931). Piaget, on the other hand, believed that cognition comes about from perception and action. Nowadays it is agreed that the cognitive development of children also plays an important role in the development of motor skills. This is particularly true with complex skills where not only practice of a single movement is essential, but other factors, too, such as general learning ability, the ability to use feedback, processing capacities, planning strategies, making decisions on which information is essential and which is not, etc.

The relationship between perception, action and cognition is rather complex and not completely understood. Sometimes there are astonishing discrepancies between perceptual-motor competencies and the corresponding cognitive knowledge (Frick et al 2003, Huber et al 2003, Krist et al 1993), whereas in other cases cognition and concepts guide our actions (Krist 2001).

The questions to be raised are whether conceptual knowledge guides actions, whether conceptual knowledge is derived from actions (as Piaget would argue) and whether judgments and actions represent forms of knowledge that are inseparable. One field where these questions were intensively studied is the field of intuitive physics (i.e. people's intuitive concepts about simple phenomena of motion), where knowledge expressed in perceptual-motor tasks can easily be assessed.

Krist et al (1993) investigated, for instance, children's knowledge about projectile motion. They asked children from the age of 5 years onwards to propel a ball from various heights onto a target on the floor at various distances. Besides the action condition, a judgment condition was used in which, for each combination of platform height and target distance, the speed of the ball had to be judged on a graphic rating scale. According to the laws of physics, speed in this situation is a direct function of distance (the farther, the faster), and an inverse function of height (the higher, the slower).

Children's speed productions reflected these principles very well, with virtually no age trend from the youngest children up to adults. In the judgment condition, however, 5-year-olds failed to integrate the relevant dimensions, and many 10-year-olds (and even several adults) showed striking misconceptions. Most of these children seemed to hold an inverse-height heuristic: that the ball should fall faster the higher the platform of release.

In other tasks, however, children used their concepts to drive their actions. Krist conducted a study in which children moving at constant speed were asked to hit a target on the floor by dropping a ball (Krist 2001). Those children who held the concept (assessed in a judgment condition) that an object dropping from a moving carrier falls straight down, dropped the ball significantly later (above the target) than those who had the correct knowledge that the object falls in the forward direction; these children released the ball clearly before being exactly above the target.

SUMMARY

Major developmental changes in motor control are observed in particular during the first 2 years of life. This is mainly due to the fast progression of neural development during this time. We have seen, for instance, that maturation and myelination of particular brain areas are strongly related to the development of motor control over specific body segments. Motor development in children and young adolescents can best be characterized as a fine-tuning of accuracy and speed of movement, but also as a development of movement control strategies which cause characteristic qualitative changes.

For the development of specific motor skills it has been claimed that sensory stimulation and practice are as essential for the development of neural pathways as brain maturation itself. This new multicausal view of motor development has opened a rich field of research investigating the different influences and effects of various environmental, biomechanical, cognitive, perceptual, and neural factors on motor development.

However, a profound understanding of their relative importance is still missing. In this respect, the field of developmental cognitive neuroscience is a particularly vigorous and rapidly growing field of research (Nelson 2001). Scientists have used various approaches for a better understanding of neural correlates of motor development. Neuroimaging techniques are not well adapted to the study of movement skills and they are often not suitable for studying normal young human subjects. Therefore researchers study, for example, infants (many of whom are born prematurely) who have suffered perinatal brain lesions (Thelen 2000). These infants do not always attain full recovery of function, nevertheless many of them show considerable functional outcomes (see Elman et al 1996 for a review).

References

Adolph K E, Avolio A M 2000 Walking infants adapt locomotion to changing body dimensions. Journal of Experimental Psychology: Human Perception and Performance 26:1148–1166

Angulo-Kinzler R M, Ulrich B, Thelen E 2002 Three-month-old infants can select specific leg motor solutions. Motor Control 6:52–68

Ashmead D H, McCarty M E, Lucas L S, Belvedere M C 1993 Visual guidance in infants' reaching toward suddenly displaced targets. Child Development 64:1111–1127

Badan M, Hauert C A, Mounoud P 2000 Sequential pointing in children and adults. Journal of Experimental Child Psychology 75:43–69

Bernstein N A 1967 The coordination and regulation of movements. Pergamon Press, Oxford

Bushnell E W 1985 The decline of visually guided reaching during infancy. Infant Behavior and Development 8:139–155

Bushnell E W, Boudreau J P 1993 Motor development and the mind: The potential role of motor abilities as a determinant of aspects of perceptual development. Child Development 64:1005–1021

Clifton R K, Muir D W, Ashmed D H, Clarkson M G 1993 Is visually guided reaching in early infancy a myth? Child Development 64:1099–1110

Connolly K J 1968 Some mechanisms involved in the development of motor skills. Aspects of Education 7:82–100

Corbetta D, Thelen E, Johnson K 2000 Motor constraints on the development of perception-action matching in infant reaching. Infant Behavior and Development 23:351–374

Dennis W, Dennis M 1940 The effect of cradling practices upon the onset of walking in Hopi children. Journal of Genetic Psychology 56:77–86

Diamond A 1990 Developmental time course in human infants and infant monkeys, and the neural bases of inhibitory control in reaching. Annals of the New York Academy of Sciences 608:637–676

Diamond A, Lee E Y 2000 Inability of five-month-old infants to retrieve a contiguous object: A failure of conceptual understanding or of control of action? Child Development 71:1477–1494

Eliot L 1999 What's going on there ? How the brain and mind develops in the first five years of life. Bantam, New York

Elman J L, Bates E A, Johnson M H et al (eds) 1996 Rethinking innateness: A connectionist perspective on development. MIT Press, Cambridge

Frick A, Huber S, Reips U-D, Krist H 2003 Task specific knowledge about the law of pendulum motion in children and adults. Manuscript submitted for publication

Ghez C 1991 The control of movement. In: Kandel E R, Schwartz J H, Jessell T M (eds) Principles of neural science. Prentice Hall, London

Gesell A 1933 Maturation and the patterning of behaviour. In: Murchison C (ed) A handbook of child psychology. Clark University Press, Worcester, MA, p 209–235

Gesell A 1946 The ontogenesis of infant behavior. In: Carmichael L (ed) Manual of child psychology. Wiley, New York, p 295–331

Goldfield E C, Kay B A, Warren W H 1993 Infant bouncing: The assembly and tuning of action systems. Child Development 64:1128–1142

Grodd W 1993 Normal and abnormal patterns of myelin development of the fetal and infantile human brain using magnetic resonance imaging. Current Opinion in Neurology and Neurosurgery 6:393–397

Hall W G, Oppenheim R W 1987 Developmental psychobiology: prenatal, perinatal, and early postnatal aspects of behavioral development. In: Rosenzweig M R, Porter L W (eds) Annual Review of Psychology. Annual Reviews Inc, Palo Alto, p 91–128

Hatwell Y 1987 Motor and cognitive functions of the hand in infancy and childhood. International Journal of Behavioral Development 10:509–526

Hay L 1984 Discontinuity in the development of motor control in children. In: Prinz W, Sanders A F (eds) Cognition and motor processes. Springer, Berlin, p 351–360

Huber S, Krist H, Wilkening F 2003 Judgment and action knowledge in speed adjustment tasks: Experiments in a virtual environment. Developmental Science 6:197–210

Krist H 2001 Development of naive beliefs about moving objects: The straight-down belief in action. Cognitive Development 15:397–424

Krist H, Fieberg E L, Wilkening F 1993 Intuitive physics in action and judgment: The development of knowledge about projectile motion. Journal of Experimental Psychology: Learning, Memory, and Cognition 19:952–966

Lasky R E 1977 The effect of visual feedback of the hand on the reaching and retrieval behavior of young infants. Child Development 48:112–117

Lederman S J, Klatzky R L 1987 Hand movements: A window into haptic object recognition. Cognitive Psychology 19:342–368

Lockman J J 1990 Perceptuomotor coordination in infancy. In: Hauert C A (ed) Developmental psychology: cognitive, perceptuo-motor, and neuropsychological perspectives. North-Holland, Amsterdam, p 85–111

McCarty M E, Ashmead D H 1999 Visual control of reaching and grasping in infants. Developmental Psychology 35:620–631

McDonnell P 1975 The development of visually guided reaching. Perception and Psychophysics 18:181–185

McGraw M B 1945 The neuromuscular maturation of the human infant. Hafner, New York

McGraw M B 1946 Maturation of behavior. In: Carmichael L (ed) Manual of child psychology. Wiley, New York, p 332–369

Nelson C 2001 Handbook of developmental cognitive neuroscience. MIT Press, Cambridge

Newell K M 1986 Constraints on the development of coordination. In: Wade M G, Whiting H T A (eds) Motor development in children: aspects of coordination and control. Nijhoff, Boston, p 341–360

Pellizzer G, Hauert C A 1996 Visuo-manual aiming movements in 6- to 10-year-old children: Evidence for an asymmetric and asynchronous development of information processes. Brain and Cognition 30:175–193

Penfield W, Rasmussen T 1950 The cerebral cortex of man: a clinical study of localization of function. Macmillan Press, New York

Piaget J 1973 Das Erwachen der Intelligenz beim Kinde. Klett, Stuttgart

Piaget J 1975a Das Erwachen der Intelligenz beim Kinde; Gesammelte Werke, Studien-Ausgabe. Vol 1. Klett, Stuttgart

Piaget J 1975b Der Aufbau der Wirklichkeit beim Kinde. Klett, Stuttgart (originally published 1937)

Prechtl H F R 1985 Ultrasound studies of human fetal behaviour. Early Human Development 12:91–98

Prechtl H F R 1993 Principles of early motor development in the human. In: Kalverboer A F, Hopkins B (eds) Motor development in early and later childhood: Longitudinal approaches. European Network on Longitudinal Studies on Individual Development (ENLS). Cambridge University Press, New York, p 35–50

Rabinowicz T, Leuba G, Heumann D 1977 Morphologic maturation of the brain: A quantitative study. In: Berenberg SR (ed) Brain, fetal and infant. Martinus Nijhoff, The Hague, p 28–53

Robin D J, Berthier N E, Clifton R K 1996 Infants' predictive reaching for moving objects in the dark. Developmental Psychology 32:824–835

Savelsbergh G J P, van der Kamp J 1994 The effect of body orientation to gravity on early infant reaching. Journal of Experimental Child Psychology 58:510–528

Shirley M M 1931 The first two years, a study of twenty-five babies: I. Postural and locomotor development. Univerity of Minnesota Press, Minneapolis, MN

Spelke E S, von Hofsten C 2001 Predictive reaching for occluded objects by six-month-old infants. Journal of Cognition and Development 261–282

Sporns O, Edelman G M 1993 Solving Bernstein's problem: A proposal for the development of coordinated movement by selection. Child Development 64:960–981

Staudt M, Krägeloh-Mann I, Grodd W 2000 Die normale Myelinisierung des kindlichen Gehirns in der MRT – eine Metaanalyse. [Normal myelination in childhood brains using MRI – a meta analysis]. Fortschritte auf dem Gebiet der Röngtenstrahlung und der Neuen bildgebenden Verfahren 172:802–811

Streri A, Spelke E 1988 Haptic perception of objects in infancy. Cognitive Psychology 20:1–23

Streri A, Spelke E, Rameix E 1993 Modality specific and amodal aspects of object perception in infancy – the case of active touch. Cognition 47:251–279

Thatcher R W, Walker R A, Giudice S 1987 Human cerebral hemispheres develop at different rates and ages. Science 236:1110–1113

Thelen E 1994 3 month old infants can learn task-specific patterns of inter-limb coordination. Psychological Science 5:280–285

Thelen E 1995 Motor development – a new synthesis. American Psychologist 50:79–95

Thelen E 2000 Motor development as foundation and future of developmental psychology. International Journal of Behavioral Development 24:385–397

Thelen E, Fisher D M, Ridley-Johnson R 1984 The relationship between physical growth and a newborn reflex. Infant Behavior and Development 7:479–493

Thelen E, Skala K, Kelso J A S 1987 The dynamic nature of early coordination: Evidence from bilateral leg movements in young infants. Developmental Psychology 23:179–186

van der Fits I B M, Klip A W J, van Eykern A, Hadders-Algra M 1999 Postural adjustment during spontaneous and goal-directed arm movements in the first half year of life. Behavioral Brain Research 106:75–90

von Hofsten C 1980 Predictive reaching for moving objects by human infants. Journal of Experimental Child Psychology 30:369–382

von Hofsten C 1982 Eye-hand coordination in the newborn. Developmental Psychology 18:450–467

von Hofsten C 1983 Catching skills in infancy. Journal of Experimental Psychology: Human Perception and Performance 9:75–85

von Hofsten C 1989 Mastering reaching and grasping: The development of manual skills in infancy. In: Wallace S A (ed) Perspectives on the coordination of movement. North-Holland, Amsterdam, p 223–258

von Hofsten C 2002 On the development of perception and action. In: Valsiner J K, Connolly J (eds) Handbook of developmental psychology. Sage Publications, London

von Hofsten C, Lindhagen K 1979 Observations on the development of reaching for moving objects. Journal of Experimental Child Psychology 28:158–173

von Hofsten C, Rönnqvist L 1988 Preparation for grasping an object: A developmental study. Journal of Experimental Psychology: Human Perception and Performance 14:610–621

von Hofsten C, Feng Q, Vishton P, Spelke E S 1994 Predictive reaching and head turning for partly occluded objects. In: International Conference on Infant Studies, Paris

von Hofsten C, Vishton P, Spelke E S, Feng Q, Rosander K 1998 Predictive action in infancy: tracking and reaching for moving objects. Cognition 67:255–285

von Hofsten C, Feng Q, Spelke E S 2000 Object representation and predictive action in infancy. Developmental Science 3:193–205

White B L, Castle P, Held R 1964 Observations on the development of visually guided reaching. Child Development 35:349–364

Wilkening F, Krist H 1998 Entwicklung der Wahrnehmung und Psychomotorik. [Perceptual and motor development]. In: Oerter R, Montada L (eds) Entwicklungspsychologie, Psychologie Verlags-Union: Weinheim

SECTION 2

Clinical insights

SECTION CONTENTS

Chapter 7

Birthing interventions and the newborn cervical spine

D. Ritzmann

INTRODUCTION

Why should an obstetrician write a chapter in a book about manual therapy? As we know today, problems in newborn babies, children and adults can have their roots in pregnancy and birth, and the risk of damage to the newborn brain during birth has been the target of research for many years. Amongst manual therapists and obstetricians, pathologists and neurologists there is now growing interest in the newborn cervical spine and its possible damage during birth.

This introductory section outlines different views on childbirth; the next two sections describe the development of obstetric research and inventions in Europe and the research on the function of the pelvis during birth. This is followed by an explanation of risky situations and interventions during birth. The final section looks at the special anatomical and physiological situation of the newborn head and spine and the possible damage to these structures during birth.

To give birth and to go through birth is a fundamental experience for both mother and child. We know today that successful childbirth depends on other factors as well as the anatomy of the pelvis, the diameters of the child's head and the power and timing of the contractions. For more than a hundred years, researchers have been working on the function of the pelvis during birth, the movements of the joints, the stretching of the ligaments and the interdependent changes in the movements of the mother and the unborn child. More recently, researchers have also been looking at the psychological dimensions of giving birth and of being born. We are learning more and more about this subtle teamwork between mother and unborn child, especially how to empower and how not to disturb it.

There are many different views on giving birth. Some of the most important are the following three:

- Giving birth and being born is fundamentally a mechanical problem between the pelvis of the mother and the head or breech of the child (traditionally European).
- Giving birth and being born is fundamentally a problem of rhythm and of disturbances of rhythm (traditionally shamanistic approach).
- Giving birth and being born is fundamentally a problem of not being disturbed (new and very old views of Christian belief).

Because this chapter is concerned with birthing interventions and their effects on the newborn cervical spine, we will concentrate on the traditional Western view of mechanics. All the same we should not forget that in practical obstetrics the rhythm and the absence of disturbances is much more important. Gradually this finding has led to the now more widely held view that there is no sense in measuring the outer pelvis with a pelvimeter, or the inner pelvis using hands, X-ray or MRI (magnetic resonance imaging) to assess the prospects for giving birth. It is only in the situation of a breech presentation that clinics prefer an X-ray or MRI of the pelvis to help in planning the birth.

SHORT HISTORY OF EUROPEAN OBSTETRICAL RESEARCH AND INVENTIONS

In Europe, a change occurred in obstetric practice during the sixteenth and seventeenth centuries. Alongside a decline in female knowledge as a result of politics and church prosecution, male obstetricians entered this field which until then had been the domain of 'wise women' (the French term for midwife 'sage-femme' – 'wise woman' literally translated – reflects this). New instruments were invented and introduced. At the end of the seventeenth century, two members of the English family Chamberlen (Hugh and Paul) spoke of an instrument that would enable every woman to give birth to a living child, but there is no picture of this instrument. In 1721 the renowned Belgian surgeon Johannes P. Palfijn (1650–1730) showed a new instrument, which was called 'the iron hands of Palfijn'. It was the first known and depicted obstetric forceps.

During the eighteenth century there was a growing interest in the medical community in learning more about the female pelvis during birth. William Smellie (1697–1763) wrote in 1754 about the possibility of learning more about the inner pelvis by touching during birth. He described how it was possible to turn the child's head with gentle pressure during birth. He also postulated that the unborn child usually enters the pelvis transversally, the only person to do so for about 150 years. This fact was not accepted until the beginning of the twentieth century, when Christian Kielland (1871–1941) came to the same conclusion (Parry Jones 1952). His instrument, the Kielland forceps, is still used today.

In 1934 Dr Eugene W. Caldwell (1870–1918), professor of radiology in New York, used X-rays to prove that Smellie and Kielland were correct. During the nineteenth century, especially in France, a number of obstetricians tried to construct better forceps to obtain the best traction direction. There was much sophisticated work in this field. But the same famous men did not accept the minimal hygienic standards proposed by Dr Ignaz Semmelweis, the famous trailblazer for hygiene in surgical wards, nor did the high mortality of mother and child in connection with interventions lead them to be careful in promoting their use.

As pathology and radiology developed, the female pelvis became a target of research. Four types of female pelvic forms have been described since the nineteenth century, and were classified in 1934 by Caldwell and Moloy: the gynecoid type, the android type, the platypeloid type and the anthropoid type. This classification of female pelvic types is still used today.

The gynecoid pelvis

This is the typical transversally large inlet. The baby's head enters the pelvis in the transverse position. In obstetric books, it is considered the most usual female pelvis. Nevertheless Borell and Fernström found it in only 25–30% of a northern European population during birth. We can see here the typical way of entering the pelvis transversally in *Homo sapiens sapiens*. It seems that for 4 million years starting with *Australopithecus* the pelvis has been getting a transversally larger inlet in females. With this usual birth position at the pelvic inlet the unborn baby has to turn 90 degrees with head, shoulders and rump. This screwing movement is typical for human birth. In four-footed animals the pelvis is straight and no screwing movement is necessary.

The android pelvis

This is the typical male pelvis. Borell and Fernström found it in about 10–20% of women during birth. The baby's head enters the pelvis in the oblique diameter.

The anthropoid pelvis

Anthropoid relates to the primates who have this typical large sagittal inlet of the pelvis. Radiologically it is found in between 5 and 73%, the wide range indicating the clashes of opinion on how to define it. The baby's head enters the pelvis in the sagittal diameter.

The platypeloid pelvis

This is the typical flat pelvis, found in women with rickets. It has a gynecoid form, but is very narrow in the sagittal diameter. It is found in varying frequencies from 1 to 56% (note, again, the wide range of reported incidences). Often the baby's head cannot enter the pelvis, as the radiographic analysis might suggest. If it can enter, it lies in the oblique diameter.

Research on the different forms of female pelvis decreased as cesarean sections became more frequent. Some special pelvic forms have been thought to be associated with special risks during birth, for example the so-called long pelvis described by Kirchhoff. Later studies showed that these pelvic forms are frequent in normal births as well, so the postulated risk is not proven (Borell and Fernström 1957) With the reduction in rickets and poliomyelitis in Europe, the pelvis is very seldom a problem for birth.

RESEARCH ABOUT THE FUNCTION OF THE FEMALE PELVIS

At the end of the nineteenth century, researchers started to describe the function of the pelvis, and were particularly interested in the joints and ligaments. Walcher (1889) and von Küttner (1898) described a sagittal opening of the pelvis of about 8 to 12 mm through stretching and bending of the hips of dead mothers (Borell and Fernström 1981). They concluded that the sacroiliac joints allow this opening. During pregnancy there is a relaxation of the sacroiliac joints which can lead to recurrent blockages of these joints with painful consequences. To study these joint movements during birth is nowadays nearly impossible. From manipulations during birth to get blocked sacroiliac joints back to their normal function we can assume that the movement in the sacroiliac joints is important for a normal birth. In human birth, all the space between the pelvis and head of the baby is needed. When a joint cannot move smoothly the birth can be disturbed.

The relaxation of the pelvic ligaments and joints is triggered by the hormone relaxin. This hormone also has an influence on the ripening of the cervix and on the connective tissue in vessels and the skin (Sherwood 1994). Radiological examinations in the middle of the twentieth century demonstrated a relaxation of the sacroiliac joints of some millimeters and a relaxation of the symphysal joint from about 4 mm to usually 8 mm at the end of pregnancy (Borell and Fernström 1981). This is reversible 3 to 5 months after birth.

The movements of the pelvis during birth are described by Borell and Fernström: when the baby's head enters the pelvis, the symphysal joint descends. In midpelvis the symphysal joint moves cranially and at the pelvic outlet even more. This cranial movement can reach several centimeters.

To allow the pelvis to move in such a way during birth it is essential that the mother is as undisturbed as possible. It seems that the Indian way of birthing (described by Moysés Paciornik in 1985) in the squatting position reduces the necessity for interventions to a minimum. Paciornik reports a frequency of under 5% for forceps delivery. In the squatting position the pelvis is 'freely hanging'. It is logical that the joint movements can work undisturbed in this position.

The movement of the pelvis during birth seems to be related to the posture of the mother and to the tightness of the muscles, which are influenced by fear and psychological tension. This would explain why it is important to give support throughout birth so that the level of operative interventions is kept to a minimum.

RISKY SITUATIONS DURING BIRTH

To give birth and to go through birth is a fundamental experience for both mother and child. There are situations that by themselves are risky for mother and child or are followed by risky maneuvers by the obstetricians or midwives. We now take a closer look at the impact of these situations and interventions, especially for the newborn cervical spine.

Risky situations are:

- arrested parturition
- extremely rapid delivery
- breech delivery
- delivery of children with deflected heads.

Arrested parturition

Arrested parturition is a very frequent situation, especially in obstetric clinics. Often it leads to interventions such as hormone injections to accelerate the frequency of contractions or to instrumental or cesarean deliveries. Different underlying problems can lead to an arrest, but often the cause is not clear. In this situation the obstetrician uses the term 'disproportion between pelvis and head'. More research is needed in this field. Often it is not clear why the contraction forces vanish, why the unborn baby does not enter deeper into the pelvis or why a normal birth turns suddenly into an arrest.

Could factors such as changes in staff, lack of intimacy, or ongoing disruption of this very intimate process of giving birth due to the technical controls and the emotionally uninvolved staff be the cause of the immense problem of disturbed births?

There is always an underlying problem that leads to an arrest of birth. This could be a maternal problem such as:

- weak labor (exhausted mothers, mothers in fear or grief, disturbed mothers)
- uncoordinated labor pains (induced births, preterm births, pain and fear)
- anatomical problems of the pelvis (seldom).

Arrested birth can also be due to a problem concerning the unborn baby such as:

- transverse or breech presentation
- dorsoposterior presentation
- a deflected head.

Extremely rapid delivery

Extremely rapid delivery can cause problems to the baby because of the immense power the contractions exert on the baby's head and neck. The baby can rush through the pelvis, pushed by continuous contractions. A certain percentage of babies with problems related to the cervical spine have this birth history.

Breech delivery

Breech deliveries are special deliveries. Even in communities far away from modern obstetrics (as e.g. in the countryside of Nepal) women do not give birth alone with mother and husband if there is a breech delivery. A midwife will be present at birth in this situation.

The risk of a higher morbidity and mortality relates not only to the baby but also to the mother, especially in poorer countries where no antibiotics or instrumental interventions are available. Breech deliveries are often more protracted than vertex deliveries and have a higher risk of arrest and damage to the baby.

Interestingly, Leonardo da Vinci drew only dead mothers with unborn babies in breech presentation because he had to base his anatomical research on autopsies of mothers who died during childbirth.

The delivery of children with deflected heads

Unborn babies with deflected heads usually lie in the dorsoposterior vertex presentation. The dorsoposterior presentation describes an unborn baby with its spine turned towards the mother's spine. In this position the head is often deflected and is less able to bend during parturition. Quite often the birth takes much longer than usual or is eventually arrested. In this unfavorable situation the labor forces cause more stress to the unborn baby and the risk of injury increases. Frequently it is necessary to deliver the baby by forceps, so the risks of this intervention augment the overall risk of the deflected head. Babies in breech presentation with deflected heads have a very high risk of morbidity. Nowadays this is an indication for a cesarean delivery.

RISKY INTERVENTIONS DURING BIRTH

All interventions during birth are risky, if not done carefully and with respect for the special situation of the mother and the unborn child.

Risky interventions are the following:

- pressure from above
- traction from beneath
- all rotatory forces.

Pressure from above

Pressure from above can increase in fast deliveries, but also through all kinds of interventions in arrested births. These interventions can be the traditionally exerted external direct forces by means of cords and bags, in Western obstetrics the so-called 'Kristeller fundal pressure'. Initially Samuel Kristeller (1820–1900) proposed a soft pressure by hand, nowadays it is most often a very powerful pressure. In the original publication, this maneuver was advocated as an aid for multiparae where the abdominal muscles were atrophied and thus not functioning normally any more. The most frequently used augmentation of contraction forces nowadays is labor-inducing medication.

Traction from beneath

Traction from beneath has a long history: Before 1700 there had been nets and strings to get the child from beneath. In the early eighteenth century the newly invented obstetric forceps sometimes replaced these older traction forces. In 1954 Tage G. Malmström proposed a new traction instrument, the vacuum extractor. This instrument is now replacing the obstetric forcipes.

At the beginning of the twentieth century, Hermann Johannes Pfannenstiel (1862–1909) and John Martin Munro Kerr (1868–1960) invented new surgical techniques to make cesarean sections safer. At the end of the same century, Michael Stark proposed a shorter and less traumatic surgical option, the so-called 'soft cesarean'.

All these different interventions have their particular risks to the newborn spine and head, even the cesarean section. Problems with the newborn spine can result from a long birthing process which in the end is terminated by an instrumental delivery or a cesarean section, but there are also sometimes problems if the baby has been delivered by a planned cesarean section. Often to get the baby out of the uterus the incision needs quite a powerful pressure from above. So even this intervention can be harmful to the baby. It would be best to prevent all types of interventions, but here we need more research.

Rotatory forces

Rotatory forces are now seldom exerted. If the head of the unborn baby does not turn in the best position and stays in the wrong diameter, it may be possible to turn the head by hand as Smellie proposed in the seventeenth century or by Kielland forceps as proposed in the early twentieth century, but this must be done without force. If any force is exerted on the head, the cervical spine can be injured and the result can be deleterious. Rotatory interventions are difficult and dangerous.

Today the distribution of modern techniques depends more on politics and tradition than on medical reasoning. The cesarean section rate varies from under 6% in Italy to over 50% in Brazil; it also varies from region to region and from hospital to hospital. The vaginal intervention rate is 1–2% in Italy but more than 15% in Switzerland. There are countries with low intervention rates and others with higher rates but with similar newborn morbidity or mortality rates.

There has been an overall lowering of newborn mortality and morbidity in the last century, but independently of the frequency of instrumental interventions. It seems more connected to the health situation of women in rich Western countries.

THE DANGERS FOR THE NEWBORN CERVICAL SPINE

We can differentiate between pressure forces, traction forces and bending forces. These different types of forces have different effects on the newborn cervical spine and head.

Pressure forces

During normal birth the unborn baby is protected from direct forces by the amniotic fluid. The fluid causes a distribution of the uterine muscle forces. With the opening of the amniotic cavity, by itself or by intervention, the forces exerted on the baby lead to a direct pressure on head and neck in the vertex presentation. If the baby is turning correctly through the pelvis, it will not get stuck and will move slowly downwards. If there is an arrest in labor, the contraction forces will press the spine against the suboccipital region.

These pressure forces, whether due to strong contractions, manual pressure (Kristeller), or hormonal augmentation of the natural contractions, can occasionally lead to a subluxation of the atlas into the foramen magnum with disruption of the cerebellum. The atlas of the neonate is much smaller in relation to the foramen magnum than in adults. With pressure, it can protrude into the foramen magnum.

Axial pressure is the force usually encountered in a normal birth. The neonate's anatomy and biomechanics correspond to the special requirements of birth. The cervical spine has horizontal joint facets, enabling better adaptation to bending forces; the small processi uncinati do not hinder the compensating movements of the vertebrae during birth. The center of rotation of the cervical spine in sagittal movements is the high cervical region C_2–C_4, not the deeper one as in adults – C_5–C_6 (see Chapter 3). This situation allows the unborn baby to hold the neck quite stretched with a flexed head. On the other hand, the region C_2–C_4 is more vulnerable to traction and rotatory forces in the newborn baby. If the head is in an extremely flexed position (as in dorsoposterior flexed vertex presentation) the high cervical region is under massive pressure (Sacher 2002; see also Chapter 8).

If other forces than axial pressure are exerted during birth – e.g. rotatory or traction forces – the weak ligaments cannot prevent the spinal cord, the vessels and nerves from being damaged. The ligament of the dens axis is weak and cannot protect the brainstem from extension.

Traction forces

Traction forces during birth can lead to damage to the spinal cord, the spinal nerves, the vessels of the cervical spine and the brain. Often no damage to the osseous structures is seen on radiography, but there is extensive damage to the soft tissue of the spinal cord, the nerves, vessels or even the brain. Modern techniques of MRI or PET can reveal these lesions more precisely.

The arteriae cerebri mediae and the sinusoidal veins are at special risk under traction forces. They can rupture and cause intracerebral and subdural bleeding. If this happens, they can bleed profusely or create adhesions, which can squeeze the spinal cord.

What extent of traction power is exerted on the newborn cervical spine?

Few physicians since Samuel Kristeller have investigated this question. Kristeller, in 1861, measured an average traction power of 15.9 kg by forceps. A hundred years later Laufe (1969) reported an average of 7.7 to a maximum of 19 kg by forceps. Interestingly in 1990 Justus Hofmeyr reported exactly the same traction force by the metal suction cap of the vacuum extractor as Samuel Kristeller: 15.8 kg (Hofmeyr et al 1990). The weaker silicon suction cap exerted a somewhat smaller power.

In 1874 Duncan examined the spines of newborn dead babies and reported the following data: the vertebral spine of a newborn dead child can suffer an extension of 5.6 cm before it breaks, but the spinal cord can only withstand 0.7 cm extension before it ruptures. It is about 100 years since we saw fractured vertebrae during childbirth, but spinal cord damage is nonetheless possible. A description of spinal cord injuries without radiographic abnormality in children has been published by Osenbach and Menezes (1989).

Rotatory forces

The special anatomy of the newborn cannot protect the spinal cord, the vessels and nerves from rotatory forces. These are the most dangerous manipulations done during birth.

The horizontal joint facets of the cervical vertebrae allow more movement possibilities during birth, but are not adapted at all to rotatory movements. The interconnected nerves and vessels in the cervical spine and the weak ligaments can lead to a disruption or stretching of these structures. The arteriae basilares are especially at risk from rotatory forces. If stretched or ruptured, subdural and intracerebral bleeding can result.

As different structures may be involved in cervical spine injury and brainstem damage, the symptoms vary in signs and extent. The main symptoms of intracerebral bleeding are early death, breathing depression and epileptic cramps. Nowadays ultrasound of the brain allows early diagnosis.

The leading symptom complex of spinal cord injuries is the so-called 'spinal shock'. Early symptoms can be early neonatal death, respiratory depression, gasping and hypotonic muscles. Late symptoms can be spasticity, paraplegia and an atonic bladder. Injuries of the upper cervical spine can also lead to gastrointestinal kinetic problems such as spasms of the pylorus, gastroesophageal backflow and hypotonic jejunum. A possible effect can be relapsing pneumonia, a symptom that can lead to the diagnosis of high cervical injury (see Chapter 8).

If the spinal nerves are stretched or ruptured, paralysis of the plexus brachialis (cervical plexopathy) can result, very often combined with torticollis on the same side (Suzuki et al 1984). They are the main symptoms of damage in the upper cervical spine. This can be the more frequent Erb–Duchenne upper plexopathy with injuries to neural structures C_5/C_6 or the less frequent Klumpke caudal plexopathy with injuries to spinal nerves C_7/T_1, sometimes combined with a Horner syndrome.

The real incidence of damage to the upper cervical spine and brainstem structures is not known. Some authors have published data on the frequency of missed diagnosis in child neurology and pathology, which are quite high (10% to over 50%) (Towbin 1964, Rossitch and Oakes 1992). Studies of newborn babies that had a special interest in high cervical function revealed a high frequency (about 30%) of functional impairment. This seems to be connected with traction forces and special risks as mentioned above such as

breech presentations, twins, arrested births and deflected heads during birth (Buchmann and Bülow 1983, Seifert 1975, Biedermann 1999).

CONCLUSION

We begin to understand how vulnerable the structure of the newborn cervical spine is. Further insight into this complex problem will surely influence the way we regard birthing. Giving birth under water or in a squatting position, for example, alters the stress exerted on the cervical spine. Not to disturb the rhythm and the intimacy of giving birth is an important issue in reducing the incidence of arrested births and therefore the risk of damage to the newborn. These are just two of many areas where the work of obstetricians intersects with the work of those engaged in manual therapy.

References

Biedermann H 1999 Biomechanische Besonderheiten des occipito-vervicalen Überganges. In: Biedermann H (ed) Manualtherapie bei Kinder. Enke, Stuttgart, p 19–28

Buchmann J, Bülow B 1983 Funktionelle Kopfgelenksstörungen bei Neugeborenen im Zusammenhang mit Lagereaktionsverhalten und Tonusasymmetrie. Manuelle Medizin 21:59–62

Borell U, Fernström I 1957 The movement at the sacroiliac joints and their importance to changes in the pelvic dimensions during parturition. Acta Obstetrica Gynecologica Scandinavica 36:42

Borell U, Fernström I 1960 Radiologic Pelvimetry. Acta Radiologica. Supplementum 191

Borell U, Fernström I 1981 Schwangerschaft und Geburt. Urban & Schwarzenberg, Munich

Caldwell W E, Moloy H C 1933 Anatomical variations in the female pelvis and their effect in labor with a suggested classification. American Journal of Obstetrics and Gynecology 26:479

Hofmeyr G J et al 1990 New design rigid and soft vacuum cups. British Journal of Obstetrics and Gynaecology 97:681–685

Laufe E L 1969 Crossed versus divergent obstetric forceps. Obstetrics and Gynecology 34(6):853–858

Osenbach R K, Menezes A H 1989 Spinal cord injury without radiographic abnormality in children. Pediatric Neuroscience 15:168–175

Paciornik M 1985 Let the Indians show you how to live

Parry Jones E 1952 Kielland's forceps. Butterworth, London

Rossitch E, Oakes W J 1992 Perinatal spinal cord injury: clinical, radiographic and pathologic features. Pediatric Neurosurgery 18:149–152

Sacher R 2002 Geburtstrauma und Halswirbelsäule. Unveröffentlichtes Dokument

Seifert I 1975 Kopfgelenksblockierung bei Neugeborenen. Rehabilitacia, Prague (Suppl) 10:53–57

Sherwood O D 1994 'Relaxin'. In: Physiology and Reproduction

Suzuki S et al 1984 The aetiological relationship between congenital torticollis and obstetrical paralysis. International Orthopaedics SICOT 8 175–181

Towbin A 1964 Spinal cord and brainstem injury at birth. Archives of Pathology 77:620–632

von Küttner O 1898 Experimentell anatomische Untersuchungen über die Veränderlichkeit des Beckenraumes Gebärender. Beitrage zur Geburtsh Gynäkogie 1:210

Walcher G 1889 Die Conjugata eines engen Beckens ist keine konstante Grösse, sondern lässt sich durch die Körperhaltung der Trägerin verändern. Zentralblatt für Gynäkologie 13:892

Further reading

Achanna S et al 1994 Outcome of forceps delivery versus vacuum extraction. Singapore Medical Journal 35:605–608

Annibale D J et al 1995 Comparative neonatal morbidity of abdominal and vaginal deliveries after uncomplicated pregnancies. Archives of Pediatric and Adolescent Medicine 149:862–867

Avrahami E et al 1993 CT demonstration of intracranial haemorrhage in term newborn following vacuum extractor delivery. Neuroradiology 35:107–108

Bhagwanani S G et al 1973 Risks and prevention of cervical cord injury in the management of breech presentation with hyperextension of the fetal head. American Journal of Obstetrics and Gynecology 115(8):1159–1161

Biedermann H. 1993 Das KISS-Syndrom der Neugeborenen und Kleinkinder. Manuelle Medizin 31:97–107

Bjerre I et al 1974 The long term development of children delivered by vacuum extraction. Developmental Medicine and Child Neurology 16:378

Bresnan M J et al 1974 Neonatal spinal cord transection secondary to intrauterine hyperextension of the neck in breech presentation. Journal of Pediatrics 84(5):734–737

Brey J et al 1956 Vacuum extractor with special reference to early and late infantile injuries. Gebhilfe und Frauenheilkunde 22:550

Buchmann J et al 1992 Asymmetrien in der Kopfgelenkbeweglichkeit von Kindern. Manuelle Medizin 30:93–95

Cardozo L D et al 1983 Should we abandon Kielland's forceps? British Medical Journal 287:315–317

Carmody F et al 1986 Follow-up of babies delivered in a randomised comparison of vacuum extraction and forceps delivery. Acta Obstetrica Gynecologica Scandinavica 65:763–766

Chalmers J A 1989 Commentaries (The obstetric vacuum extractor is the instrument of first choice for operative vaginal delivery). British Journal of Obstetrics and Gynaecology 96:505–509

Chiswick M L 1979 Kielland's forceps association with neonatal morbidity and mortality. British Medical Journal i:7–9

Dell DL et al 1985 Soft cup vacuum extraction: a comparison of outlet delivery. Obstetrics and Gynecology 66:624–628

Drife J O 1996 Commentaries (Choice and instrumental delivery). British Journal of Obstetrics and Gynaecology 103:608–611

Fall O et al 1986 Forceps or vacuum extraction? Acta Obstetrica Gynecologica Scandinavica 65:75–80

Gachiri J R et al Fœtal and maternal outcome of vacuum extraction. East Africa Medical Journal 1991; 68:539–546

Garcia J et al 1985 Views of women and their medical and midwifery attendants about instrumental delivery. Journal of Psychosomatic Obstetetrics and Gynaecology 4:1–9

Gilles F H et al 1979 Infantile atlantoccipital instability. American Journal of Diseases of Children 133:30–37

Glazener C M A et al 1995 Postnatal maternal morbidity: extent, causes, prevention and treatment. British Journal of Obstetrics and Gynaecology 102:282–287

Govaert P et al 1992 Vacuum extraction, bone injury and neonatal subgaleal bleeding. European Journal of Pediatrics 151:532–535

Govaert P et al 1992 Traumatic neonatal intracranial bleeding and stroke. Archives of Disease in Childhood 67:840–845

Graig W S 1983 Intracranial hemorrhage in the newborn. A study of diagnosis and differential diagnosis based upon pathological and clinical findings in 126 cases. Archives of Disease in Childhood 13:89–123

Greis J B et al 1981 Comparison of maternal and fetal effects of vacuum extraction with forceps or caesarean deliveries. Obstetrics and Gynecology 57:571–577

Hibbard B M et al 1990 The obstetric forceps – are we using the appropriate tools? British Journal of Obstetrics and Gynaecology 97:374–380

Hillier C E M et al 1994 Worldwide survey of assisted vaginal delivery. International Journal of Gynecology and Obstetrics 47:109–114

Jensen T S et al 1988 Perinatal risk factors and first year vocalizations: influence on preschool language and motor performance. Developmental Medicine and Child Neurology 30:153–161

Johanson R et al 1989 North Staffordshire/Wigan assisted delivery trial. British Journal of Obstetrics and Gynaecology 96:537–544

Johanson R et al 1993 A randomised prospective study comparing the new vacuum extractor policy with forceps delivery. British Journal of Obstetrics and Gynaecology 100:524–530

Johanson R et al 1999 Maternal and child health after assisted vaginal delivery: five year follow up of a randomised controlled study comparing forceps and ventouse. British Journal of Obstetrics and Gynaecology 106:544–549

Johnson N et al 1995 Variation in caesarean and instrumental delivery rates in New Zealand hospitals. Australia and New Zealand Journal of Obstetrics and Gynaecology 35:6–11

Lasbrey A H et al 1964 A study of the relative merits and scope for vacuum extraction as opposed to forceps delivery. South African Journal of Obstetrics and Gynaecology 2:1–3

Lasker M R et al 1991 Neonatal diagnosis of spinal cord transsection. Clinical Pediatrics 30(5):322–324

Leijon I 1980 Neurology and behaviour of newborn infants delivered by vacuum extraction on maternal indication. Acta Paediatrica Scandinavica 69:625–631

Ludwig B et al 1980 Postpartum CT examination of the head of full term infants. Neuroradiology 20:145–154

MacArthur C et al 1991 Commentaries (Health after Childbirth) British Journal of Obstetrics and Gynaecology 98:1193–1195

MacArthur C et al 1997 Faecal incontinence after childbirth. British Journal of Obstetrics and Gynaecology 104:46–50

MacKinnon J A et al 1993 Spinal cord injury at birth : diagnostic and prognostic data in twenty-two patients. Journal of Pediatrics 122(3):431–437

Martyn C 1996 Not quite as random as I pretended. Lancet 3347:70

Meniru G I et al 1996 An analysis of recent trends in vacuum extraction and forceps delivery in the United Kingdom. British Journal of Obstetrics and Gynaecology 103:168–170

Menticoglou S M et al 1995 High cervical spinal cord injury in neonates delivered with forceps : report of 15 cases. Obstetrics and Gynecology 86(4):589–593

Meyer C et al 1972 Regarding neuropsychic residua of infants delivered by a Swedish ventouse. Rev Neuropsychiatr Infant 20:343

Middle C et al 1995 Labour and delivery of normal primiparous women. British Journal of Obstetrics and Gynaecology 102:970–977

Moolgoaker A A 1979 Comparison of different methods of instrumental delivery based on electronic measurements of compression and traction. Obstetrics and Gynecology 54:299

Nelson K B et al 1984 Obstetrical complications as risk factors in cerebral palsy or seizure disorder. Journal of the American Medical Association 252:1843–1848

Nilsen S T et al 1984 Boys born by forceps and vacuum extraction examined at 18 years of age. Acta Obstetrica et Gynecologica Scandinavica 63:549–554

Notzon F C et al 1990 International differences in the use of obstetrical interventions. Journal of the American Medical Association 263:3286–3291

O'Discroll K et al 1981 Traumatic intracranial haemorrhage in firstborn infants and delivery with obstetric forceps. British Journal of Obstetrics and Gynaecology 88:577–581

Parazzini F et al 1994 Vaginal operative deliveries in Italy. Acta Obstetrica et Gynecologica Scandinavica 73:698–700

Plauché W C et al 1979 Fetal cranial injuries related to delivery with the Malmstroem vacuum extractor. Obstetrics and Gynecology 53:750–757

Punnonen R et al 1986 Fetal and maternal effects of forceps and vacuum extraction. British Journal of Obstetrics and Gynaecology 93:1132-1135

Pusey J et al 1991 Maternal impressions of forceps and silc-cup. British Journal of Obstetrics and Gynaecology 98:4887–4888

Ruggieri M et al 1999 Spinal cord insults in the prenatal, perinatal and neonatal periods. Developmental Medicine and Child Neurology 41:311–317

Shah P M 1991 Prevention of mental handicaps in children in primary healthcare. WHO Bulletin OMS 69: 779–789

Simon L et al 1999 Letters to the Editor (Clinical and radiological diagnosis of the spinal cord birth injury). Archives of Disease in Childhood. Fetal and Neonatal Edition 81:F235–236

Sultan A H et al 1993 Anal-sphincter disruption during vaginal delivery. New England Journal of Medicine 329:1905–1911

Takahashi I et al 1994 Rotational occlusion of the vertebral artery at the atlantoaxial joint: is it truly physiological? Neuroradiology 36:273–275

Taylor H C 1948 Breech presentation with hyperextension of the neck and intrauterine dislocation of cervical vertebrae. American Journal of Obstetrics and Gynecology 56(2):381–385

Towbin A 1969 Latent spinal cord and brainstem injury in newborn infants. Developmental Medicine and Child Neurology 11:54–68

Vacca A et al 1983 Portsmouth operative delivery trial. British Journal of Obstetrics and Gynaecology 90:1107–1112

Vojta V et al 1983 Der geburtstraumatische Torticollis myogenes und seine krankengymnastische Behandlung nach Vojta. Zeitschrift für Krankengymnastik 35(4):191–197

Volpe J 1974 Neonatal intracranial hemorrhage: iatrogenic etiology? New England Journal of Medicine 291: 43–45

Wilhelm R 1955 Die Frühbehandlung der Skoliose, eine dringliche Forderung. Zeitschrift für Orthopädie 86:221

Williams M C et al 1991 A randomised comparison of assisted vaginal delivery. Obstetrics and Gynecology 78:789–794

Young R S K et al 1983 Focal necrosis of the spinal cord in utero. Archives of Neurology 40:654–655

Chapter 8

Birth trauma and its implications for neuromotor development

R. Sacher

We begin by outlining the risks to the infant cervical spine as a result of birth trauma from the gynecological point of view, and then proceed to examine aspects of manual therapy.

When considering injuries and dysfunctions of the spine and its associated structures, the significance of birth trauma is often underestimated, and the resulting symptoms frequently misinterpreted. The consequences of trauma to the baby during birth and in the months immediately preceding and following the birth are thus of concern not only to gynecologists and pediatricians, but also to practitioners of manual therapy in a wide range of specialties, who have begun to study the risks associated with pregnancy and delivery.

The aspects to be considered therefore include not only the specific stresses on the infant spine associated with pregnancy and birth, its particular anatomical and biomechanical features, and the neurophysiological mechanisms of the cervical region, but also such matters as developmental physiology.

THE INFANT CERVICAL SPINE

Anatomical aspects

The spine of the fetus and young child has a number of special biomechanical and anatomical features to enable it to adapt to the physiological demands of the birth process. It is largely cartilaginous. The size and weight of the head after birth result in an increased inertia load on the upper cervical spine (Baily 1952, Fielding 1984, Papavasilou 1978, Townsend and Rowe 1952). But during birth, too, the large head inevitably means an increase in the leverage exerted on the craniocervical transition zone and in the demands placed on it, which may involve rotation, anteflexion and retroflexion (cephalic presentation of occiput or face).

The horizontal orientation of the joint surfaces in the frontal plane, especially in the upper cervical region, allows greater translational mobility (Catell and Filtzer 1965, Melzak 1969, Papavasilou 1978). In the sagittal plane, however, the joint surfaces – in terms of the individual vertebrae – in the newborn are more steeply aligned than in the young child, resulting in a more inclined positioning of the cervical spine (von Kortzfleisch 1993). Meanwhile, the articulating surfaces of the vertebral bodies, and the joints, are still relatively small and so increase segmental instability. The wedge shape of the vertebral bodies and the still incompletely formed uncinate processes give greater adaptability to the demands imposed by the mechanics of the birth process, but these features, combined with the weak muscles and ligaments of the newborn, produce a greater tendency to subluxation (Babyn et al 1988, Catell and Filtzer 1965, Fielding 1984, Menezes 1987). The spinal cord structures and meninges are eight times as vulnerable as the postural connective tissue structures, owing to a lack of elasticity during longitudinal traction (Leventhal 1960), a force that is not anticipated in the physiological features designed to withstand the birth process. This may be one of the reasons that many injuries of the spinal cord from birth trauma produce radiographic studies with no visible evidence of injury to the spinal column (spinal cord injury without radiographic abnormality – SCIWORA (Osenbach and Menezes 1989)).

The suboccipital region also has various special morphological features; the height of the occipital condyles in the newborn and in early infancy is about 50% of the adult measurement, and the axial angle of the atlanto-occipital joint (Fig. 8.1) is consequently considerably flatter than in adults (153° versus 124° in men and 127° in women) (Sacher in press, Schmidt and Fischer 1960). The angle formed by the axis of the atlanto-occipital joint with the sagittal plane (the average orientation) is markedly more obtuse (Fig. 8.2) (Lang 1979).

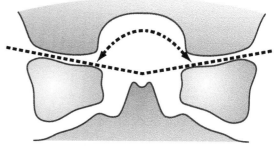

Figure 8.1 Angle of condyloid joint axis C_0/C_1.

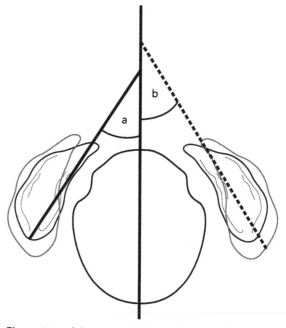

Figure 8.2 Atlanto-occipital axis in the sagittal plane; dotted lines show situation in the adult (a = 35.5°), black in the newborn (b = 28°).

Biomechanical aspects

There are four main biomechanical features:

- on lateroflexion (frontal plane) the atlas does not normally move into the concavity as it does in adults, but into the convexity (Biedermann 1999)
- the infant cervical spine appears much more extended in the sagittal plane (von Kortzfleisch 1993)
- the main pivot for movements in the sagittal plane is not in the C_5/C_6 segment as in the adult, but at $C_2/C_3/C_4$ (Catell and Filtzer 1965, Hill et al 1984, Nitecki and Moir 1994)
- paradoxical tipping of the atlas: anteflexion of the head occurs only in the craniocervical joints when nodding, accompanied by ventral sliding of the atlas (Biedermann 1999).

This biomechanical adaptation must have the purpose of providing protective mechanisms for the associated nerve structures. The question as to whether such features are already effective in the newborn has been little investigated as yet. However, the radiological findings of Ratner and Michailov (1992) suggest the existence of such a link.

The cranial shifting of the main pivot for movements in the sagittal plane enables optimum transmission of forces during labor, exerted by the axially directed contractions on the head as it moves downwards in cephalic presentations. This enables a much more extended positioning of the lower cervical spine. Meanwhile, increased anteflexion at C_2/C_3 causes increased ventral tipping of the dens axis, which makes it necessary for the atlas to slide ventrally.

The upper cervical spine has to absorb directly the adaptations in head position brought about by the dynamics of the birth process and at the same time to transmit the major part of the expulsion forces to the head. The direction producing the greatest tissue tension of the cervical spine is anteflexion of the head, while retroflexion produces the least. The upper cervical spine is therefore subjected to particular stress in the occipitoposterior presentation (Fig. 8.3).

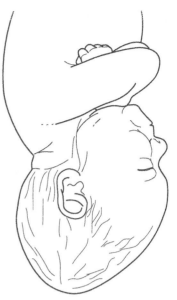

Figure 8.3 Occipitoposterior presentation.

There are also particular features associated with breech presentations, owing to the increased traction stresses on the spinal structures. Since the upper cervical spine mainly has to deal with the biomechanical demands of the head position, it is now the cervico-thoracic transition zone that has to respond to the demands placed on it by the presenting parts of the fetal anatomy. Again the decisive factor is the higher location of the rotational axis for anteflexion and retroflexion. The spinal structures of the lower cervical spine and the cervico-thoracic transition zone have only so much resilience, and the limits are soon reached. Additional traction or rotation will quickly exhaust the reserves of tension in this area. The most unfavorable situation is that of breech presentation with hyperextension of the head.

'CLASSICAL' INJURIES TO THE (CERVICAL) SPINE FROM BIRTH TRAUMA

Frequency of occurrence

The incidence of injuries to the spinal column and spinal cord from birth trauma is still not fully known. One reason for this may be the clinical picture, as the diagnosis is not always easy (Menticoglou 1995). Rossitch and Oakes (1992) have documented how rarely trauma to the structures of the spinal column is considered. They report false diagnoses (including pediatric neurology) in four out of five cases where there was severe injury to the spinal cord. The fact that the structures of the spinal cord are also not routinely included in autopsy is equally surprising (Ratner 1991b, Towbin 1969). Towbin (1970), in an autopsy study on this question ($N = 600$), found relevant injuries to the spinal cord and brainstem in 10% of cases. These consisted of spinal epidural hemorrhages, meningeal tears and injuries to blood vessels, the muscles and ligaments, and the nerve and bone structures.

Damage of this sort can also be observed in normal births, where it is hardly expected to occur (Ratner 1991b). There is considerable variation in the pattern of clinical symptoms on account of the vascularization in the region of the vertebral artery, and for this reason it is easily overlooked.

Mode of delivery

The spinal column is subjected to a variety of different stresses by longitudinal traction or compression of the spinal column and associated structures, especially if combined with torsion, flexion and hyperextension, depending on the mode of delivery (Towbin 1964). It is not possible at the present time to distinguish with certainty the role played by the 'normal stress' of the particular delivery mode and that of inadequate or inappropriate technique in assisting delivery.

Approximately 30% of the peripartum spinal column injuries described in the literature were observed in deliveries of cephalic presentations (Allen 1970, Shulman et al 1971).

A major British/Irish study (Ruggieri et al 1999) found no significant differences with regard to mode of delivery and the location of spinal column injuries. It also drew attention to the signifi-

cance of damage to the thoracolumbar spinal cord. Over 55% of the children in their patient cohort developed injuries to the spinal cord in the thoracic and lumbar regions of the spine. This, however, included children who had undergone catheterization of the umbilical artery that could have caused damage to the spinal cord by thromboembolism.

Injuries to spinal structures at the lower cervical or upper dorsal levels are more frequently found in breech deliveries (Bresnan and Abroms 1973, Caterini et al 1975, MacKinnon et al 1993). The hyperextension of the fetal head plays a particular role in these injuries, and is seen in about 5% of all breech deliveries. Up to 25% of these vaginally delivered babies developed spinal cord injuries (Bhgwanani et al 1973, Bresnan and Abroms 1973, Caterini et al 1975). Even when the child was delivered by cesarean section, a small proportion suffered serious complications at the upper cervical level (Cattamanchi et al 1981, Maekawa et al 1976, Weinstein et al 1983). In these cases it remains to be shown how far intrauterine injuries resulting from subluxation and dislocation in the upper cervical region could have caused blood vessel damage to the vertebral arteries (Gilles et al 1979, Maekawa et al 1976, Weinstein et al 1983).

Forceps deliveries may involve an increased risk of injury to the upper cervical spinal column and spinal cord (Mackinnon et al 1993, Pschyrembel 1966, Rossitch and Oakes 1992, Ruggieri et al 1999). The misapplication of these and similar extraction aids (forced traction/rotation; in the worst case, rotation in the wrong direction) can cause upper cervical complications.

There is presumably a limit to iatrogenic structural damage caused by vacuum extraction, as the vacuum device becomes dislodged if too much force is applied.

Additional risk factors

Further risk factors for spinal column and spinal cord injuries occurring at or around the time of birth appear to be: intrauterine position, premature birth, precipitate delivery, multiple fetuses, limb prolapse, shoulder dystocia, hypoxia, birthweight above 4000 g and postmaturity (De Souza and Davis 1974, Hasanov 1992, Menticoglou et al 1995, Ratner and Michailov 1992, Ruggieri et al 1999, Towbin 1969).

The clinical picture

The extent and location of the spinal cord injury determine the clinical picture (Adams et al 1988, Allen 1970, Babyn et al 1988, Bresnan and Abroms 1973, Mackinnon et al 1993, Ratner and Michailov 1992, Ratner 1991a). Severe injury to the upper cervical spinal cord is associated in particular with respiratory insufficiency, hypotonia, quadriplegia, absence of pain reactions in the dermatomes below the lesion, areflexia, and in certain cases also insufficiency of the anal sphincter after birth. Absence of the grasping, sucking and corneal reflexes may indicate involvement of the brainstem.

Towbin (1964) points out that newborn babies are not necessarily dependent on the presence and function of the brain, since anencephalic infants can live for weeks and even months. The decisive factor is the integrity of the upper cervically located vital centers.

Breathing dysfunction during the first 4 weeks of life is therefore seen as the cardinal symptom of injuries in this location. If segment C_4 is involved, paralysis of the phrenic nerve with raised diaphragm can occur.

Hypoxia following trauma in the cervico-occipital transition zone has been described in other states as well as birth trauma. Around three-quarters of deaths following shaking traumas were caused by apnea (Coghlan 2001). (The Apgar score to assess respiratory effort, heart rate, muscle tone, response to stimulation, etc. in the delivery room is in essence a neurological assessment, primarily to test the irritability of or the presence of injuries to the brainstem and upper spinal cord (Towbin 1964).)

In their clinical and animal studies, Michailov and Aberkov (1989) found associated gastrointestinal signs in cases of upper cervical birth traumas. Disruptions of vertebrobasilar circulation produce secondary spastic-hypotonic dyskinesia of the small intestine, pylorospasm and gastroesophageal reflux. Michailov and Aberkov found swallowing disorders, constant regurgitation and frequent nausea as well as aspiration pneumonia. Where there are recurring infections of the respiratory system, the possibility of a spinal cord lesion should therefore be considered. The same applies to repeated infections of the urogenital tract.

Significant lesions of the upper cervical spinal column and cord are associated with a high postnatal mortality (Babyn et al 1988, MacKinnon et al 1993, Menticoglou et al 1995). Infants who survive this type of trauma of the spinal medulla develop related neurological patterns over a period of months suggesting involvement of the first and second motor neuron. The neurological diagnosis indicates the segment involved.

It is for example possible to diagnose conditions involving the area of the trigeminal nuclei (extending to C_2/C_3) and injuries to the upper brachial plexus (Erb–Duchenne palsy) (Fig. 8.4), where the C_5 and C_6 nerve roots are damaged, immediately after birth. Lesions of the lower plexus (C_7–T_1) (Klumpke's palsy) are rarer and sometimes occur together with lesions of the sympathetic nervous system (Horner's syndrome – Fig. 8.5).

Thorburn's posture represents a particular form, in which a lesion of the lower cervical cord also leads to hypertonia of the interscapular muscles – or to bilateral abduction of the upper arm and weakness of elbow flexion (Renault and Duprey 1989).

Diagnosis and differential diagnosis

The significance of spinal cord injuries for differential diagnosis in peripartum asphyxias and the development of cerebral paresis has been emphasized by several authors (Clancy et al 1989, Morgan and Newell 2001, Sladky and Rorke 1986).

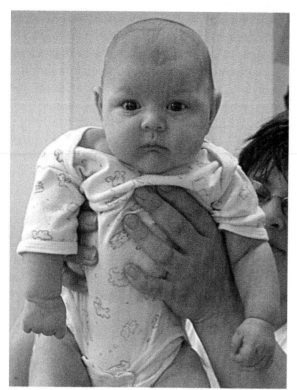

Figure 8.4   Erb–Duchenne palsy (right hand side).

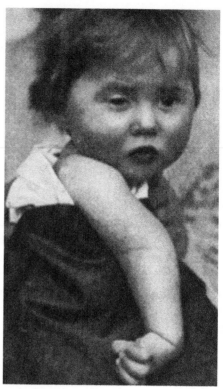

Figure 8.5   Klumpke's palsy and Horner's syndrome (from Bing 1953).

The pediatric neurological examination is useful across a wide range of conditions and the neurological patterns observed can be identified with increasing precision with the advancing age of the child. Laboratory tests, muscle biopsies and electromyography (Allen 1970, Lanska et al 1990, Ruggieri et al 1999) are mainly of use in differential diagnosis.

Opinions are divided on the use of imaging procedures. Plain film X-rays, myelography and computed tomography (CT) (Adams et al 1988), magnetic resonance imaging (MRI) and ultrasound are all used. Lanska et al (1990) emphasize the value of MRI, whereas Rossitch and Oakes (1992) point to false negative results obtained by MRI. An ultrasound examination of the perimedullary structures should be carried out to provide additional information or as an alternative (Babyn et al 1988, De Vries et al 1995, MacKinnon et al 1993, Simon et al 1999).

FUNCTIONAL BIOMECHANICAL DISORDERS OF THE UPPER CERVICAL SPINE

The spine has a number of functions: support, posture, perception, movement and protection. This means that peripartum traumas to the spine may have either a direct effect, by destroying skeletal structures, or an indirect effect by causing secondary reactions in the spine.

It must at least be concluded that pronounced hemorrhage (Babyn et al 1988, MacKinnon et al 1993, Menticoglou et al 1995), atlanto-occipital dislocations (Adams et al 1988, Allen 1970, Menticoglou et al 1995, Rossitch and Oakes 1992), ruptures of the spinal cord (Babyn et al 1988, Lanska et al 1990, Menticoglou et al 1995) and dislocated fractures of the spinal column (MacKinnon et al 1993, Menticoglou et al 1995) will lead to local muscular reactions and in certain cases forced postures. Although such neuro-orthopedic findings have not been described, it is not clear whether such symptoms were not present or simply not recorded. Ratner (1991b) is the only author to report forced attitudes (torticollis) and paravertebral muscular reactions in association with moderate and mild lesions of the spinal column and cord.

We must also ask whether the special anatomical and biomechanical characteristics of the infant cervical spine with which we began might not, in combination with the problems of childbirth and assisted delivery mentioned above, be capable of causing isolated injuries and/or dysfunctions of the spine.

Slate et al (1993), in a study of congenital muscular torticollis, describe 12 cases with upper cervical subluxations and negative neurological findings. The authors traced these subluxations to problems of intrauterine position or birth trauma. However, no details were given of the timing of the neurological examination.

Craniocervical blockages in newborn and infants

Mechanical obstructions of the functioning of vertebral joints, termed 'blockages', occur in all age groups, with infants and the newborn being no exception. Among this group, injuries from birth trauma are most frequently discussed as the cause.

Seifert (1975) found 298 individuals with dysfunctions in the craniocervical region among 1093 randomly selected newborn infants. A significant correlation with postural asymmetries was found.

Buchmann and Bülow (1983) found upper cervical dysfunctions in about one-third of newborn infants ($N = 683$) studied. The incidence of craniocervical blockages in those with forceps deliveries was greater than can be accounted for by chance. Information on problems of intrauterine position or indications for cesarean delivery was not available. This, together with the small number of cases, makes it difficult to draw even a cautious conclusion about the connection between the birth process and dysfunction of the spinal column.

Biedermann (1999) was also able to demonstrate a connection between birth traumas or forced intrauterine positions and the occurrence of reversible arthrogenous dysfunctions of the spine in infants and the newborn in the course of his extensive investigations. Artificial means of assisted delivery (forceps, vacuum extraction), multiple pregnancies, breech presentations, prolonged expulsion period and transverse lie are particular risk factors.

The craniocervical transition zone in embryology and developmental anatomy

A brief look at the phylogeny of the craniocervical joints will help give an insight into their nature.

Vertebrates evolved in water, and at that stage they possessed a comparatively unarticulated notochord or spine rigidly connected to the head with no intervening joint. Head and body formed a single functional unit, and the control of functions such as orientation and balance was entirely directed by the sense organs located in the head (Hassenstein 1970). As differentiation progressed and the joint connection between trunk and body developed, it became necessary to acquire proprioceptive information about the relative position of head and body, and to integrate control mechanisms. This task fell primarily to the craniocervical region, which includes the occipital condyles, atlas, axis and the C_2/C_3 motor segment together with its associated structures. In humans, the special place of the craniocervical transition zone is partly a consequence of embryonic development. Cells from the neural crests of this zone colonize parts of the gastrointestinal tract, the primordial heart, the urogenital tract (Wolff's duct), and the thymus. A similar process underlies the development of the musculature of the tongue, pharynx, larynx, esophagus and thoracic girdle (Christ et al 1988). Numerous special features are also found in the neurophysiology of this region (Abrahams et al 1990, Tayler and McCloskey

1988, Traccis et al 1987, Wolff 1996, Zenker and Neuhubber 1994). In this context the exceptionally dense provision of muscle spindles in the suboccipital musculature and the close link with the sympathetic trunk (superior cervical ganglion) and the trigeminal nuclei (extending to C_2/C_3) are relevant.

Neurophysiological aspects of upper cervical dysfunctions

The spontaneous motor development that takes place in the first year of life involves tactile, proprioceptive and vestibular information, since these types of perception are directly connected with movement, as well as forming the basis for establishing the ideal pattern of movement and proprioception, and for subsequent differentiation, not only of the motor system but of the sensory system, too. The afferent impulses of the cervical receptor region are integrated into the motor system for control of body support (Wolff 1996). For infants, including the newborn, these tonic reflexes of position and support are particularly important (other aspects of perception being still immature). These reflexes are an expression of the genetically programed motor repertoire on which individual learning is based.

The neurophysiological system here, together with the immaturity of the sensorimotor system in (early) infancy, means that craniocervical blockages in infants and the newborn have special potency. There is an association with reactions of the afferent aspect of proprioception, in which the impairment of receptive performance and the difference in the flow of information to the receptors from each side caused by the blockage must play a part (as is the case in the labyrinths) (Hülse et al 1998). Blockage also leads to the known nociceptive, vegetative and myofascial reactions and effects on joint mechanics. Predisposed infants develop a set of symptoms that extends beyond the local effects of craniocervical blockage, known as KISS syndrome.

CLINICAL INVESTIGATIONS

A study involving 403 infants confirmed that the risk profiles given above for the classical cervical spine injuries caused by birth trauma are also responsible for causing craniocervical blockages of early infancy in symptomatic individuals (Sacher 2003).

The details recorded included the route (vaginal/cesarean section) and mode of delivery (spontaneous/assisted extraction; elective/emergency cesarean section), birthweight >4000 g, post-term (>41 weeks) or premature birth (<37 weeks), abnormal fetal position during pregnancy or birth, occipitoposterior cephalic presentation, short expulsion period, prolonged labor (>24 hours), and use of Kristeller's maneuver.

Spontaneous birth

Barely 30% of the infants with craniocervical blockages who fell into this category had no previously suspected risk factors. Three infants in this group had fractures of the clavicle as evidence of force affecting the fetus during birth, one in combination with Erb's palsy and one with cephalhematoma. Two further infants had pronounced cephalhematomas. Spontaneous birth does therefore hold a potential for trauma that should not be underestimated, even when there are no other known risk factors.

Risk factors were found in more than two-thirds of the spontaneous deliveries. The main risk factor was the use of Kristeller's maneuver, which was applied in more than half the deliveries in this category. This maneuver was originally designed to be used in multiparous women whose lax abdominal wall (diastasis recti abdominis) meant that they were no longer able to exert proper abdominal muscular pressure. It is dangerous to apply it to a uterus that is not in labor or where the abdominal wall is tensed hard (Rockenschaub 2001).

The effect of Kristeller's maneuver is to increase the intra-abdominal expulsion pressure to such an extent that the presenting part of the fetus is pushed out past any hindrances or resistance that may be present. In a normal birth with no extra-corporeal augmentation of pressure, the head passes through the birth canal by means of slight repetitive sideways inclination of the head which forces it gradually deeper – a physiological process known as asynclitism (Rockenschaub 2001). If Kristeller's maneuver is applied, this gradual, force-reducing downward movement of the presenting fetal part will no longer happen, and the potential for trauma rises.

High birthweight and short expulsion period were further risk factors frequently encountered. Five infants suffered trauma consisting of lesions of the upper brachial plexus as a consequence of spontaneous delivery; two of these infants were above normal birthweight, two were born after a short expulsion period, with shoulder dystocia in one case. Kristeller's maneuver was used in the delivery of one infant with an upper brachial plexus lesion.

Extraction aids

In 38 cases it was necessary to use artificial means of extraction for vaginal deliveries. It is worthy of note that Kristeller's maneuver was applied in 71% of these cases.

The risk of birth trauma appears to increase when extraction aids are used, especially if there are additional risk factors. Three newborns (two with birthweight >4000 g) had fractures of the clavicle. Kristeller's maneuver had been used.

Cesarean section

Cesarean delivery had been performed in 35% of the cases.

The main risk factor in elective section was abnormal fetal position, which occurred in 40% of the infants delivered by this means. However, 30% of the group under study exhibited none of the assumed risk factors (e.g. elective cesarean section) but still developed dysfunctions of the craniocervical joint. Assuming an average rate of cesarean section of 18–19% in Germany (Schücking 1999), an above-average number of infants delivered by cesarean section appeared in the study cohort. The large number of cases of abnormal fetal position may account for this.

Another reason for the high proportion of cesarean sections is the vulnerability of the upper cervical structures when traction tension is applied. The physiology of the birth process does not allow for traction in the upper cervical area, and so the human fetus does not have adequate protective mechanisms for this. However, every cesarean section involves considerable traction force on the spine and its associated structures, regardless of whether the fetus is taken out by the head or the legs.

The conclusion must be drawn that elective cesarean section seems to increase rather than reduce the risk of developing craniocervical blockages of infancy (as opposed to severe upper cervical injuries).

The most severe birth injuries were observed with emergency cesarean section. During the delivery of one post-term infant with excess birthweight, the uterus was ruptured when Kristeller's maneuver was performed and an emergency cesarean followed. One infant was later found to have a brainstem hemorrhage. Another infant was delivered by emergency cesarean section without any further risk factors being present, yet peripartum upper cervical trauma was strongly suspected.

Additional risk factors

Additional risk factors were present in a large number of births.

Breech presentations

First deliveries appear to be a predisposing factor for breech presentations (Boos 1994, Rayl et al 1996). It is therefore assumed that the firm abdominal wall of primiparous women and the fact that the uterus has not previously been stretched make spontaneous turning more difficult. Multiparous women are at similar risk for the opposite reason: low tension of the uterus wall and too little pressure from the abdominal wall muscles offer too little resistance to support the turning movement, aided by the extremities (Feige and Krause 1998).

Abnormal fetal position is often associated with intrauterine forced positions on account of lack of space, which can lead to dysfunctions in the craniocervical transition zone (Biedermann 1999). However, four infants with such abnormalities of lie during pregnancy were delivered spontaneously and without complications with cephalic presentations. They nevertheless had craniocervical blockages. It is interesting to note in this connection a circumstance that has been known for some years: that breech delivery infants have often developed 'congenital torticollis'. In these cases, too, the cause was assumed to be intrauterine forced positions (Martius 1964). The author further believes that the Mauriceau–Smellie–Veit maneuver in vaginal deliveries predisposes to developing this type of birth injury.

Another explanation may be that the different birth presentation in turn affects the mode of delivery and adds a potential further risk to the upper cervical transition zone. Almost 80% of the 48 cases of abnormal fetal position during pregnancy or birth were delivered by cesarean section.

Intubation

When infants have been intubated after birth, the procedure (i.e. intubation) itself and the resultant trauma can be considered as possible causes of craniocervical blockages. Also, problems of respiratory distress may signal the presence of a lesion of the cervical spine caused by birth trauma and/or the consequence of other types of central nervous damage.

Prolonged labor (>24 hours)

Prolonged delivery is frequently associated with increased birth risks that can result in an abnormal mechanical stress for the fetus (e.g. abnormalities of the pelvis or of engagement) (Schmitt-Matthiesen 1992) and so involve greater risk to the craniocervical transition zone.

Short expulsion period (<10 minutes)

Here, too, an increase in the mechanical stress on the fetus is probably brought about by strong contractions (Schmitt-Matthiesen 1992), exerted particularly on the presenting parts of the fetus and the upper cervical transition zone. There is no exact quantitative time definition of precipitate birth with a short expulsion period, with reference simply being made to delivery with 'few labor pains' (Martius and Rath 1998). In establishing a history it is difficult to verify such details of the final stage of childbirth, and the solution chosen when recording the data was to use information about the length of the expulsion period.

Birthweight above 4000 g

More than 13% of the infants with craniocervical blockages had a birthweight in excess of 4000 g, and delivery of these infants was more often artificially assisted or carried out by emergency section, in line with the percentage of these high birthweight infants within the particular mode of delivery. High birthweight was the only risk factor for half the infants assessed as being in the high weight category.

Premature births

Premature birth was recorded in 42 cases (approximately 10%). Assuming a premature birth rate of 6–8% in German-speaking countries (Goerke and Valet 2000, Pschyrembel and Dudenhausen 1991), this represents only a slightly increased rate in the study cohort. The proportion of infants who had been born prematurely and had craniocervical blockages after elective cesarean section was relatively high. This is possibly connected with the indications for elective section as opposed to vaginal delivery, which are fairly generously framed for the premature birth group. Another point is that four premature infants were intubated following elective section, making postnatal causes a possibility.

Children born considerably before term spend some time without full head control. Increased postnatal inertia load on the upper cervical structures can therefore be considered in such cases. However, the small number of premature babies delivered spontaneously and without further risk factors contradicts this as an explanation. At 5% this percentage was within the expected range for premature births. It is more probable that infants whose gestation period is markedly shorter are more likely to develop craniocervical blockages on account of the risks associated with this.

Post-term births

Normal term was exceeded in just 11 cases. This risk factor was only encountered once on its own in combination with elective cesarean section; in most instances these post-term births were accompanied by high birthweight (a total of 4) or the delivery called for manual and/or artificial assistance.

Occipitoposterior position

A total of 10 infants presented in the occipitoposterior position, a figure that was just 3% of all included infants with cephalic presentations. However, from its incidence in the average population, one would expect to find the occipitoposterior position in 0.5–1% of all cephalic presentations (Pschyrembel and Dudenhausen 1991). Since the position is unfavorable for the upper cervical region, this aspect may once more constitute a predisposing factor here.

Limb prolapse/presentation

It was difficult when taking the history to differentiate between actual prolapse of arm or hand and presentation of the extremity, or between complete and incomplete prolapse of the fetal extremity, and

this group was therefore recorded together. Most of the 10 cases assigned to this group must have involved uncomplicated instances, since the care records did not document the fact. The comparatively high incidence (2.5%) of this feature in our study cohort was, however, surprising. Such events are described as happening in 0.05–0.1% of all births (Mändle et al 1995). Infants born to multiparae are reported to be particularly affected.

Conclusion

In conclusion, each mode of delivery contains its own specific risks to the upper cervical region, irrespective of the presence of additional risk factors.

Additional risk factors for the development of craniocervical blockages in infancy could be assumed in more than two-thirds of all symptomatic infants. These include the use of Kristeller's maneuver, high birthweight (>4000 g), short expulsion period, intrauterine forced or abnormal positions, occipitoposterior position or prolonged delivery (>24 hours), prolapse or presentation of an extremity, shoulder dystocia and postpartal traumas such as intubation. Premature birth, post-term delivery and twin pregnancies appear to be co-factors that often occur together with the above risk factors.

The contention that birth trauma plays the predominant role in the pathogenesis of craniocervical blockages of early infancy (i.e. that perinatal traumas are the main cause) is not without its critics (Buchmann and Bülow 1983). As in adults, other causes for dysfunctions of this type are logically possible and may in fact be responsible. In particular, the cause may be reactions that are visceral or static-dynamic in nature; or the dysfunctions may stem from cerebral errors in the control of the motorsensory system. The young age of the study cohort, however, makes these causes less likely.

If the risk profile for the development of classical upper cervical lesions, which was mentioned at the beginning, is compared with the risk factors presented here for the occurrence of reversible articular dysfunctions of the craniocervical joints in symptomatic infants, the common elements cannot be ignored. Where the causative mechanism is the same, only the degree of trauma or additional individual factors will determine the extent of the cervical lesion.

IMPLICATIONS FOR PRACTICE

Each mode of delivery carries individual risks, both in itself and in the implications for obstetrics, calling for appropriate obstetric skill. Knowledge of these risks makes it possible to avoid them in the context of preventive obstetrics, and also enables improved assessment of the birth trauma involved, with the necessary type of aftercare.

Birth is attended by risk of trauma independently of the mechanism of childbirth and even obstetric practice in strict conformity with accepted principles can do no more than minimize the risk. Seen in this light, obstetrics becomes both the price of our evolution and the challenge with which it presents us.

References

Abrahams V C, Rose P K, Richmond F J R 1990 Properties and control of the neck musculature. In: Binder M, Mendell L (eds) The segmental motor system. Oxford University Press, New York, p 58–71

Adams C, Babyn P S, Logan W J 1988 Spinal cord birth injury. Value of computed tomographic myelography. Pediatric Neurology 4:105–109

Allen J P 1970 Birth injury to the spinal cord. Northwest Medicine 5:323–326

Babyn P S, Chuang S H, Daneman A, Davidson G S 1988 Sonographic evaluation of spinal cord birth trauma with pathologic correlation. American Journal of Roentgenology 151:763–766

Baily D K 1952 The normal cervical spine in infants and children. Radiology 59:712–719

Bhgwanani S G, Price H V, Laurence K M, Ginz B 1973 Risk and prevention of cervical cord injury in the management of breech presentation with hyperextension of the fetal head. American Journal of Obstetrics and Gynecology 115:1159–1161

Biedermann H 1999 Manualtherapie bei Kindern. Enke, Stuttgart

Bing R 1953 Kompendium der topischen Gehirn-und Rückenmarksdiagnostik. Schwabe, Basel

Boos R 1994 Die Beckenendlage – Analyse der perinatologischen Daten, ultrasonographische Befunde und antepartales Verhalten. Habilitationsschrift, Medizinische Fakultät der Universität des Saarlandes, Homburg

Bresnan M J, Abroms I F 1973 Neonatal spinal cord transsection secondary to intrauterine hyperextension of the neck in breech presentation. Fetal and Neonatal Medicine 84:734–737

Buchmann J, Bülow B 1983 Funktionelle Kopfgelenksstörungen im Zusammenhang mit Lagereaktionen und Tonusasymmetrie. Manuelle Medizin 21:59–62

Catell H S, Filtzer D L 1965 Pseudosubluxation and other normal variants in the cervical spine in children. A study of 160 children. Journal of Bone and Joint Surgery 47:1295–1309

Caterini H, Langer A, Sama J C, Devanesan M, Pelosi M 1975 Fetal risk in hyperextension of the fetal head in breech presentation. American Journal of Obstetrics and Gynecology 123:632–634

Cattamanchi G R, Tamaskar V, Egel R T et al 1981 Intrauterine quadriplegia associated with breech presentation and hyperextension of fetal head: a case report. American Journal of Obstetrics and Gynecology 140:831–833

Christ B, Jacobs H, Seifert R 1988 Über die Entwicklung der zervico-occipitalen Übergangsregion. In: Hohmann D (ed) Neuro-Orthopädie 4. Springer, Berlin

Clancy R R, Sladky J T 1989 Rorke L B. Hypoxic-ischemic spinal cord injury following perinatal asphyxia. Annals of Neurology 25:185–189

Coghlan A, Le Page M 2001 Gently does it. New Scientist 16:4–5

De Souza S W, Davis J A 1974 Spinal cord damage in a new-born infant. Archives of Disease in Childhood 49:70–71

De Vries E, Robben S G, van den Anker J N 1995 Radiologic imaging of severe cervical spinal cord birth trauma. European Journal of Pediatrics 154:230–232

Feige A, Krause M 1998 Beckenendlage. Urban & Schwarzenberg, Munich

Fielding J W 1984 Injuries of the cervical spine in children. In: Rockwood C A Jr, Wilkins K E, King R E (eds) Fractures in children. Lippincott, Philadelphia, p 683–705

Gilles F H, Bina M, Sotrel A 1979 Infantile atlanto-occipital instability: the potential of extreme extension. American Journal of Diseases of Children 133:30–37

Goerke K, Valet A 2000 Kurzlehrbuch Gynäkologie und Geburtshilfe. Urban & Fischer, Munich

Hasanov A A 1992 Das Geburtstrauma des Neugeborenen (rus). University of Kasan, Kasan.

Hassenstein B 1970 Biologische Kybernetik. Quelle & Meyer Heidelberg

Hill S A, Miller C A, Kosnik E J et al. 1984 Pediatric neck injuries. A clinical study. Journal of Neurosurgery 60:700–706

Hülse M, Neuhuber W L, Wolff H D 1998 Der kranio-zervikale Übergang. Springer, Berlin

Lang J 1979 Kopf. Teil B; Gehirn-und Augenschädel. In: von Lanz T, Wachsmuth W (eds) Praktische Anatomie. Springer, Berlin

Lanska J M, Roessmann U, Wiznitzer M 1990 Magnetic resonance imaging in cervical cord birth injury. Pediatrics 85:760–764

Leventhal H R 1960 Birth injuries to the spinal cord. Journal of Pediatrics 56:447–453

MacKinnon J A, Perlman M, Kirpalani H et al 1993 Spinal cord injury at birth: diagnostic and prognostic data in twenty-two patients. Journal of Pediatrics 122:431–437

Maekawa K, Masaki T, Kokubun Y 1976 Fetal spinal cord injury secondary to hyperextension of the neck: no effect of cesarean section. Developmental Medicine and Child Neurology 18:229–232

Mändle C, Opitz-Kreuter S, Wehling A 1995 Das Hebammenbuch. Schattauer, Stuttgart

Martius G, Rath W 1998 Geburtshilfe und Perinatologie. Thieme, Stuttgart

Martius H 1964 Lehrbuch der Geburtshilfe. Thieme, Stuttgart

Melzak J 1969 Paraplegia among children. Lancet 45–48

Menezes A H 1987 Traumatic lesions of the craniocervical junction. In: Van Gilder J C, Menezes A H, Dolan K (eds) Textbook of craniovertebral junction abnormalities. Futura, Mount Kisco

Menticoglou S M, Perlman M, Manning F A 1995 High cervical spinal cord injury in neonates delivered with forceps: report of 15 cases. Obstetrics and Gynecology 86:589–594

Michailov M K, Akberov R F 1989 Röntgensemiotik und Differentialdiagnostik der funktionellen Undurchgängigkeit des Verdaungstraktes im Kindesalter, bedingt durch Geburtstraumen der Wirbelsäule und des Rückenmarks. Radiologica Diagnostica 30:669–674

Morgan C, Newell S J 2001 Cervical spinal cord injury following cephalic presentation and delivery by Caesarean section. Developmental Medicine and Child Neurology 43:274–276

Nitecki S, Moir C R 1994 Predictive factors of the outcome of traumatic cervical spine fracture in children. Journal of Pediatric Surgery 29:1409–1411

Osenbach R K, Menezes A H 1989 Spinal cord injury without radiographic abnormality in children. Pediatric Neuroscience 15:168–175

Papavasilou V 1978 Traumatic subluxations of the cervical spine during childhood. Orthopedic Clinics of North America 9:945–954

Pschyrembel W 1966 Praktische Geburtshilfe. Walter de Gruyter, Berlin

Pschyrembel W, Dudenhausen J W 1991 Praktische Geburtshilfe. Walter de Gruyter, Berlin

Ratner J 1991a Spätfolgen geburtstraumatischer Läsionen des zentralen Nervensystems. Der Kinderarzt 22: 385–391

Ratner J 1991b Zur perinatalen Schädigung des zentralen Nervensystems. Der Kinderarzt 22:29–34

Ratner J, Michailov K 1992 Klinisch-röntgenologische Befunde bei geburtstraumatischen Verletzungen der Halswirbelsäule. Der Kinderarzt 23:811–822

Rayl J, Gibson P J, Hickok D E 1996 A population based case-control study of risk factors for breech presentation. American Journal of Obstetrics and Gynecology 174:28–32

Renault F, Duprey J 1989 La posture de Thorburn. Archives Françaises de Pediatrie 46:273–275

Rockenschaub A 2001 Gebären ohne Aberglaube. Facultas-Univ.-Verlag, Vienna

Rossitch E, Oakes W J 1992 Perinatal spinal cord injury: clinical, radiographic and pathologic features. Pediatric Neurosurgery 18:149–152

Ruggieri M, Smarason A K, Pike M 1999 Spinal cord insult in the prenatal, perinatal and neonatal periods. Developmental Medicine and Child Neurology 41:311–317

Sacher R 2003 Die geburtstraumatische Gefährdung der infantilen (Hals-) Wirbelsäule. päd – Praktische Pädiatrie 3:222–225

Sacher R (in press) Arbeit in Vorbereitung

Schmidt H, Fischer E 1960 Die okzipitale Dysplasie. Thieme, Stuttgart

Schmitt-Matthiesen H 1992 Gynäkologie und Geburtshilfe. Schattauer, Stuttgart

Schücking B A 1999 Kaiserschnitt auf Wunsch. Österreichische Hebammenzeitung 5:14–15

Seifert I 1975 Kopfgelenksblockierungen bei Neugeborenen. Rehabilitacia (Suppl) 10/11:53–56

Shulman S T, Madden J D, Esterly J R et al. 1971 Transection of spinal cord. A rare obstetrical complication of cephalic delivery. Archives of Disease in Childhood 46:291–294

Simon L, Perreaux F, Devictor D, Millotte B 1999 Clinical and radiological diagnosis of spinal cord birth injury. Archives of Disease in Childhood/Fetal and Neonatal Edition 81:F235

Sladky J T, Rorke L B 1986 Perinatal hypoxic/ischemic spinal cord injury. Pediatric Pathology 6:87–101

Slate R K, Posnik J C, Armstrong D C, Buncic J R 1993 Cervical spine subluxation associated with congenital muscular torticollis and craniofacial asymmetry. Plastic and Reconstructive Surgery 91:1187–1195

Tayler J L, McCloskey DI 1988 Proprioception in the neck. Brain Research 70:351–360

Towbin A 1964 Spinal cord and brainstem injury at birth. Archives of Pathology 77:620–632

Towbin A 1969 Latent spinal cord and brainstem injury in newborn infant. Developmental Medicine and Child Neurology 11:54–68

Towbin A 1970 Central nervous system damage in the human fetus and newborn infant. American Journal of Diseases of Children 119:529–542

Townsend E H Jr, Rowe M L 1952 Mobility of the upper cervical spine in health and disease. Pediatrics 10:567–573

Traccis S, Rosati G, Patraskakis S et al 1987 Influences of neck receptors on soleus motoneuron exciticity in men. Experimental Neurology 95:76–84

von Kortzfleisch P 1993 Zur Biomechanik der kindlichen Halswirbelsäule. Inaugural-Dissertation, Universität Köln, Institut II für Anatomie

Weinstein D, Margalioth E J, Navot D 1983 Neonatal fetal death following cesarian section secondary to hyperextended head in breech presentation. Acta Obstetrica Gynecologica Scandinavia 62:629–631

Wolff H D 1996 Neurophysiologische Aspekte des Bewegungssystems. 3rd edn. Springer, Berlin

Zenker W, Neuhuber W L 1994 Feinbau von Rückenmark und Spinalganglien. In: Benninghoff (ed). Anatomie, 15th edn, vol 2. Lehmann, Munich

Differential diagnosis of central and peripheral neurological disorders in infants

L. Babina, H. Biedermann, S. Iliaeva

Small children, before undergoing manual therapy, have to be thoroughly examined as their symptoms are so diverse at the time of the first encounter. One of the biggest problems for those active in this field is to achieve a valid differential diagnosis in order to distinguish between a functional and/or truly central (i.e. cerebrospinal) origin of the clinically observed situation. Neuropediatric and neuro-orthopedic procedures can help to improve the level of this still difficult distinction. We have to accept the fact that most of the small children we examine and treat suffer from a combination of those two types of problems. Combined with the injuries and irritations acquired during delivery or in utero are genetically determined ailments and other morphologically fixed disorders.

A sharp separation between the three groups (genetic, central and functional) is by no means as simple as one would like it to be, but up to a point we are able to define probabilities which help to sort out those children with a mainly central (i.e. neuromorphological) problem and those where the predominant part of the pathology can be attributed to a functional disorder in the arthrovertebral region. This differentiation does not imply that children with a primarily neuromorphological disorder cannot be treated with manual therapy and profit from such a treatment. As we point out in Chapter 25, patients with cerebral palsy improve markedly after manual therapy.

But the primary cause of a given problem has to be evaluated as well as possible in order to define our treatment goals realistically.

This diagnostic canon does not yet exist. One of the main reasons is the fact that most neurologists and pediatricians do not recognize that functional disorders of the vertebral spine may make an important contribution to their patients' problems. Until now it was the cerebrum where one looked in order to find the cause of neurological problems. As the role of the spinal system has been neglected there is no incentive to pay much attention to this differential diagnosis. This is the situation in the West, at least until very recently. In Russia, on the other hand, a long-established tradition exists of examining this area situated between neurology and orthopedics.

To establish a diagnostic base we use observation of the spontaneous movements, examination of the primitive reflexes and Vojta's screening tests (Fig. 9.1) (Vojta and Peters 1992). These tests show abnormal movement patterns with a multitude of causes:

- disharmonious maturation of an otherwise intact cerebrum
- cerebral trauma
- perinatal injury of the spinal cord
- perinatal injury of the vertebral spine
- lesion of a peripheral nerve
- neuromuscular disorder
- endocrine disorder.

Differentiation between these possibilities is not easy with the standard tests, let alone an assessment of where the problem originates. Here the work of Ratner comes into play. Until his premature death in 1992 he was head of the neuropediatric clinic in Kazan (Ratner and Bondarchuk 1990, Ratner and Michailov 1992) and published prolifically on pediatric neurology and perinatal injuries of the spinal column. Based on this work a more precise procedure is possible.

Assigning a neurological finding to a neuropediatric category or a neurological syndrome and/or a functional vertebrogenic disorder offers some important possibilities to a manual therapist, as it is the base from which to decide about further diagnostic tests and the ensuing therapy. To compile this information, neurologists, pediatricians and manual therapists have to work together. This is easier said than done, as these different specialties use a different vocabulary. Here we have tried to bridge this gap and offer an initial version.

Figure 9.1   A: Peiper–Isbert-reaction. B: Vojta test. The correct interpretation of these tests has to take into account the developmental age of the child. The two pictures show a normal reaction pattern for a 3-month-old.

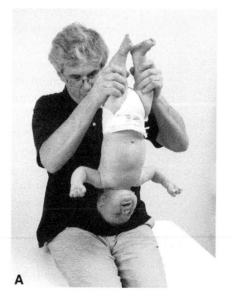 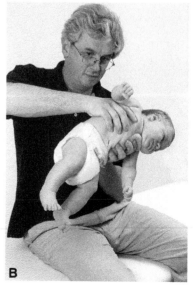

A   B

We do hope to improve on this using the comments of our readers.

MEDICAL HISTORY

The history starts with the family history and the health situation of the mother. One main focus is on the risk factors before and during pregnancy:

- Which (if any) medications and/or drugs were taken?
- Infectious diseases, e.g. cytomegalic inclusion disease and rubella, or endocrine disorders, e.g. hyperthyroidism, dysfunction of the suprarenal gland. The third group are cardiovascular problems, e.g. valvular defects. Problems in these fields increase the probability of a more 'central' neurological problem.

Problems immediately before or during birth:

- premature labor
- transverse presentation
- placental anomalies
- delayed delivery
- twin pregnancies
- lengthy labor
- oversized child
- vacuum extraction, forceps or other extraction aids.

All these items make functional problems more probable.

Our questionnaire covers these items and the completion of this form helps the parents to remember these details. It is astonishing (and has to be taken into account in the evaluation of the questionnaire) the extent to which the details of the delivery are forgotten by the parents – and how sketchy the documentation of the delivery often is. We saw several callused clavicular fractures in children whose birth was described by parents and documentation as 'quite normal'.

Sensorimotor development of the child: children with retarded motor development due to a central problem often have retarded psychic development, too. In KISS children there is often a marked difference between the apparently normal mental and the slower sensorimotor side of development. Parents often talk about the unhappiness of their (KISS) children who want to do things they cannot achieve, thus becoming discontented, unhappy and angry.

There are many variants in the motor development which are interpreted differently depending on the viewpoint of the examiner.

Most neuropediatric specialists tend to consider a child's preference to shove on the buttocks (Fig. 9.2) instead of crawling a normal variant of motor development. Seen from the viewpoint of manual therapy, this preference indicates problems with the sacroiliac (SI) joints and/or the occipitocervical (OC) region.

For most parents the moment when their child starts walking is much more important than the period during which the child crawled. Almost all professionals, on the other hand, put the emphasis

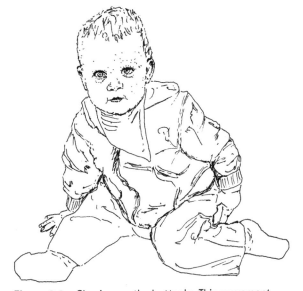

Figure 9.2 Shoving on the buttocks. This movement pattern is often used by babies who cannot master the difficulties of crawling. Its pathological significance is often underestimated. These children are able to develop normally, but having left out the crawling phase makes them susceptible to other coordinative disturbances.

on this detail of motor development, as it is a very good indicator of a child's motor competence. Crawling is by far the most important step in the acquisition of bipedal gait and – skipped over – the lack of this coordination level tends to render the further coordinative successes more fragile (Birrer and Levine 1987, Loovis and Butterfield 1993, Patel et al 2002). So it is important to get information about other 'milestones' (Ayres 1979) in the child's development as well.

All these observations should be complemented by reports of others, especially those who are already in professional contact with the child, e.g. physiotherapists or crèche staff. Another aid to verify the statements of the parents are photographs. To that end we ask the parents to bring pictures of the first years of their child. The quality of these photographs varies widely, but more often than not they offer at least a base for further questions to the parents. Quite a few parents are themselves surprised to what an extent one can see a stereotype posture in these albums.

Sometimes when you look at the siblings and remark on their individual postural pattern the ensuing discussion leads to the discovery of related problems in these children.

JACK BE NIMBLE, JACK BE QUICK: OBSERVATION AND APPRAISAL OF MOVEMENT AND POSTURE

Almost all books on pediatric neurology offer a fairly comprehensive overview of the tests and observations appropriate for a specific age, and this is not the place to list them (Dubowitz et al 1999, Fenichel 2001, Swaiman 1994). It should be emphasized that the neurological examination of all children, and especially newborn and toddlers, has to be smooth and as quick as possible in order to succeed. Before one even touches the baby, a calm and trustful atmosphere has to be established. Enough space, no external noise and a well-lit and warm environment may sound like a matter of course, but in practice these basic pre-

conditions are not always met. It is important that the child is well rested and neither hungry nor ill.

An experienced therapist starts grasping vital diagnostic information the moment the family comes into the room – which is one of the reasons we strongly advise being present when the baby is brought into the examination room. This enables the therapist to evaluate the reaction of the child to the room's setting and to use this background information to gauge the reaction to the tests performed on and with the child.

The first aim in dealing with a new young patient should be to open up to the *Gestalt* of the disorder, i.e. use one's professional prejudices. This is an intentionally provocative remark, but – especially for the beginner – the over-supply of available tests tends to hide the basic truth that a clinical diagnosis was and will be an act of intuition. If this was not the case we could indeed program computers to take care of diagnostics – and treatment, too, for good measure. But this first impression needs to be verified, questioned and fine-tuned to the individual situation in order to give us a meaningful base to proceed from.

Our examination of the small child has to be quicker than the evaporation of patience of the little patient – which takes place quite rapidly. It is not realistic to ask all relevant tests to be applied in order to get a valid diagnosis. Having gained a first hunch by observing the child on the arm of its parent, we apply the most important tests first and continue from there as far as the patient allows us to go, keeping in mind that we need a minimum of compliance for the treatment, too.

The observation of the child's spontaneous movements is the principal source of information for the examiner; all tests serve to standardize the hunches one gets from the examination of the baby before one even touches it. And the more the child is in distress, the more the watching parents will get nervous – which feeds back onto the child's behavior immediately. The amount of distress is of diagnostic interest, too, and one should keep in mind at what time of day the child is presented. The younger the child, the more the diurnal rhythm plays a part, and at noon almost every child is much more irritable than between 9 and 11 a.m. So it does make sense to note the time of the examination routinely.

It is useful to make the transition of the baby from the parent's lap into our hands as smooth as possible. At the end of the initial conversation we sit next to the parents and help them to undress the child while it is still on their lap. How far we go with this undressing is open to discussion: in the beginning of our work with small children we routinely undressed them completely, the way we were taught at university. Later on we realized that there is a trade-off between the area of skin visible and the mood of the little patient. So we use a bit of *realpolitik* and mostly leave the underwear on, at least in the beginning. It is easier to examine a moderately cooperative baby in its underwear than a naked baby stiff with anger.

Examination in the dorsal position

We start the examination in a dorsal position, trying to get into visual contact with the child. Some important points: does the child seem to be happy, relaxed? Were we able to pick it up from the parent's lap without too much adverse reaction? Sometimes a total lack of negative reaction is a pathological sign, too. How does the child react? Does it avert its gaze or do the eyes follow movements? If we get eye contact, does the child follow with its gaze in all directions?

From month 4 on we can offer toys to grasp and examine.

We observe if there are appropriate motion patterns, stereotype gesturing, tremor or myoclonal movements.

How is the posture on the examination table? Is there a constant or intermittent opisthotonos?

How does the child react to noise (Moro test and similar maneuvers, Fig. 9.3).

Examination of the head should consider the following: micro- or macrocephaly, fontanelle prominent or caved in, how are the cranial sutures?

Adduction and pronation of the arms and/or extension and inside rotation of the legs are symptoms of central nervous problems. KISS children, on the other hand, often show unilateral fisting, mostly on the concave side of the body, together with fewer (or less differentiated) movements of the extremities on that side. After manipulation, this often changes rather quickly and the ability to grasp things improves.

Children in whom there is a risk of cerebral palsy do not show such an improvement.

We also look to see if there is a 'cervical' pattern to the child's symptoms. Facial asymmetry, unilateral enophthalmos, marked folding of the neck skin (often clammy) and a laterally fixed posture of the head are signs which direct our attention towards a functional problem of the (cervical) spine. In children with a fixed retroflexion (KISS II) a marked persistence of the Moro test is typical. These children react with a marked and Moro-like movement to noise and change of position well beyond the age of 5 months.

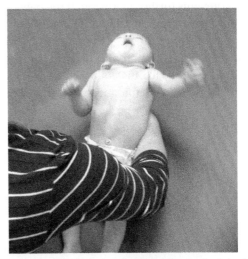

Figure 9.3 Moro reaction. This reaction is physiological till the third month. Later on its persistence is pathological. The differential diagnosis between a functional or central origin is not easy. Persistence till adolescence may be one reason for coordination disorders (Goddard Blythe and Hyland 1998). In this case the lack of head support and the asymmetry of the hands are pathological.

Examination of the form of the thorax and the abdomen is important, too. Children with a paretic diaphragm have a retracted lower rib case which is fixed in an exhalation position. A reduced muscle tone of the abdominal muscles can have a multitude of different origins which have to be checked.

Examination in the ventral position

Next is the examination in the ventral position (Fig. 9.4). First and foremost we are interested in the posture and movement of the head and the coordination of the arm muscles. From the age of 4 months the child can support head and shoulders, albeit still a bit wobbly, in a neutral and symmetrical position and is able to direct head and eyes towards a stimulus.

KISS I (fixed lateroflexion) children often have delayed head control and an asymmetrical posture. If the stimulus comes from the 'right' – i.e. convex – side they are able to fixate the stimulus and they will follow it with their eyes till the point when the limited movement range of their cervical joints prevents further following. If the baby is in a mood to be sufficiently cooperative this allows for a repetitive test of the range of movement. It is evident that this restriction of movement is frustrating (and painful) for the child and *one* reason for the fits of rage these children sometimes display.

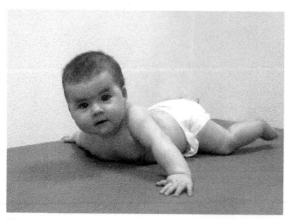

Figure 9.4 Ventral examination: inadequate prop of the shoulders. This baby cannot bring the right arm into a supportive position.

Sometimes the child compensates for the restricted range of movement by lifting the shoulder. By pulling up the shoulder the distance between origin and insertion of the sternocleidomastoid muscle is minimized. In those cases where – through treatment or by its own means – the child is unable to overcome this condition, there is a chance that the muscle reacts to this long-term shortening by fibrotic transformation. This transformation of the muscle results in a thin, piano-wire like remnant of the sternocleidomastoid. These cases cannot be effectively treated by means of a functional therapy, be it manual therapy or other physiotherapeutic means. In most cases a myotomy offers the best chances of improvement.

Children with a basically functional problem display a mild form of absence of head control; a basic muscular tonus is present and this tonus can be reinforced by repeatedly testing it. If the muscular tonus is severely reduced or completely absent, a central origin of this condition is probable.

KISS II children display hyperextension of the head in the ventral position and a fixated thoracic hyperkyphosis. Because of the hyperactivity of the neck extensors, the shoulders are often protracted and the child cannot bring the elbows into a ventral position (see p. 287). We call this posture 'the dying swan' (Vasilyeva et al 2001). An additional test is to check for hypersensitivity of the neck area, especially the insertions at the occiput.

It is essential to distinguish between the hyperextension due to functional and arthrogenic problems and the classic opisthotonos caused by central nervous problems, e.g. meningitis.

Examination of cranial nerves and eye muscles

We also examine the quality of the cranial nerves and the functioning of the eye muscles. Eye movement can be tested by establishing eye contact and moving one's head in front of the child. Alternatively a toy or a colored object might be moved in front of the child's eyes. A strabismus convergens (nervus abducens) or divergens (nervus oculomotorius) has to be excluded. The optico-facial reflex gives a rough idea about the strength of vision (nervus opticus), as the auro-palpebral reflex allows testing of the infant's hearing.

The evaluation of the functioning of the facial nerve distinguishes between a central paresis affecting the muscles of the lower half of the face and a distal paresis which affects the entire face. The caudal group can only be examined and evaluated indirectly (nervus vagus, nervus glossopharyngeus, nervus hypoglossus.). In a newborn baby with swallowing difficulties, injury to these nerves has to be considered after other possibilities have been excluded.

Testing the muscular tonus

The neonatal automatisms and the muscular tonus are the next steps in the test battery.

First and foremost we are interested in whether the different muscle groups display a regular muscular tonus, comparing the upper and lower extremities and the left and right side as well as the tonus of the ventral and dorsal muscle groups. The tonus can be normo-, hyper- or hypotonic and regionally different. KISS children without additional neurological problems have a normal muscular pattern.

If an elevated muscular tonus is found we have to look for articular disorders. A hip dysplasia with reduced abduction results in a heightened muscular tonus of the adductor and the psoas muscles, but a blockage of the iliosacral (IS) joint can cause the same phenomena. Additional differential diagnosis is always necessary in these cases.

A hip dysplasia can be verified by sonography and/or radiography, an IS blockage is associated with local trigger points and a palpable dysfunction of the joint; it should subside shortly after successful treatment, either locally or at the OC junction.

If these two causes can be excluded, a central coordination disorder becomes the most probable reason. In this case we expect to find additional signs, e.g. fixed extension and inversion of the foot/feet and spasticity of the biceps surae muscle.

In the quite frequent case of a combination of IS blockage and a dysfunction of the central nervous system, the normalization of the joint function leaves the reduced abduction as the persisting 'central' sign.

Muscle reflexes

The routine control starts with ASR (L_5/S_1), PSR(L_3/L_4), BSR(C_5/C_6) and TSR(C_7/C_8). We register the amount of response, and possible enlargement of the zone, and compare the reactions on both sides.

Positive Babinski and Rossolimo reactions are pathological from the fourth month on. KISS children without neurological problems display normal and symmetrical reflexes without these signs.

Primitive reflexes

For the examination of the primitive reflexes we use Ratner's methodology (Ratner and Bondarchuk 1990).

Search reflex

Slight touch of a cheek induces a search movement of the mouth and slight rotation of the head to the side of the stimulus. The neuronal chain includes the nervus trigeminus as its afferent and the nervus facialis (mouth movement) and the nerves of the upper cervical segments (head rotation) as the efferent part. If the child does not sense the touch we suspect a cerebral problem; if the head rotation is reduced a cervical disorder is most probable.

Sucking reflex

If a nipple or a finger is found with the mouth, a sucking movement begins. This neuronal chain goes via nervus trigeminus. nervus facialis, nervus vagus and nervus hypoglossus. This reflex is purely cerebral.

In a few cases the sucking response improved very quickly after cervical manipulation. A possible explanation might be found in an increased perfusion of the vertebral artery with a consequent improvement of brainstem function.

Babkin reflex

The baby is in a dorsal position and the palms of its hands are pushed with the thumb of the examiner. The normal reaction is an opening of the mouth. This is a purely central reflex.

Grasping reflex

The forefinger touches the palm of the hand, coming from the wrist. The ensuing grasp reflex is assessed qualitatively and in comparison with the other side. The neurological chain of this reflex uses the segment levels C_5–C_8. This reflex is purely spinal and a cerebral or high cervical lesion leads to a marked amplification of the response on the traumatized side. In cases of plexus paresis and lesion of the lower cervical structures, this reflex is attenuated.

KISS I children without signs of neurological impairment often show a diminished reaction to that stimulus on the side where the muscles are shortened, a phenomenon we explain by the reduction in muscular strength on the concave side due to the inhibition of these muscles on the segmental level.

Moro reaction (see Fig. 9.3)

The child is placed in a half-sitting position and fixated at the back and the head. A slight passive retroflexion of the head sets off a generalized movement of the arms. The neuronal chain of this reflex runs through the cervical level C_5/C_7. Attenuation of this reaction can be the result of a central muscular hypertension, a lesion of the lower cervical area or a trauma to the plexus brachialis. KISS I children without additional neurological problems show, in most cases, an asymmetrical reaction to

this test. In KISS II children this reflex persists for a long time, disappearing rapidly after successful treatment (i.e. 1–3 days later).

Galant reaction

During this test the child is held in a ventral – and strictly horizontal – position supported under its belly by the hand of the examiner. Starting from the lower scapular angle the paravertebral skin is stimulated by gently stroking it. This elicits in normal cases a slight contraction of the muscles of this side resulting in a side-bending of the trunk to this side. The head follows this movement.

If the Galant reflex is missing a spinal lesion is probable; central lesions do not seem to influence this test. We often see a asymmetrical reaction in KISS I children.

Foot-grasp reflex

The examiner places his thumb on the sole of the baby's foot close to the toes. More or less rapidly a 'grasping' reflex is elicited. The quality of this reaction can be classified as normal, intensified or reduced. The neural chain of this reflex involves the lumbar segments L_5–S_2.

This reflex is attenuated in cases of cerebral palsy and more frequently due to lesions of the lumbar spinal cord, e.g. in babies born in the breech position.

Walking automatism

The reflex chain of this test runs along the spinal segments; in spasticity and after trauma to the lumbar spinal cord this reflex is diminished. In cases of athetosis, this automatism persists after the third month.

The tonic neck reflex

The elucidation of this reflex peaks between the second and third months, but it can be found earlier. If it persists after the third month, this is considered to be a sign of a central lesion, and certainly if present after the sixth month. We see this reflex in children with KISS aged 6 months and older without any other signs of a central lesion and the pathological pattern subsides after manual therapy of the suboccipital structures.

Vojta's reactions

These standardized tests (Vojta 1988) are a handy screening tool when examining the state of the sensorimotor system during the first year. Our impression is that we have to re-evaluate the significance of these tests according to the influence of the suboccipital structures on the smooth functioning of the motor patterns involved. To illustrate these considerations we shall focus on the first four tests.

Traction reaction

This test figures centrally in our examination of small children. The traction reaction yields a lot of information about the degree of coordination in the dorsal position. Especially interesting are the posture of the head and the legs and the relative movements of shoulder and pelvis.

Any analysis of the functioning of the muscles supporting the head can at the most be summary.

KISS I children often show an asymmetric posture of the head (Fig. 9.5), less frequently a weakness of these muscles. KISS II children show a characteristic reaction pattern. Recognizing this pattern can make it easier to find a functional disorder of the OC junction even when other signs are less clearly discernible.

The anteflexion of the head proceeds in two phases. Initially the nodding movement is initiated by the activation of the short flexors of the neck. This movement takes place exclusively in the upper cervical spine (i.e. C_0/C_2) without any involvement of the rest of the cervical spine, which becomes activated in the second phase of the anteflexion. Now the long flexors and the entire cervical column (i.e. to T_3) take part in the movement. These muscles are innervated by the spinal nerves caudal to C_3. The short flexors are innervated via nerves originating in the craniocervical junction, which renders them irritable by disturbances of the functional equilibrium of this level. This irritability is twofold, as it can be caused directly by mechanical irritation of the local nerve fibers and via the spinal/pontal processing of faulty input from this region, a phenomenon we could validate experimentally (Vasilyeva et al 2001). This makes it especially important to examine the two phases of head anteflexion separately.

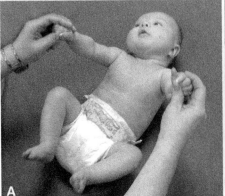 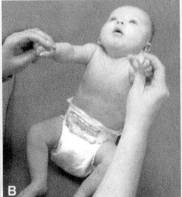 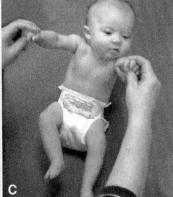

Figure 9.5 Traction reaction. This child has a marked weakness in supporting its head in the first phase (A) pulling the chin to the chest. Afterwards the head is thrown back (B) and pulled forward asymmetrically (C). Differential diagnosis with a central tonus disorder: the muscular tonus of the rump is normal, only the short flexors of the neck are weakened. Together with the asymmetry of the head posture in C, this is typical for KISS.

For this differentiated examination we use Janda's method (Janda 1983), which we modified slightly for the examination of small children:

To examine the function of the short flexors of the neck the child is put on its back and a bright toy is held in front in such a way as to attract the child's attention. After the child has fixed the toy with its eyes we move it cranially in order to force the child's neck into a retroflexion. Only then is the toy moved caudally; the child will react to that by activating the short flexors (nodding) and later on by using the entire neck muscles to bend the head forward in order to follow the moving toy with its eyes.

Babies with a fixed retroflexion cannot nod. In the first phase of the anteflexion the head is instead hyperextended or not included in the movement at all. We call this a dove's move (Vasilyeva et al 2001). In the second phase the child catches up and in using the long flexors the head is indeed brought up.

If the baby has a unilateral blockage of an IS joint we observe an asymmetry of the bending phase of the legs or an asymmetry of the rotation of the legs. This movement pattern has to be distinguished from the early signs of a cerebral palsy. The latter shows a fixed extension of the leg in inner rotation of the leg at the affected side. Here the leg is held in an extended posture with predominance of the triceps surae muscle, and scissoring of the legs and toe stance. Sometimes a similar picture can be observed in children with a bilateral blockage of the IS joints. In these cases the fixation of such a posture diminishes soon after the successful manipulation.

Landau reaction

We look at the posture of the spine as a whole together with the positioning of head and extremities. In cases of KISS I the asymmetry of the neck and skull is immediately distinguishable. A hypotonia of the trunk is rather rare in these cases.

KISS II children show a typical position, too. The shoulders are retracted and the edges of the shoulder blades approach each other, the head is hyperextended and the cervical and dorsal spine are in hyperlordosis. The head founders after a few minutes toward the support. The dystonia between the attenuated flexors and the hyperactive extensors which we found in KISS II children (Vasilyeva et al 2001) helps to explain this pattern.

Axillary suspension response

The child is held in a vertical position with its back to the examiner. To get reliable results one has to take care to hold the trunk without irritation of the trapezius muscle (this would provoke an extension of the lower limbs).

A blockage of the IS joint results in an increased or diminished flexion of the relevant leg, depending on the relative position of the sacrum and ilium. Fixed extension of the legs with scissoring and toe stance are certain signs of a spastic lesion.

Vojta reaction (lateral tilt maneuver) (see Fig. 9.1B)

The child is initially held in a vertical position from which it is tilted laterally into a horizontal position. Care should be taken to have the child's hands open when starting the tilt, as closed hands, especially in early infancy, might provoke an artificially abnormal flexed posture of the arm.

In examining the reaction of the child we have to pay attention to the upper half of the body, i.e. the posture of the trunk and head and the upper two extremities. KISS I children have an asymmetrical posture of head and body. The positioning of the head is markedly clumsy on the side of the dysfunction, the hand often in a fisted position on the opposite side. The posture of the legs is mostly asymmetrical, too.

KISS alone does not lead to adduction of the legs or forced extension of the feet. If these signs are present, an at least partially central genesis of the problem is very likely.

Children with a KISS II symptomatology may show a Moro-like reaction after the age of 5 months. Hyperextension of the head, retraction of the shoulders and a (reactive) hypotonia of the trunk are part of this clinical picture, too.

THE DIFFERENTIAL DIAGNOSIS: FUNCTIONAL VERTEBROGENIC VERSUS CENTRAL/SPINAL

Having completed the whole neuropediatric examination, we have the necessary means at our disposal to reach a conclusion as to how many symptoms are caused by a functional vertebrogenic problem (i.e. a KISS sensu stricto), by a more centrally situated disorder or by a traumatic lesion of a region of the spinal cord. It should not be forgotten that this differential diagnosis, necessary as it may be for our assessment of the long-term prognosis of that child, does not alter the actual therapy too much. The combination of rehabilitative measures is more determined by the response of the young patient to the different therapeutic approaches than by the eventual diagnosis.

The one paramount conundrum of neuropediatrics lies in the fact that an exquisite arsenal of diagnostic tools – even correctly used – leads more often than not to roughly the same therapeutic protocols. Ultimately the outcome depends more on the initiative and personality of the individual therapist and the supportive environment at home than on the fine print of this diagnosis.

This is by no means a request to drop diagnostics and fall back on a purely pragmatic 'how-to' approach to rehabilitation – far from it. But one should keep in mind that the eventual result of all these therapeutic efforts cannot be predicted with any precision.

This caveat should be kept in mind when one gives a long-term prognosis to the parents, who do naturally enough insist on it. The justified request of 'tell us everything' has to elicit a balanced response which avoids the pitfalls of drawing too dark a picture or seeking refuge in an all too rosy future. The former extreme is more comfortable for the doctor involved, as it is always possible then to say 'I told you so' – but there is a high probability that this pessimistic picture discourages and demotivates family and caregivers, thus weakening the support our young patients need so urgently. If we are too optimistic, on the other hand, we are in danger of losing the confidence of the parents and with it any influence and compliance.

A central coordination disturbance in combination with functional vertebrogenic disorders is probable if the following dysfunctions are observed (see also Table 9.1):

Table 9.1 Differential diagnosis

Clinical symptomatology	1	2	3
Asymmetry of movements	+	+	+
Dysfunctioning of cranial nerves	−	+	−
Muscular hypotonia	−	+	+
Increased muscular tonus or asymmetry	−	+	+
Asymmetry of myotatic reflexes	−	+	+
Persistence of Babinski and Rossolimo/Starling sign	−	+	+
Asymmetry of primitive reflexes	+	+	+
Persistence of primitive reflexes	[a]	+	±
Vojta tests: asymmetry		[c]	[c]
In execution	[b]	+[b]	+[b]

1, KISS without neurological co-symptoms.
2, Combination of KISS and a central coordination disorder.
3, KISS combined with a cervical/spinal irritation.
[a] Besides Moro sign and ATNR.
[b] 'Functional' pattern.
[c] 'Central' (i.e. spastic) or hypotonic pattern.

- dysfunctions of cranial nerves
- missing early childhood reflexes or their persistence (with the exception of the Moro reaction, the asymmetric tonic neck reflex (ATNR) in KISS II children)
- seizures of all types
- central muscular hypotonia
- retardation of psychological development
- retardation of language acquisition
- central disturbances of movement, e.g. spinal palsy or disorders of the pyramidal tracts
- dyskinesia and extrapyramidal and/or cerebellar motion disorders.

In our daily contact with these children we became aware of the fact that a spastic dystonia is in many cases accompanied by a functional problem of the OC junction on the side of the hemiplegia. In cases of tetraplegia the blockage of the OC junction is mostly found on the side of the more pronounced symptoms. Due to this combination it can be difficult to distinguish between a mostly functional vertebrogenic problem and an athetotic/-dyskinetic disorder. Of course, children with a central disorder can have problems of this kind at the same time. From the viewpoint of manual therapy it seems to be practical to check if there is a functional problem with a vertebrogenic origin, as this can be dealt with much more easily.

These vertebrogenic components of the clinical picture are peripheral to the main problem, but in the context of a centrally triggered disorder, these functional problems gain a disproportionate impact on the clinical situation. The role of manual therapy in these cases is not central – physiotherapy and training have a more important role. But manual therapy offers an uncomplicated adjuvant therapy which in some cases is prerequisite to a successful rehabilitation effort using physiotherapeutic techniques.

In many cases we found a combination of functional vertebrogenic disorders with an irritation of the spinal cord. Taking into account the anatomical situation and the close proximity and interdependence of these structures, it seems plausible

that a trauma of the spinal cord during delivery results in a rather variable clinical picture.

On the cervical level the situation resembles closely that of cerebral palsy. A close examination of the delivery history (forceps, vacuum extractor, breech presentation) and the presence of other signs of cervical irritation may help to clarify the predominant cause of the problems observed.

Signs of an irritation of the cervical part of the sympathetic nerve can be present, too. This group of symptoms comprises unilateral enophthalmia, microsomia and flattening of the occipital part of the skull.

In most cases of KISS I we find an irritation of the cervical autonomous system on the contralateral side of the functional impairment. In cases of KISS II this observation is very rare. To this day we do not have the corresponding scientific investigations at our disposal, but some interesting details are starting to emerge. In papers on sudden infant death syndrome (SIDS), Doppler sonographic research showed that rotation and reclination of the head often leads to a decreased perfusion of the contralateral vertebral artery; this might be a starting point for further research (Saternus 1982).

Traumatic lesions of the lower cervical segments (C_5/C_7) show another clinical picture. If it is only the motor neurons in the anterior horn that are involved, the child shows a peripheral mono- or paraparesis of the arm(s). The differential diagnosis of a plexus lesion, Erb–Duchenne, needs to be excluded in these cases. If further neurological examination reveals signs of spastic symptoms, the diagnosis of a medullar base of the ensuing problems is facilitated. Our experience with these cases indicates that vertebrogenic functional disorders and the mechanical irritation of the spinal cord are etio-pathogenetically intertwined, which is why manual therapy is the most comprehensive approach in these cases.

Most of the symptoms are greatly alleviated 2–3 weeks after treatment. As this therapy does not demand a lot of effort or cooperation from children and parents, we recommend starting with a test manipulation as soon as acute destructive processes or tumors have been excluded. Minimizing the influence of functional vertebrogenic problems clarifies the clinical picture and helps to optimize the rehabilitation, at least in part because of the encouragement the improved situation conveys to the parents and therapists.

Injuries of the thoracic medulla are very rare at birth. The defects are more often situated more caudally, i.e. at the lumbar level and here involving the pyramidal tracts. This leads to a spastic paresis of one or both legs. Other probable causes (spinal stenosis, tumors or an isolated para-sagittal cerebral trauma) are much less frequently found.

The more massive traumas of the lumbar spinal cord are quite as rare as those of the thoracic level. These children display a mono- or diparesis of the legs. In most cases, a typical anamnesis can be found with breech (pelvic) presentation and a difficult and/or forced delivery.

In both cases, these primarily central neurological lesions are accompanied by blockages of the OC and IS joints. These functional disorders are not at the root of the clinical problem, but aggravate the situation further. Their treatment can facilitate the 'classic' rehabilitation and has to be repeated regularly (i.e. 3–4 times a year). This accompanying therapy is very motivating for the families and for the physiotherapists, as it makes progress possible which otherwise would be beyond the reach of the therapists.

CONCLUSION: STANDING ON TWO LEGS

We hope to have shown here that the manual therapy approach differs somewhat from that of traditional neurology. In examining newborn babies and toddlers the additional information obtained by looking for signs of birth trauma in the spinal structures opens the view to a wider range of possible pathologies than the 'classic' approach which attributes almost everything to disorders of the intracranial structures.

Manual therapy – applied sparingly – can ease rehabilitation and thus motivate everybody involved in this long-term endeavor. It is quite common to find a clearer clinical picture after the functional problems of vertebrogenic origin have been taken care of – at least temporarily.

If the neurological component of the problem at hand is dominant we have to surmise that the treatment has to be repeated. In our experience it suffices to do that 2–3 times a year, at least in the continental European context of a close-knit collaboration between manual therapy, physiotherapy and rehabilitation (e.g. logopedics, remedial education).

Adding this new dimension to the therapeutic arsenal improves the future prospects of our young patients without imposing too much effort on them – and in many cases we can provide the little step forward that was missing.

References

Ayres A J 1979 Sensory integration and the child. Western Psychological Services, Los Angeles

Birrer R B, Levine R 1987 Performance parameters in children and adolescent athletes. Sports Medicine 4(3):211–227

Dubowitz L, Dubowitz V, Mercuri E 1999 The neurological assessment of the preterm and full-term newborn infant. Clinics in Developmental Medicine 148:1–155

Fenichel G 2001 Clinical pediatric neurology. Saunders, Philadelphia

Goddard Blythe S, Hyland D 1998 Screening for neurological dysfunction in the specific learning difficulty child. Journal of Occupational Therapy 61(10):459–464

Janda V 1983 On the concept of postural muscles and posture. Australian Journal of Physiotherapy 29:83

Loovis E M, Butterfield S A 1993 Influence of age, sex, balance, and sport participation on development of catching by children grades K-8. Perceptual and Motor Skills 77(Pt 2):1267–1273

Patel D R, Pratt H D, Greydanus D E 2002 Pediatric neurodevelopment and sports participation. When are children ready to play sports? Pediatric Clinics of North America 49:505–531

Ratner A, Bondarchuk S V 1990 [Neurologic evaluation of unconditioned reflexes in the newborn]. Pediatriia 4:38–41

Ratner A J, Michailov M K 1992 Klinisch-röntgenologische Befunde bei geburtstraumatischen Verletzungen der Halswirbelsäule. Kinderarzt 23:811–822

Saternus K-S 1982 Lageabhängige zirkulationsbedingte cerebrale Hypoxämie – eine Erklärungsmöglichkeit des plötzlichen Kindstodes. Zentralblatt Rechsmedizin 24:635

Swaiman K 1994 Pediatric neurology. Mosby, St Louis

Vasilyeva L F, Ilewa S, Biedermann H 2001 EMG – Veränderungen bei der Manualtherapie von Kleinkindern. Manuelle Therapie 5:122–126

Vojta V 1988 Der zerebralen Bewegungsstörungen im Säuglingsalter. Enke, Stuttgart

Vojta V, Peters A 1992 Das Vojta-Prinzip. Springer, Berlin

Chapter 10

Manual therapy from a pediatrician's viewpoint

H. Kühnen

I work as a pediatrician in a semi-rural area of Germany close to the Dutch border. Our task is the primary provision of pediatric care. This brings a lot of children to our practice whose diverse problems were not easily attributable to our standard classification of pediatric problems. These cases included many children who were classified as 'hyperactive' or 'having problems with their sensory integration'. In quite a few cases, I accompanied these young patients through the years without being really able to offer specific help and the only resort was to send these children to a physiotherapist. It was through this contact that my attention was oriented towards manual therapy as a specific treatment for these problem cases. After some quite impressive improvements achieved by manual therapy (Kühnen 1999) more and more of these schoolchildren were referred to us. I thus had the opportunity to examine the development of children who display symptoms of KISS but had not yet been specifically treated.

In our practice, the sensorimotor development of the children was documented routinely during the first years while performing the regular preventive medical check-ups. These files provided the database for a retrospective evaluation of those cases where we decided to apply manual therapy at a later time. After getting to know more about manual therapy, I noticed astonishing changes with infants in their sensorimotor

Table 10.1 The routine checks on children during their first years

Check-up number	Age at check-up
U1	At birth
U2	3rd to 10th day
U3	4th to 6th week
U4	3rd to 4th month
U5	6th to 7th month
U6	10th to 12th month
U7	21st to 24th month
U8	3 to 4 years
U9	after the 5th birthday

development. Now I was curious to know what had happened to all the children with KISS who had not been treated.

In Germany there are five obligatory preventive medical check-ups during the first year of a child. Another check-up is done at the end of the second year, one during the fourth and one in the fifth year (Table 10.1). I especially focused on schoolchildren who came to see me because of abnormal behavior, problems in school or perception disorders. These children had difficulties in writing and reading, struggled in minute motor activities (fine motor manipulations) and had difficulties in concentrating. Often they were outsiders in school, 'daydreamers', hyperactive and enjoyed neither sports nor playing games. They had difficulties in their social surrounding, struggled with social contacts or they were loners. Often they were only focused on one single friend. Clumsiness and slowness prevail in these cases and the technical term used is dyspraxia.

METHODS

To assess the problem at hand we use a standard procedure which consists of the following items.

Case history of the parents or caregiver

Review of the documentation, which was made during the preventive medical check-ups during the first year of the child, plus additional checks (Vojta Schedule (Vojta and Peters 1992), Muenchener Funktionelle Entwicklungsdiagnostik (Allhoff and Rennen-Allhoff 1984), Denver (VanDevoort and Lee 1984, Fleming 1981), test battery for the diagnosis of minimal cerebral motor disorders (Pediatric Center, Munich)).

Neurological examination

Included are the results of physiotherapy, occupational therapy and orthopedic examination. Also taken into account are the vestibular function, proprioception, tactile perception, coordination and auditory perception.

Clinical examination

Ballgames

Task: catch the ball with both hands and throw it with one hand.
Observation: eye movement, ability to focus on the ball, catching with both hands or with support of the forearms and the whole body, supporting the posture by holding the arms close to the body, crossing the middle-line, ability to stand firm, but at the same time to change positions.

Football

Task: kick the ball with one leg.
Observation: which leg kicks, hemispheric specialization, associated movements, does the child need support, does he have to hold on to something, is he able to deal with a moving ball or does he have to set up the ball in a certain position before kicking it.

Line-walking

Task: first, move one foot after the other forward. Second, walk the same way backward, walk forward again, but without looking down to the line.
Observation: does the child walk with feet pointing inward or outward, oscillation and posture of arms, asymmetry, posture of the spine, shoulders and pelvis (stretch or flex), posture of the head, associated movements.

Shoving on knees

Observation: movement of the pelvis, ability to stretch and flex the pelvis, movement pattern of feet, lifting up of the lower leg, fixed posture of the head, associated movements.

Stamping

Observation: asymmetries, especially with eyes closed, posture of spine and shoulders.

Alternation of the weight load on both buttocks

Task: while kneeling, move the bottom alternately to the right and to the left.
Observation: flexibility of the pelvis, posture of the body, the feet and lower legs, heel.

Diadochokinesia exercise

Task: circle with the hand around your wrist. This movement is supposed to be quick and easy and shows the ability alternately to supinate and pronate.
Observation: isolated movements of the wrist, without engaging the rest of the arm, position of the arm, posture of the head and associated movements.

Thumb–finger-test

Task: press your thumb against each finger of the same hand, backwards and forwards, with and without eye contact; movements should be done one after another.
Observation: reliability of thumb–finger opposition, progression, posture of fingers.

Standing on one leg

Task: stand on one leg for as long as possible. Then do the same thing with outstretched hands and finally with closed eyes. A 4-year-old should be able to stand on one leg for at least 10 seconds.
Observation: asymmetries, constant asymmetrical bent of the body to one side, regardless of the leg engaged, synkinetic movements, e.g. closed hands or hands in palmar flexion with extended fingers, athetoid movements, posture of the uncharged leg, ability to hold the balance, preference of one leg.

Jumping on one leg

Observation: jumping on one leg, on the same spot (for small children) and for children 4 years and older we look at jumping on one leg backwards and forwards.

We look at the way of jumping and of charging the foot. Does the child jump with a flat foot or does he bounce or walk on tiptoes; associated movements, such as posture of head and shoulders, integrating the hand and showing a mimical reaction, on one or both sides.

Tiptoeing

Observation: posture of the upper part of the body, tension of shoulders, lifting of shoulders unilaterally or on both sides, posture of the head, associated movements of hands and fingers.

Heel-walk

Observation: narrow or wide based, tension of legs, posture of pelvis and body, moving the mouth, opening the mouth, tongue showing, posture of arms and hands, associated movements.

Jumping jack

Task: stretching the arms while straddle jumping and bringing the arms back in again while jumping.
Observation: posture of knees, head, coordination.

Oscillation

Task: march, goose-stepping.
Observation: movements of the arms, either reciprocal or homonymous hand at the same time moving ahead of the leg.

Movements with both hands

Task: sweep with one hand and tap with the other hand.
Observation: is the child able to do different movements at the same time, nuances of muscular tension, nuances of the movement.

Standing

Task: stand up straight, with hand stretched out in front.
Observation: posture of body, shoulders, head, asymmetries in posture and/or forward tilt of pelvis, kyphosis, lordosis, side-bending of the spine, constant asymmetries, posture of feet, toes and knees.

Bowing

Task: bend body forward with stretched knees.
Observation: side-bend of the spine, distance between fingertips and surface, development of spine, pain when the spine is tapped.

Romberg test

Task: stretching out forward, hand and arms in supine position, with eyes closed and eyes open.

Then still standing, turn head to the right and to the left, backwards and forwards.
Observation: asymmetries, does the head stay on a middle-line while moving forwards and backwards, do the hands stay in the same position while the head is moving.

The next test battery is done on the examination table.

Sitting upright

Task: sitting on a bench with legs stretched out.
Observation: posture of body, legs and feet, is the child able to sit up straight alone, does he integrate shoulder movements, lifting up of shoulders, asymmetries, do legs and knees stay stretched, abduction and bending of knee joints, plantarflexion of feet, differences in effective length of legs.

Supine

Observation: asymmetries in posture of head, lordosis in the lumbar part of spine, difference in effective length of legs.

Lasègue

Task: the examiner lifts up the stretched leg in supine.
Observation: bending of knee joint to 90 degrees, rotation of leg, asymmetries.

Suboccipital trigger points

Singly or bilaterally hyperesthetic evaluation of the pain threshold in the craniocervical area.

Sitting with dangling legs

Observation: posture of body and head, asymmetries, weight carried on both buttocks.

Flexibility of the tongue

Observation: reaction of the pupils, nystagmus, esotropia, eye movement while head moving around, associated movements, integrated movements in mouth area, lower jaw and tongue movements.

Yawning

Symmetry of teeth, overbite, open bite, crossbite, prognathia, progenia, difficulty swallowing.

Testing of auditory abilities

- Clapping: two beats, three beats, syncopes, longer sequences.
- Nonsense verses: repeat for example, 'sim salabim bamba saladu'.
- Numbers: repeat: up to five numbers.

These tests are the standard procedure for almost all children and their documentation allows us to compare the development of these children in comparison with others of their age group, but also their individual development without manual therapy and later on when manual therapy was applied.

Some of these children are presented in the following case histories.

By giving the following examples we would like to demonstrate the connection between the observations of development during the infant years and sensorimotor problems at school age.

There is no such thing as a definitive test which gives a clear-cut decision as to where to apply manual therapy and where not. Several factors influence this decision, and these items have to be seen and evaluated together. Three 'markers' stand out in this context:

- problems during labor
- non-standard development during the first year, especially skipping of the crawling phase

- signs of problems with the sensorimotor system, most often with a distinct 'sidedness'.

In our experience it is often worthwhile to test the effect of manual therapy, even more so as the outcome can be evaluated after one, or at the most two treatments. We tried for years to develop a score in order to have a simple tool for the evaluation of candidates for manual therapy, but in real life this does not work and the decision has do be done on a case-by-case basis.

Case studies

Maik (age 8 years, 5 months)
The pregnancy was without pathological findings; the presentation was cephalic, right hand coming first; there was extensive episiotomy because of narrowness of the birth channel.

Maik was very anxious as an infant, always kept close to his mother and was often ill with infections of the upper respiratory tract.

Clinical findings: the traction reaction test showed delayed head control. At the age of 6 weeks the Landau reaction was still completely hypotonic. There were slight signs of a hemiplegia on the right side, the Vojta reaction on the right side was retarded, and there was retraction of the shoulders during the Landau test. He often cried during examinations in the consulting room. Maik liked crawling and started to walk after 14 months.

At the age of 4–5 the notes of the preventive medical check-up (U8 and U9) included the following entries: Maik showed conspicuous deficits in sensory integration and had problems with his proprioception and balance. Nonetheless, he did not have any problems getting good grades in school, but he did struggle on the social interaction level. Because of his weak body posture, physiotherapy was prescribed (which he did not like at all). He even refused to swim.

Examination at the age of 8: limited ability to turn head to the left, limited head anteflexion, hypotonia of the abdominal muscles.

Line-walking: his legs were rotating outwards, without looking at the line, he made big steps with supporting steps in between, very unsteadily. Standing on one leg was better on the right leg than on the left. With closed eyes he nearly stumbled. Examined in standing position, the thoracic area of the spine displayed a left bend with counterswing at the lumbar level. Suboccipital pain points on both sides.

Because of his clumsiness and postural problems he was sent for examination (and treatment) by a specialist in manual therapy.

Three weeks after his treatment we examined him again. Maik was much more relaxed and more easygoing with his family and in school. He was less aggressive. His mother was delighted that it was possible for her to hug her son for the first time.

Maik's movement patterns were much smoother, his energy is much more focused now and he has got himself much better under control. He stops now as soon as he gets tired and he is able to walk along the line without looking at it. Although standing on one leg is still better on the right leg than on the left, his overall performance improved markedly. He still has a slight asymmetry and a weak posture.

Conclusion: Maik's problem was his asymmetry *and* his weak posture.

Florian (age 6 years, 4 months)

The pregnancy was without pathological findings; face presentation. The delivery was very quick, so that the father nearly missed the birth. Afterwards Florian suffered from colic with lots of vomiting, regular respiratory infections with asthmatic bronchitis, eczema, sleep disorders with trouble falling asleep.

At the age of 6 weeks, there was retarded head control on the traction reaction test, and retraction of the shoulders on the Landau test. At the age of 18 weeks, there was orofacial hypotonia on the traction test and fisting on the Vojta test. The collis horizontalis test (to assess the reaction of the trunk and extremities when the infant is lifted) showed a slight lateralization to the left. Later on he did not crawl much, but started walking at the age of 1 year.

Shortly after his fourth birthday (U8): weak balance and problems with kinesthesia. He could only stand on one leg if he was holding onto something. He was just able to jump on one leg one or two times and fell over doing the jumping jack test. Walking along the line backwards was only possible for him by looking at the line.

At that age we prescribed psychomotor therapy.

A good year later he came for the next routine check-up (U9): His general posture was hypotonic and he had problems balancing.

At the age of 6, he could not walk along the line without problems, legs were pointing inward. He had to 'feel' his way, especially with the left foot. Standing on one leg was better on the right, as was jumping on one leg. He walked very clumsily, with a slapping movement of his feet. In standing, his spine showed a left-side deviation in the thoracic region. He had difficulties sitting with his legs straight. In a sitting position he had a pronounced thoracic kyphosis. If asked to sit straight, his legs were rotated inwards. Hypotony of the abdominal muscles.

Changes after therapy: Florian now plays more independently, he has much more patience with his Lego. His hoarseness after kindergarten disappeared and he can control his articulation better. Before he needed to build up his muscular tonus by shouting; obviously he does not need this any more.

Jonas (age 7 years, 1 month)

Jonas was a 'restless baby' during pregnancy so that his mother could hardly sleep at night. The delivery took a long time. Weight after birth was 4260 grams, height was 59 cm and his head circumference was 37 cm.

Jonas was already lifting up his shoulders while in the incubator and he did not like to be touched. During his infant years he cried a lot, hardly moved and drank very hastily. He had to be carried around a lot and the stroller had to be rocked almost constantly. Jonas was very demanding on his mother and the rest of the family. His sister frankly said one time it would be best to give him back.

At the routine check at the age of 6 months he showed several signs of clumsiness, e.g. on the Vojta test and the axillary suspension. His period of crawling was very short, and he started walking at 9½ months.

At the age of 2 years his behavior was difficult and often very aggressive; he often tumbled. He shouted frequently and had a very loud voice.

At 3 years, he was still walking clumsily with a very stamping gait and a lot of associated movements. He was very attached to his mother. In addition, he kept throwing himself on the ground in fits of tantrum. At that age we started out with sensory integration therapy, which could not be continued because of his mother's new pregnancy.

A few months later at the routine check (U8): while line-walking, his legs pointed inwards. He did not like walking backwards. When asked to sit with his legs in front of him, he was not able to sit straight. While jumping on one leg, he pulled his knee up very high. He had many proprioception difficulties. Even though he started physiotherapy before going to primary school he still had these difficulties, especially with memorizing certain activity patterns.

Starting at primary school was a stressful time. Intellectually, Jonas was absolutely ready to enter school, but his sensory integration was not up to the exertions of school. Nonetheless, he got through the first year of school, but only with hard work. He was very aggressive during that time at home. He was sad about himself, cried a lot and also complained about his dyspraxia.

Examination at the age of 7: He could not talk and play with the ball at the same time. His way of doing the jumping jack was very uncoordinated. Walking along the line, his right shoulder was pointing forward. He could only do it by looking at the line and only very fast. He stopped walking as soon as he hit something. While standing on one leg, he lifted the other out to the back, as though imitating an airplane.

The manual therapy started a few months later (two sessions). The changes in Jonas' behavior were very impressive: he was now able to do two things at the same time. His movements became quicker and more fluent. He acted more spontaneously. His dyspraxia improved and he was able to concentrate much longer. He has his hair longer now and does not wear only black clothes anymore. At the school's sports meeting, he was the best of his school in long jump. And now he even thinks about joining the soccer team.

Check-up 4 months later: standing on one leg is absolutely fine and so is the jumping jack. He is able to cross in the midline, his level of sensory integration is completely age-appropriate now. The coordination of his movements is very good.

He does not need any additional information anymore, like for example visual clues, higher muscular tonus or other additional stimuli. A slightly higher muscular tonus on the left side has persisted.

Especially surprising is the success of the therapy regarding general behavior and complex movement patterns. These improvements were not achieved with any other form of therapy.

Simon (age 15 years, 6 months)

Pregnancy and delivery were without pathological findings, apart from the mother having insomnia during the pregnancy. Up to the fifth month, Simon did not move or turn around and he was very weak. In the traction reaction test the head control lagged behind; in the Landau maneuver he did not straighten up completely.

During his sixth month his development speeded up and he started to show signs of verticalization. He started crawling at 8 months, and also started pulling himself up until he was able to stand up and slowly started walking, but always had to hold onto something. At 10 months he was able to walk independently. No asymmetries noticed.

At the U8 check-up, there were anomalies in doing the diadochokinesia exercises and with standing on one leg. His anxious and jealous behavior was described as rather cute during his infant years and it was tolerated while he was in kindergarten. In school, Simon became an outsider, was very lonely due to his hyperkinetic behavior. He had no friends and was very aggressive; he even hurt himself.

He had a very bad reputation in school, the teachers gave up on him and threatened to expel him from school. Simon started psychotherapy, remedial education, and the family tried methylphenidate medication in combination with occupational therapy over many years.

At the age of 15, Simon had an excessive thoracal kyphosis when sitting with outstretched legs, a misaligned spine and could not cross the middle line in his movements. On examination a marked hyperesthesia on the suboccipital points came to attention.

His situation escalated when his half-brother committed suicide. Because Simon was in an identity crisis and he was suicidal, too, the parents planned to send him to a psychiatric hospital.

Coincidentally, it was possible to apply manual therapy just before his hospitalization, which had to be scheduled a long time in advance. After one manual treatment his behavior changed completely. He became much more talkative and easygoing. At home as well as in school, he became much more stable. He also now avoids contact with drug addicts. This was a tremendous change, not only for Simon, but also for his parents, who were quite skeptical of the manual therapy at first.

It was the combination of his hyperactivity and the persistently conspicuous findings during the routine check-ups which induced us to propose this last-minute attempt.

Elisabeth (age 9 years, 4 months)

Elisabeth is the fifth child in her family. The pregnancy was quite complicated, because of premature labor, pelvic presentation with rotation immediately prior to delivery. Weight after birth was 3200 grams, height was 51 cm and head circumference 34 cm.

At the age of 6 weeks, respiratory infection with obstructive bronchitis began. At 9½ weeks, a near SID (sudden infant death): weak, cyanotic whining while lying in face-down position in the stroller, apparently found just in time.

Elisabeth cried a lot as an infant. Her muscular tonus was low and there were signs of a hemiparesis on the right side. She was prone to tantrums, did not like to get dressed, but she liked to be touched.

At the age of 2, Elisabeth was still very anxious, her language development was retarded, especially compared to other aspects of her development. Considering her personality as a whole, Elisabeth seemed to be quite clever, even though she did not achieve 'good' scores in some of the tests.

At 4 years, she only played by imitating others and was not very creative or very sensitive. She was scared of everything new, everything needed to be explained to her. She had weak posture, she stood knock-kneed and with a hollow back. There was a conspicuous Romberg reaction as she moved her arms when turning her trunk. She needed a lot of visual control and encouragement from her mother.

I examined Elisabeth again when she was in the third grade of primary school. She had above all problems with logical thinking. She was amazed by things which she should have known already. So she was very inflexible, rigid, with a very constricted train of thoughts. She had insomnia (especially difficulties falling asleep) and hardly ever slept through the night. She was very unbalanced in her eating habits and there were a lot of tensions during meals. Elisabeth had problems sharing things with others and mostly kept the bigger part for herself. At 8³/4 she still needed a lot of motivation from her mother.

Her posture was still marked by an excessive lumbar lordosis; balancing on one leg was much easier on the right than on the left leg, as was jumping on one leg. When doing the diadochokinesia exercises, she moved her other hand as well. There was hypotony of the abdominal muscles. While sitting with straight legs, her back was bent in a dorsal right-shift of the spine, and there were pronounced trigger points suboccipitally.

Because of the difficulties in school there had already been a psychological examination. Both of Elisabeth's parents were very skeptical about manual therapy, but as a last resort they agreed to it.

After the manual therapy (two sessions) they were very surprised how much Elisabeth's behavior had changed and how fast her attitudes matured. Her mother described the changes as Elisabeth being much more awake and open than before. Even her teacher at school noticed the differences.

At the neurological check-up, Elisabeth still had a slight difference of the muscular tonus and an asymmetry in her posture, but her improvement continued. She graduated successfully from secondary school without further intervention.

Conclusion: all the symptoms, such as the asymmetry of posture, the restlessness, the details of the case history (near SIDS) and the weakness in her posture, were symptoms of a functional vertebrogenic disorder – and the impact of the manual therapy astonished everyone.

Kathrin (age 11 years, 8 months)

Kathrin was the first child; her mother was early in labor and had to stay in bed to avoid premature labor. Towards the end of the pregnancy the pelvic presentation turned into a face presentation. The delivery took 5 hours; during the extrusion phase the mother had two to four travails. Weight at birth was 3600 grams, her length was 53 cm and head circumference 33 cm.

Kathrin was a very calm baby, and she slept a lot. At 3 months, a tendency for fisting was noticed. On her baby pictures, Kathrin's head always tended to lean to the left, she had very big, open eyes and enjoyed sitting up.

In kindergarten (5 years) she integrated a lot of mimic movements into her regular movements. Nonetheless, she had difficulties in understanding certain words and had a deficit in visual awareness, especially in three-dimensional perspectives.

Even though she got enrolled in primary school a year later than usual, she still struggled. Her story-telling was sometimes incomplete, and she was not very flexible. She had very low self-esteem.

At the neurological check-up at the age of 10, Kathrin had asymmetry with left-side deviation of the spine. She also had hypersensitivity to midline percussion over the thoracic spine and at the suboccipital trigger points. While walking along the line, she dropped her left shoulder. Standing on one leg was better on her right leg than on the left; jumping on one leg was still very clumsy. She could only do the jumping jack after practising it a few times and even then she did it very slowly and stiffly, with her mouth open. The thumb–finger test on her left side was very weak.

She started with the manual therapy at almost 12 years of age. Within 4 weeks, she had changed completely. All of a sudden she was able to get up early in the morning. She had more self-esteem. Her writing was much better, she was not frightened of exams any more, and her grades got better. These improvements lasted without further therapy.

Sarah (age 6 years, 11 months)

Sarah was the first child and the pregnancy was inconspicuous. As the mother had an asymmetrical pelvis as a consequence of a car accident, a cesarean section was planned even though the child was in a normal position.

After birth she cried a lot and had to be carried around in a vertical position to soothe her, which was so time-intensive that the parents took shifts. The diagnosis of a pes equinovarus led to the prescription of physiotherapy at the age of 5 months. She was a very mobile child with a strong tendency to verticalize. She crawled for only a very short time and started walking at the age of 11 months.

From the beginning, Sarah had problems with falling asleep which led to the establishment of elaborate 'sleep-rituals'; her linguistic development was rather delayed – 'she took her time'. As a whole she appeared to be a bit behind in her general development, active, but cautious and guarded.

In kindergarten she had many friends and was very popular.

At the age of 5 another series of physiotherapy exercises was prescribed as her motor patterns still seemed to be a bit lateralized. In general her motor development was described as clumsy, with a lot of falling and stumbling.

In primary school she tired quickly during lessons, and after the third lesson she was hardly able to concentrate. Sarah had problems splitting her attention between two things. At the beginning she wrote in mirror image, then from left to right, letters as much as digits; initially she had problems in dealing with numbers up to 20.

At that point in time she was sent to a specialist in manual therapy. The radiograph showed a bifid arch of C_1 and the functional examination a blockage at the level C_1/C_2. The ensuing manual therapy was administered even more carefully than usual.

A follow-up 1 year later showed a markedly improved situation with no signs of postural asymmetry. The situation in school was much more relaxed and her mathematical capabilities improved. Homework, before a big stress, was done well and without complaints.

A year later she fell from her double-decker bed and hurt her neck. A short time later she complained of headaches and a neurological and ophthalmological examination was sought which produced no pathological findings (EEG, CT, etc.). No further treatment ensued.

A few months later she came back to see me because of the restlessness in her legs. She could not find sleep anymore and complained of dysesthesia in her elbow and knees. Her father had a history of restless leg complaints.

The examination showed a marked hyperlordosis of the lumbar spine, a high muscular tonus of the pelvic area and a blockage of both iliosacral joints. There were no signs of irritation of a segmental nerve but there was bilateral impairment of the Lasègue-sign indicating contraction of the hamstrings. The mother reported that her handwriting had got worse and she had concentration problems in school.

The functional examination of the spine revealed – almost as expected – a blockage of both the iliosacral and occipitocervical junctions. After their removal the headaches subsided and the school situation improved.

STATISTICAL RESULTS

Between 1996 and 1998 we examined 104 schoolchildren. All of them were examined and treated with manual therapy. Out of these 104 children, 69 showed a definite improvement, i.e. no more treatment was necessary and they had a successful school career. They had clearly improved when we examined them again at the neurological check-up.

With 22 of the children we could not do the follow-up examination, because they never got back to us.

Thirteen children did not show any improvements at all.

All the children examined were conspicuous during their infant years: they all had postural asymmetry with either fixed lateralization or retroflexion of the head. We looked for signs and symptoms of functional vertebrogenic disorders in the case histories of these children. This was the main clue for thinking of manual therapy as a possible solution to the children's problems.

The cases presented here are meant to give an idea of which combination of anamnestic and clinical findings are suggestive of functional problems of the vertebral spine as at least a contributing factor in a particular case. In almost every case, these vertebrogenic problems were not the only ones, often not even the most important ones. But their successful treatment gave these children more room to maneuver and thus enabled them to overcome their otherwise insurmountable difficulties. In all these cases, two to three sessions of manual therapy sufficed.

References

Allhoff P, Rennen-Allhoff B 1984 [Problems with developmental diagnostic procedures]. Monatsschrift Kinderheilkunde 132(9):674–679

Fleming J 1981 An evaluation of the use of the Denver Developmental Screening Test. Nursing Research 30(5):290–293

Kühnen H 1999 Erfahrungen mit der Manualmedizin in der neuropädiatrischen Landpraxis. In: Biedermann H (ed) Manualtherapie bei Kindern. Enke, Stuttgart, p 187–198

VanDervoort R L, Lee E B 1984 Use of Denver Developmental Screening Test. Pediatrics 74(3):445–446

Vojta V, Peters A 1992 Das Vojta-Prinzip. Springer, Berlin

Chapter 11

The influence of the high cervical region on the autonomic regulatory system in infants

L. E. Koch

INTRODUCTION

The craniocervical region plays a very important role in human ontogeny, especially in sensorimotor development. Disturbances of this region in infancy are manifold and their influence on the smooth progress of the biomechanical capabilities of the newborn can hardly be overestimated. It reaches far beyond the mobility of head and neck, influencing basic regulatory mechanisms situated in the brainstem (Ramirez 1998).

To distinguish between a purely central (neurological) and primarily peripheral (functional) etiology is difficult. If a peripheral origin of the pathology is established and the appropriate manual therapy is applied to the upper cervical spine, marked vegetative (autonomic) reactions can frequently be observed. Alterations in the heart rate and other vegetative reactions (flush, apnea and sweating) were monitored after the application of a unilateral impulse to the high cervical spinal cord (manual therapy). One of the main benefits of manual therapy in newborn babies is situated precisely at this transition zone between motional and regulatory control. A sound and undisturbed sleep or a baby who does not over-react to any unexpected sensory stimulus after successful treatment – these effects show the impact of a dysfunctional craniocervical junction on the autonomic regulatory system. In many regards, these results of our therapy are more important to the

125

child and parents than an improvement in the range of head mobility.

While treating the babies we encountered sometimes quite intense vegetative reactions following manipulation of the suboccipital structures. Although we never saw any severe side effects while manipulating babies following the guidelines of the European Workgroup for Manual Medicine (more than 20 000 babies treated by our members – Schmitz and Ewers 2002), these reactions aroused our interest and we decided to set up a study.

Using observations from case reports, a systematic study of these effects was designed. This study is based on a survey of 695 infants between the ages of 1 and 12 months. A notable change in the heart rate was evident in 47.2% of all examined infants. In 40.1% of these infants the change in heart rate was characterized by a heart rate decrease of 15–83% compared to control conditions. Infants in their first 3 months of life responded more often with a severe bradycardia (50–83% decrease), older infants (7–12 months) more often with a mild bradycardia (15–49.9% decrease). In 12.1% ($n = 84$) of the infants the bradycardia was accompanied by a temporary apnea.

We know that anatomical and functional mechanisms are involved in the development of disturbed postural and motor patterns and that these mechanisms have a specific component originating from the upper cervical spine. In addition to that we have a non-specific reaction which is characterized as a change in vegetative reaction patterns. The quantity and quality of these reactions are difficult to define, but it seems probable that a mechanical irritation of the upper cervical region serves as a trigger (a long-term potentiation (LTP) (Aroniadou-Anderjaska and Keller 1995) and has great influence on the organization of optimal movement patterns, the development of sensory capabilities and the proper functioning of the autonomic regulatory system.

In this study we examined whether a mechanical irritation of the atlanto-occipital region can cause a bradycardia or other vegetative reactions. A mechanical stimulation of the atlanto-occipital region is *essential* in manual therapy in newborn and the study of its effects on the autonomic system could therefore provide insights into the age-dependence of these processes.

A marked sensitivity of the atlanto-occipital region was first noticed during routine manual therapy of newborn babies. This therapy included an impulse applied to the atlanto-occipital region which was often associated with vegetative responses. Our study included only infants that were diagnosed with asymmetries in the horizontal and sagittal plane of body posture and motion (Biedermann 1991, 1992, 1996, Buchmann et al 1992). The diagnosis and therapy was performed according to the guidelines set by the European Workgroup for Manual Medicine (EWMM) and the German Society for Manual Medicine (DGMM).

PATIENTS AND METHODS

We evaluated the impulse-induced changes in the heart rate, the occurrence of flush and apnea in a group of children ranging from 1 to 12 months of age. The study included only infants with the diagnosis of KISS (365 males and 330 females). The infants examined here were born between the 28th and the 42nd week of pregnancy; 100 were born before the 37th week (premature), 176 were born after the 40th week of pregnancy. The weight at birth ranged from 1.3 to 5.1 kg, and body size from 41 to 57 cm. At the time of therapy the weight ranged from 4.0 to 11.5 kg, and body size from 59 to 80 cm.

All infants showed some kind of deficits in neuromuscular coordination as well as asymmetry such as wryneck and C-scoliosis. Asymmetry in the atlanto-occipital C_0/C_2 region was determined following X-ray examination using the technique described by Gutmann and Biedermann (1984). X-ray analysis revealed a slight predominance of left-sided asymmetry (382 left, 313 right) in the examined infants. Those examined also showed a pathological pattern of neuromuscular development tests (Vojta and Peters 1992). One hundred and twenty infants experienced an intrauterine mal-posture; 305 of the 695 infants had some sort of traumatic birth (vacuum extraction, forceps delivery, Kristeller's maneuver, cesarean section, prolonged labor, etc.); 83 infants suffered from developmental disorders of the hip and feet. Hypertonia of paravertebral back muscles was common (575 of the 695). Infants with neurological disorders were excluded from the study (idiopathic cerebral palsy, floppy babies, vitium cordis, basilar impression, assimilation of atlas, or other anomaly of the spinal column and spinal cord).

The therapeutic impulse used to treat KISS consisted of a short, gentle thrust administered onto the suboccipital region with the inner side of the interphalangeal portion of the second digit. Representative impulses were measured as ranging between 30 and 70 N (Koch and Girnus 1998). It should be noted in this context that so far no serious incidents have been reported (more than 20 000 babies treated by members of the EWMM – Schmitz and Ewers 2002).

For the manual therapy the infants were positioned on their back while the chiropractor was sitting perpendicular to the child's head. Great care was taken that the infant was comfortable before administering the impulse. The child's body was relaxed and any rotation of the spine was avoided. The impulse was applied to the side of the asymmetry.

Characterization of the vegetative responses

In every case, changes in heart rate, blood pressure, frequency of breathing, oxygen saturation and the peripheral temperature were measured using a standard monitor (Datex from Engström Ltd). The frequency of breathing as well as the peripheral temperature were often unreliable because of movement artifacts. Therefore these values were not further evaluated and we concentrated in this study on changes in the heart rate.

The stable frequency at the beginning was defined as 100%. Change in frequency after impulse was measured and set in relation to the frequency at the beginning. Changes of less than 15% were excluded.

Mild bradycardia was defined as a decrease ranging from 15% to 49.9% and severe bradycardia, a decrease of 50.0% upwards. Parallel to these measurements we qualitatively observed also the presence of flush and apnea. A flush was defined as an increased blood flow resulting in an initial facial reddening, which then spread further down to other body parts. A minor and localized reddening of the cheeks was not considered a flush. Usually the flush occurred almost instantaneously following the mechanical impulse. A flush and the crying of the infant was usually associated with the outbreak of sweating. Sweating started in the head and then spread out from there to the rest of the body.

Apnea (temporary respiratory arrest) usually occurred with a delay of several seconds following irritation of the high cervical region. For ethical reasons and because this study was strictly a by-product of chiropratic therapy we did not wait for the spontaneous termination of the apnea. Instead we restored normal breathing immediately after the onset of the apnea by blowing air onto the baby's face. Therefore we defined apnea not as a cessation of breathing lasting for more than 8–10 seconds, but rather as a respiratory arrest that exceeded the duration of one normal breathing cycle (Ramirez 1998).

RESULTS

All infants (1–12 months) that were treated in Eckernförde (Germany) for signs of KISS during the period from September 1998 to April 2000 were included in this study. No attempt was made to obtain an even age distribution for our study. As demonstrated in Figure 11.1A, the distribution has a relatively sharp rise at the second month and starts to diminish after the sixth month, which reflects the age distribution of KISS cases in our consultation and may not be representative of the occurrence of KISS elsewhere. The increased number of younger children in our study suggests that these children suffered more severely from asymmetry-related symptoms. Therefore they were brought more often for treatment compared to their older counterparts. Slightly more girls than boys were treated in the later months (9–12), but otherwise there was no obvious bias in the gender distribution (Fig. 11.1B).

Measurements of the heart rate were successful in all 695 infants. In these children we compared the heart rate before (resting heart rate), during and following the impulse. Normally the bradycardia showed a standard curve: 2–14 seconds after the impulse there was a sharp decrease in heart rate. The bradycardia lasted for 3–10 sec-

onds, in rare cases up to 25 seconds, after which heart rate recovered to the same or higher frequency than the initial heart rate.

In the histogram shown in Figure 11.2 we plotted for all 695 infants the percentage heart rate changes. The changes were not normally distributed. There was a high percentage of children with bradycardia, but there was no obvious population of infants that exhibited a tachycardia. The average heart rate change was −14.1%. An increased heart rate of more than 15% occurred in only 7.3% of the children, whereas 40.1% of the children showed a heart rate decrease of more than 15%.

Figures 11.3A and 11.3B show an example of the bradycardic responses to the manual impulse in one child. The child exhibited severe bradycardia (77.8%) and responded after 7 seconds. This bradycardia was associated with apnea, flush and loss of muscle tone for 6 seconds. The heart rate recovered within 13 seconds.

As a next step we examined whether the occurrence of bradycardia was associated with a particular age. Figures 11.4A, B and C show the age distribution of all children who exhibited a bradycardia (>15% heart rate decrease).

The severity of bradycardia was assessed for different ages by comparing the number of

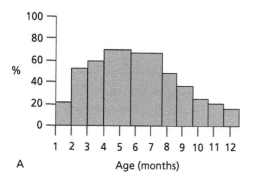

A

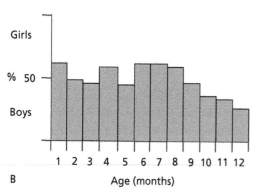

B

Figure 11.1 Age (A) and sex (B) distribution of the infants in the study.

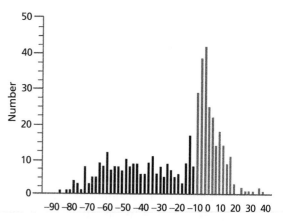

Figure 11.2 Distribution of percentage heart rate changes of the infants in the study.

A

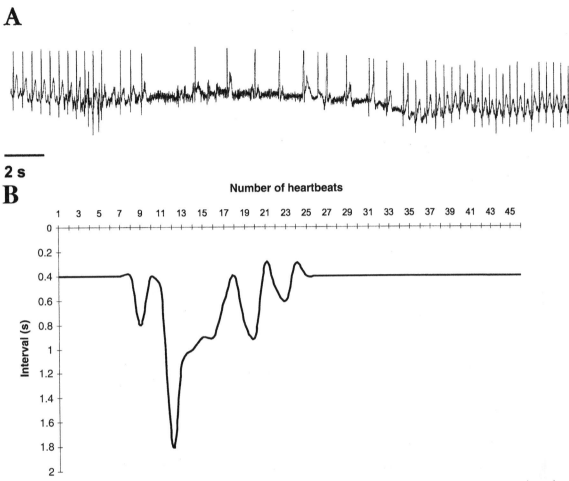

2 s

B

Figure 11.3   Example of a typical bradycardia. A: ECG obtained from a 5-month-old infant born prematurely and delivered by cesarean section. The child had the following clinical symptoms: asymmetry of motion and posture (wryneck to the left, C-scoliosis to the right), hypertension in the back muscles, positive Galant sign on the left side, Peiper–Isbert test positive, incomplete Vojta test to the left side, weak head control, circle-like loss of hair at the back of the cranium. Drinking disturbance, slobbering. Diagnosis was confirmed with an X-ray (anterior-posterior) which showed an offset at the level of C_1/C_2 to the right as referred to the occiput. Frequency before therapy was 150 heartbeats per minute. A moderate impulse was administered contralateral to the offset (in the left direction). During the impulse the infant was lying in a supine position. It responded after 7 seconds with bradycardia (77.8%) which was associated with apnea, flush and loss of tension for 6 seconds. Heart rate recovered to 165 beats per minute. B: The heart rate reaction shown diagramatically.

occurrences of mild versus severe bradycardia in children during their first 3 months ($n = 99$) and in children aged 4–12 months ($n = 180$). This comparison revealed a significantly increased occurrence of severe bradycardia in the younger age group compared to the group of children older than 3 months (chi-squared of 9.87, df = 1 and a significance of 0.0017; the Kendall tau-b

showed 0.196 with a significance of 0.0005; Table 11.1).

The occurrence of a bradycardia was often accompanied by other vegetative responses, such as apnea and flush. It was interesting that a combination of bradycardia, flush and apnea showed an age distribution similar to that seen in sudden infant death syndrome (Fig. 11.4C).

Table 11.1   Statistical data concerning mild/severe bradycardia

Age of patients	Mild	Severe	Total
1–3 months	56	43	99
4–12 months	136	44	180

Chi-squared = 9.87, df = 1, significance = 0.0017.
Kendall tau-b = 0.196, significance = 0.0005.

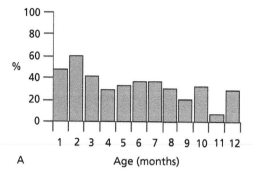

A

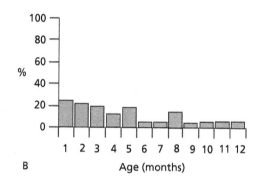

B

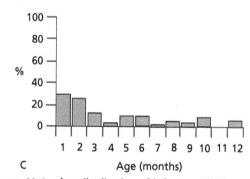

C

Figure 11.4   Age distribution of infants exhibiting bradycardia. A: All bradycardia. B: Severe bradycardia. C: Bradycardia combined with flush and apnea.

DISCUSSION

The mechanical impulse to the suboccipital region led in a significant number of cases to a decrease in the heart rate (40.1%). The distribution (classes: mild/severe) among the young infants (1 to 3 months) differs significantly from that in older infants (4–12 months).

In the young infants the number of cases of severe bradycardia is higher. Most bradycardia led to a fast recovery which was associated with a short period of tachycardia, suggesting that this sequence of events constitutes a normal and physiological response to the mechanical irritation of the suboccipital region.

The observation of this vegetative response leads to an important safety issue. How safe is manual treatment for young infants? The manual therapy has proven to be a successful technique which can be used to treat disorders, especially disturbances of motor patterns of various etiology (wryneck, C-scoliosis, irritation of the plexus brachialis), sensorimotor disturbances of integration ability (retardation of sensation and coordination), as well as pain-related entities such as excessive crying with '3 month colic' or hyperactivity with sleeplessness.

In older children, disturbances of this kind are known as retardation of development in motor patterns as well as in sensory abilities. The epidemiological prevalence of such disturbances has been estimated to be as high as 16.8–17.8% (Boyle et al 1994, Goodman and McGrath 1991). In many cases, manual therapy seems to be the most successful method for treating such disorders. It is therefore increasingly popular as a fast and efficient treatment.

Although retrospective studies about complications in manual therapy are available for adults, no data for children are available. There is a need for empirical analysis and if possible prospective as well as retrospective studies, but one has to add that no serious complications have been reported up to now. Those members of the EWMM specializing in the treatment of babies and infants report about more than 20 000 children treated without serious complications (Schmitz and Ewers 2002). We observed that the younger infants (first to third month) were more likely to respond with a marked bradycardia than the older infants (fourth to twelfth month), who were more likely to exhibit only a mild bradycardia. This finding indicates that an irritation of the cervical region will more likely lead to a severe bradycardia in the first 3 months. All children treated recovered rapidly (<25 seconds) from the bradycardia.

References

Aroniadou-Anderjaska V, Keller A 1995 LTP in the barrel cortex of adult rats. Neuroreport 6:2297–2300

Biedermann H 1991 Kopfgelenk-induzierte Symmetriestörungen bei Kleinkindern. Kinderarzt 22:1475–1482

Biedermann H 1992 Manuelle Therapie bei Kleinkindern. Orthop Praxis 28:380–385

Biedermann H 1996 KISS-Kinder. Enke, Stuttgart

Boyle C A, Decoufle P, Yeargin-Allsopp M 1994 Prevalence and health impact of developmental disabilities in US children. Pediatrics 93(3):399–403

Buchmann J, Bülow B, Pohlmann B 1992 Asymmetrien der Kopfgelenksbeweglichkeit von Kindern. Manuelle Medizin 30:93–95

Goodman J E, McGrath P J 1991 The epidemiology of pain in children and adolescents: a review. Pain 46(3):247–264

Gutmann G, Biedermann H (eds) 1984 Die Halswirbelsäule. Part 2: Allgemeine funktionelle Pathologie und klinische Syndrome. Fischer, Stuttgart

Koch L E, Girnus U 1998 Kraftmessung bei Anwendung der Impulstechnik in der Chirotherapie. Manuelle Medizin 36(1):21–26

Ramirez J 1998 The neuronal control of breathing: New insights and experimental approaches with implications for the investigation of sudden infant death (SID). In: Saternus K, Kamirow S (eds) Säuglingssterblichkeit – Plötzlicher Kindstod (SID), Schmidt-Römhild, Lübeck, p 53–65

Schmitz H, Ewers J 2002 EWMM-Workshop Antwerpen. Manuelle Medizin 40:253–254

Vojta V, Peters A 1992 Das Vojta-Prinzip. Springer, Berlin

Chapter 12

Attention deficit disorder and the upper cervical spine

R. Theiler

In recent years there has been a notable increase in work aimed at shedding light on attention deficit disorder (ADD). Neurological examination, with particular attention to motor function, plays a fundamental part in such work, and includes the need to examine both body posture and the attitude of the trunk in detail.

Even where there is no obvious evidence of abnormality, careful examination of preschool and school-age children frequently reveals indications of movement deficits of the upper cervical spine consistent with kinematic imbalances due to suboccipital strain (KISS). Such findings are also very frequent in children with suspected ADD or similar problems, primarily involving clumsiness of gross motor function and, more especially, fine motor function, difficulty in concentrating, and functional and behavioral difficulties.

During the early stages of our observation of child cases involving a combination of KISS and ADD, manual medical treatment was given solely to correct postural asymmetry. Following successful treatment of KISS, we found in many cases that improvement had occurred not only in those aspects relating directly to the postural deficit, but also in concentration and cognitive abilities.

EVALUATION

These findings led us to explore what exactly was being improved. We carried out a neurological motor examination and neuropyschological examination of children with suspected ADD. The aspects considered in the neuropsychological examination were derived from various psychological screening instruments (Frostig, Mottier test, Wettstein logopedic language comprehension test, etc.). Ruf-Bächtiger took, developed and applied various of these tests, creating an investigation procedure with 64 items (Ruf-Bächtiger and Baumann 1997) which was relatively simple to use. The procedure for arriving at the ADD diagnosis also made considerable use of the Conners questionnaires for parents and teachers (Conners et al 1998), but these were not used in the subsequent evaluation of the success of treatment. When conducting the neurological examination, particular attention was paid in assessing body posture in relation to symptoms associated with KISS syndrome.

INVESTIGATION

Manual therapy was given to 48 children (aged 6½ to 12 years, of whom 27 were boys) with ADD according to the DSM-IV criteria, and confirmed KISS syndrome. Follow-up began by testing the free mobility of the cervical spine, and then investigating those neuropsychological and neuromotor findings from the initial examination that were not age-related. If the child had recouped the developmental delay to a greater degree than could be accounted for by the time lapse since initial examination, or if the child's performance had become normal for his or her age, this was evaluated as improvement. The time intervals varied because in many cases differing amounts of time were needed between initial examination and the successful conclusion of manual therapy. The clinical diagnosis of KISS was based on segmental testing of cervical spine mobility. The radiological examinations consisted of Gutmann–Sandberg anteroposterior radiographs of the atlanto-occipital area and conventional lateral radiographs of the cervical spine (see Chapters 18 and 19). The

follow-up examination after manual therapy was clinical only; no radiological follow-up was performed.

Box 12.1 summarizes the components of the neurological and neurophysiological examinations (tests). In addition to the tests listed in Box 12.1, basal neural status was also examined.

Social maturity/competence, impulsivity/suppression of impulses, sustained effort, ability to sustain attention, and ability to concentrate were assessed as observation criteria for the purposes of these examinations, rather than by means of specific tests, and were included in the study as a means of judging the overall success of treatment.

The study was designed as a straightforward investigation. It was carried out in the context of the normal day-to-day activity of a specialized pediatric practice. It was not possible to run a control group because of a lack of comparable placebo therapies.

RESULTS

The results are summarized in Tables 12.1, 12.2 and 12.3.

Box 12.1 Tests (the items with an asterisk (*) were validated for determining the age group)

- Tactile-kinesthetic perception: gross and fine motor coordination, graphomotor test*, graphesthesia imitation*, graphesthesia choice*, Affolter tower
- Visual perception: reproduction of forms, dot picture*, vexing image, grasping of simultaneously presented points*, imitation of point sequences*, building after a photographic example, mosaic dice*, discrimination test figure-background (Frostig 7a/8a*, recognizing a fingerprint, Lang stereotest II), Visus testing
- Language perception: repetition of nonsense syllables*, choice of nonsense syllables*, repetition of sentences
- Acoustic perception: imitation of tonal patterns*, if necessary audiogram

Table 12.1   Results of the neuropsychological examination before manipulation (N = 48)

Impairment	Before manipulation: deficit in years/number of children		
	>2 years	>1 year	<1 year
Tactile-kinesthetic	20	12	16
Visual	20	15	13
Verbal	25	17	6
Acoustic	6	9	33

For the examination techniques used, see the corresponding section in the main text.

For the purposes of the study, the diagnosis of ADD involved retardation in two or more fields of perception in the neuropsychological examination (Ruf-Bächtiger 1995, Ruf-Bächtiger and Baumann 1997). A deficit of up to 1 year was regarded as still being within the normal range, so that the chil-dren accepted into the study were performing at a level appropriate to children 2 or more years below their actual age.

Abnormal performance was mainly found in items involving tasks that called upon several different modalities. Performance was most negatively affected if they were related to verbal, visual and tactile-kinesthetic perception (in that order), and least affected if they related to acoustic/auditory perception. All the children had difficulty with motor coordination, but a majority were found to have retardation amounting to less than 2 years in this area.

The results were particularly striking for items in which the information perceived then had to be translated into motor activity: repetition of nonsense syllables (Mottier test, modified by Ruf-Bächtiger), graphesthesia imitation, and the imitation of series of dots. Marked retardation in these items is often found in ADD, as

Table 12.2   Results of the neuropsychological examination after successful manipulation (children with deficits of >2 years – first row of Table 12.1)

Impairment	Before manipulation on >2 years	After manipulation: deficit in years/number of children			
		>2 years	>1 year	<1 year	Normalized
Tactile-kinesthetic	20	4	10	5	1
Visual	20	3	7	5	5
Verbal	25	4	6	10	5
Acoustic	6	2	1	3	0

Table 12.3   Results of the neuropsychological examination after successful manipulation (children with deficits of 1–2 years – second row of Table 12.1)

Impairment	Before manipulation 1–2 years	After manipulation: deficit in years/number of children		
		>1 year	<1 year	Normalized
Tactile-kinesthetic	12	4	6	2
Visual	15	3	8	4
Verbal	17	3	9	5
Acoustic	9	5	3	1

these tasks demonstrate particularly clearly any difficulties in the processing of information. However, these three tests were also the ones that showed the best response to manipulation. The performance of some of the children was normal after manipulation therapy (Tables 12.2 and 12.3). Differences were most often evident in the modified Mottier test and imitation of series of dots. Ten children with reduced visual concentration span had reading difficulties. Following completion of manipulation therapy they achieved an oral reading fluency appropriate for their age, usually in the days immediately following therapy. These children in particular reached a normal level of achievement in all the tasks that demanded normal visual intake capacity.

It appears from the results obtained that a small proportion of the children (7 out of 48) were exhibiting considerable negative effects due to the atlanto-cervical misalignment alone. Following manipulation therapy they performed normally in everyday situations, achieving levels at least appropriate to their age in concentration, sustained effort, and control of impulses, and also (for the most part) motor function. Following manipulation therapy, their concentration span was completely normal.

In the neurological examination we found an improvement in coordination, with more pronounced improvement in gross than fine motor function. This correlated with the findings in the graphesthesia imitation test, where the retardation in performance decreased by at least 1 year.

Overall, no marked improvements in results were found for acoustic/auditory perception following manipulation therapy.

Parents reported that in general the children's ability to concentrate, sustained effort, ability to sustain attention, and impulsivity had improved considerably, and that their children seemed 'more mature' ('less childish'). The follow-up tests tended to confirm this, with the children working more quickly and confidently. More detailed quantification of these observations was not carried out, for the reasons given above.

A number of children who were not thereafter included in the study later showed deterioration in some or all areas that had previously been abnormal. A recurrence of KISS was found in all but a few of these cases. The improvements recorded previously returned after manipulation therapy was repeated.

After the first follow-up tests to the manipulation therapy, the impression grew that younger children were deriving more benefit from the treatment than older ones. However, at the end, the percentage of successful treatments was roughly equally distributed across the age groups. The proportion of children between the ages of 6½ and 8 was greater, but this was not statistically significant in view of the small numbers involved.

DISCUSSION OF RESULTS

One of the main findings of the neuropsychological examination in ADS is the reduced capacity for processing information (Miller 1956); there is a reduced intake concentration span in two or more fields of perception. This is an expression of deficiencies in executive functions, which are carried out in the dopamine-dependent structures of the frontal lobe and corpus striatum and its links to the limbic system. The reduced capacity for processing information also affects the direction of impulses. The reduced ability to perceive or take in information makes it impossible to achieve periods of concentration and sustained attention appropriate to the age of the child.

According to this study, the main result following successful manipulation therapy for KISS was an improvement in intake concentration span, especially in verbal and visual perception. The deficit in terms of age usually diminished within a short period by several times the measured interval between treatment and follow-up examination. The progress could not therefore simply be due to maturation of the brain. Some of the children recovered 2 or more years' performance deficit in the course of a few weeks or months, while the majority achieved a smaller but still considerable degree of improvement. Parents reported that these improvements were often already observable in everyday life on the day that manipulation therapy had taken place, or within a few days.

The model of the 'capacity for processing information' offers an explanation for this improvement in cognitive performance through orthopedic treatment. This assumes that the brain has a set capacity to process information, and that this capacity must be available if it is to process the information received through the various means of perception. This capacity can be compared to the processing memory of a computer in that it limits in just the same sort of way the amount of information from all areas of perception that can be processed. This means that it determines how well and how quickly the constant stream of stimuli of perception can be translated into appropriate action.

As with an overloaded computer memory, so in ADD with kinematic imbalance-related dyspraxia/dysgnosia (KIDD) only part of the body of information is processed at the required time, leading eventually to the moment of total overload with decompensation due to excessive demand.

In the combination of KISS and ADD, the child has a further overload factor: in addition to having a 'processing memory' that is too small for its age, the child has to correct the information distorted by the malpositioning of the head, and this corrective work probably plays a decisive role. This malpositioning means that visual information is received crookedly, and either the information has to be straightened out in the system of visual perception, or the position of the head must constantly be corrected by controlling the angle of the trunk, both solutions requiring information processing capacity. Successful manipulation therapy brings head and trunk correction back within normal range, freeing up capacity to be used for cognitive processing and bringing about a quanti-

tative improvement in the processing of information received.

In the present study the clearest differences in findings occurred in those items of the examination that required information to be processed using a variety of modalities. In these tests, sensory information had to be translated into the performance of a motor task: repeating sounds, drawing series of dots, or tracing out with the finger a line traced on the back of the hand (graphesthesia imitation). An everyday example of such a difference was that the reading performance of children with difficulty in reading aloud became normal in what was for the parents an astonishingly short time.

On the other hand, the developmental deficit before and after therapy was considerably less in procedures requiring choice (and sometimes was not demonstrable at all). To perform these procedures correctly, the children needed to show good perceptive ability, but the demands placed on their capacities appear to have been less if all the children had to do was to identify differences between pieces of information they had heard or felt.

For the majority of the children, KISS caused a considerable limitation of information processing capacity; more importantly, this was an additional limitation of capacity. Manipulation therapy helped these children to some degree, but did not fundamentally improve the underlying problem. These children therefore needed further types of treatment, in most cases medical stimulant therapy together with supporting therapy for motor function or behavior.

KIDD

If they remain untreated, infants with KISS grow into children with KISS, with more or less pronounced associated symptoms. They exhibit not only problems of posture with neck and/or back pain, but further difficulties that cannot be clearly traced to posture. These mainly involve motor clumsiness of varying severity, ranging all the way up to ataxic movement disorder. The main problem is motor coordination, in particular fine motor function, with difficulties in graphic motor function. Other problems include variable concentration ability, which understandably results in variable performance at school and in everyday life (behavior). Inconsistency in intensity is a particular feature of behavior. The form taken by the behavioral difficulty depends on the individual child, but seldom varies for any one individual. Observation shows that decompensation may be aggressive, destructive or resigned.

If the difficulties in behavior and perception are caused by poor positioning of the atlanto-cervical joint, we apply the description 'kinematic imbalance-related dyspraxia/dysgnosia which is suboccipital in origin' (KIDD).

The possibility that children whose cognitive performance becomes normal after manipulation therapy might be suffering from an associated dopamine deficiency of the frontal lobe and frontal limbic structures is remote. Such therapy

therefore provides a method of distinguishing 'KIDD' (Biedermann 1999) from 'KISS with ADD'. This in turn means that these children can be helped without recourse to drug treatment, while the others can be helped by long-term therapies.

In its various degrees the pattern of symptoms that appears in children with KIDD is often difficult to differentiate from the problems of children with ADD. From our experience as described above we have developed the following procedure for examining children with ADS (Fig. 12.1):

If the symptoms of ADD are accompanied by limited movement of the cervical spine attributable to KISS, the manual medical therapy procedure is followed (radiological examination and manipulation therapy). Follow-up takes place about 4 to 8 weeks after manipulation therapy. If that examination reveals normal mobility of the cervical spine ('suboccipital region normal'), we evaluate the effect on the ADD symptoms and discuss the implications for subsequent

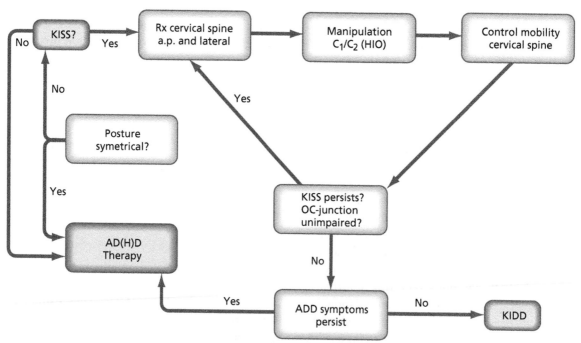

Figure 12.1 Diagnosis and therapy of KISS and ADD.

therapy. If it reveals further abnormality, we recommend that manipulation be performed a second time.

If the suboccipital region is normal and the ADD symptoms have either disappeared or been reduced to a minimum, this is interpreted as KIDD. If ADD persists when the suboccipital region is normal, we describe this as ADD with KISS.

Case studies

A.M. (female, 7 years, 2 months)

Pregnancy was uneventful, with a fast spontaneous delivery at the expected date with a birthweight of 3300 g and a length of 47 cm.

The initial development was inconspicuous: she walked at her first birthday, spoke her first sentences at her second birthday and had no major accidents or operations, apart from a fall from a swing.

The diagnosis of attention deficit hyperactivity disorder (ADHD) was made by a regional center for pediatric psychiatry: there was a very variable level of concentration depending on her interest in the topic at hand, sudden changes of mood and low frustration threshold. She showed possessive and dominant behavior while playing and in the classroom, disturbing other children or clowning around in stressful circumstances at school or in private. As she showed insufficient gross and fine motor functions, too, the psychotherapy was combined with a psychomotor therapy. She was referred for our consultation because of a persistent postural asymmetry after 1 year of this therapy schedule.

On clinical examination, we found a normal muscular tonus; lively and symmetrical muscular reflexes without pyramidal signs. In testing tiptoeing and walking on the heels, the synkinesis of the arms was notably awkward. Walking on a line was performed clumsily; she put her feet next to the line and tiptoed intermittently. In the one leg standing test the arms were used excessively to sustain balance. Jumping and clapping was uncoordinated,

and the muscular force insufficiently measured out. Finger–thumb opposition was clumsily achieved and accompanied by tonic contralateral movements.

Neuropsychological findings were as follows: if not occupied she was constantly moving around; while solving problems she became momentarily more calm, but this did not last long and she got increasingly fidgety. Her concentration span was short and she was very impulsive in tackling the assigned tasks. Her behavior got increasingly evasive with the mounting degree of difficulty of the job at hand. She tired rapidly.

Imitation of body posture was imprecise on the right side, and appropriate for her age on the left. She was unable to solve the graphesthesia imitation test (developmental age less than 5 years), repetition of nonsense syllables succeeded for groups of 3, was faulty in 4–5 (phonetic reproduction) and groups of 6 syllables could not be reproduced at all. Repetition of sentences with complex content was incomplete. Imitation of lines of points, differentiation of figure background and perception of forms was performed according to age, and acoustic perception, too.

Our diagnosis was ADHD.

Functional examination of spine revealed a marked impairment of the inclination of the head to the right and the rotation to the left with a blockage of C_1/C_2 on the left as well as a blockage of the left SI joint. The cervical spine was in a right convexity and the thoracic spine in a left convex posture. Pelvis and shoulders stood horizontally. The radiograph showed a hyperextension of the cervical spine and a lateralization of C_1 and C_2 to the left.

Treatment consisted of C_1/C_2 left (impulse technique).

In the following 3–4 days the girl complained of giddiness. Shortly afterwards the family remarked that her gait and posture became straighter and more harmonious; motor coordination improved.

Three weeks after the treatment the girl was examined again. In the motor tests she showed marked improvement while still having difficulties walking on a line. Bimanual coordination improved, though with inadequate control of power. Jumping was now performed effortlessly.

The neuropsychological tests still showed a short attention span, some impulsiveness in the search for solutions and much less evasiveness with improved perseverance. Memory span and processing capacity for tactile and kinesthetic tasks was at a level of 2 years less than her age, but verbal capacities were now normal and the visual component better than an 8-year-old, i.e. 1–2 years advanced in comparison with her age group (Fig. 12.2).

Two years later the family contacted us again as her behavior showed a relapse with increased impulsiveness, worsening of the always problematic concentration span and increased distractibility. In the meantime, an examination in pediatric psychiatry had shown her to be highly gifted. We found a recurrence of a cervical blockage and the consequent reoccurrence of the KISS symptoms. After the successful removal of the functional cervical disorders, her concentration span and control of her impulsive behavior improved again and her integration in the peer group was facilitated.

Her performance in different tests in comparison to the age average is shown in Figure 12.2.

W.S. (female, 6 years, 5 months)

Pregnancy was normal. She was born in the 42nd week with a clavicle fracture intrapartum, with birthweight of 3750 g, and a length of 48 cm. Her mother said that she was somewhat lazy drinking while being breast-fed, and when she was older always ate only what she felt like.

At examination she appeared to be a bit overweight. The psychomotor development appeared to be age-appropriate. Already at the age of 4, her clumsiness had been remarked. The development of her drawing lagged behind, with scribbling at the age of 5, and simple 'head-and-feet' figures at the age of 6. Remedial education was applied for the second kindergarten year for 1 year. She could not use scissors properly or fasten her shoes. Concentration span for things she was interested in was very good and it was almost impossible to divert her, but she did not have much stamina, especially for unfamiliar tasks, and she was prone to retreat when confronted with frustrating experiences or failure. She had difficulties sticking to the rules.

Clinical examination showed a chubby child with a reduced muscular tonus and normal and symmetrical reflex behavior, and no pyramidal pathology. Gross motor function was slightly disturbed. Jumping on one leg was impossible for her. Fine motor tasks were tackled with difficulty and tactile and kinesthetic processing was at the level of a 5-year-old (i.e. retardation of 18 months).

Neuropsychological findings showed a calm, withdrawn girl without too much energy. When the

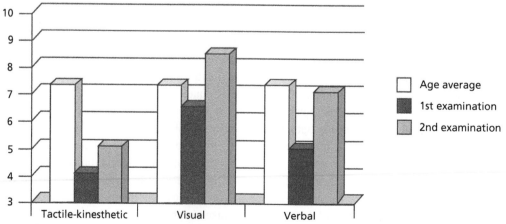

Figure 12.2   Case A.M.: performance in different tests in comparison to the age average.

tests got more complex she became more impulsive, and lost concentration and perseverance. Memory and processing capacity in all areas of perception was 1.5 years below age average. Raven Colored Progressive Matrices (CPM) corresponded to an age of 8.4–9.0 years. Summary diagnosis: ADD, inattention variant.

Functional examination of the spine revealed impaired side-bending of the head on the right side and reduction of the rotation on the left. In the sitting position, there was excessive thoracic kyphosis with reclination of the head. The orthopedic status was otherwise unremarkable. The radiograph showed a lateral displacement of C_1/C_2 to the right.

Treatment comprised manual therapy combining a sagittal impulse on C_1 and a HIO C_1/C_2 from the right side (impulse manipulation).

Two months after the manipulation, the child came back for a check-up just after her seventh birthday. The mother reported no change in any aspect. The head movements were now completely unhindered.

Neurologically, there was no significant change, albeit a few minor improvements (she was able to jump at least a bit on one leg now, for example).

Neuropsychologically, she showed a more considered way of working and was less impulsive. She was able to criticize and correct completed tasks and she could concentrate for longer. Visual memory and processing capacity were still 6 months below her age, tactile-kinesthetic processing and three-dimensional orientation 1 year below her age, and verbal memory now on the level of a 9-year-old (+2 years).

Comparing the two test results, it is clear that the girl had managed to catch up with her age group. In some aspects (e.g. visual performance) she was even able to outdo her age group considerably. Comment from the mother (after having compared the test results): 'It seems to have been effective anyway, after all!'

Further therapy involved psychomotor therapy.

Her performance in different tests in comparison to the age average is shown in Figure 12.3.

A.K. (female, 11 years, 5 months)

This girl was examined shortly before she was to enter high school ('Gymnasium'). Since her fifth school-year it had become increasingly evident that she had trouble delivering consistent results in her tests. Even accomplishing sufficient results to ensure her 'survival' in primary school seemed to be imperiled. This compelled the parents to seek an evaluation as to whether or not ADD-related problems were contributing to these difficulties.

The girl's situation in school was characterized by concentration problems and a lack of long-term attention to a given topic. In mathematics, for example, she had mostly very satisfying results with quite a few bad grades interspersed. With languages she fared even better and here the bad results were less frequent. Her behavior in school and at home was in accordance with her age and her contact with her peers unremarkable – with the normal pre-puberty edginess.

The neurological examination showed a normal muscular tonus, lively and symmetrical spinal reflexes, and no signs of pyramidal disorders. Gross motor capacities were normal; fine motor coordination degraded with increasing speed. The graph motor performance showed a similar pattern: initially normal and with a harmonious grip of the stylus, the grasp of the pen became more tensed with speedier writing and the pressure on the paper more pronounced.

Neuropsychologically, she cooperated well throughout the entire examination. The rate of errors increased with the time it took to accomplish a test, even if the level of testing was lowered. When trying to solve a more difficult task she showed more impulsive behavior and had more problems in noticing and correcting her mistakes.

In copying lines of dots and in repeating nonsense syllables, her performance was at the level of an 8–8½-year-old. The dice mosaic was copied with some effort, and losing track, she had to solve this task bit by bit. Tactile-kinesthetic perception and processing were age-appropriate.

The clinical picture showed a scoliotic posture with a cervical-thoracic left convexity and a counterswing at the thoracolumbar level. The pelvis was in a

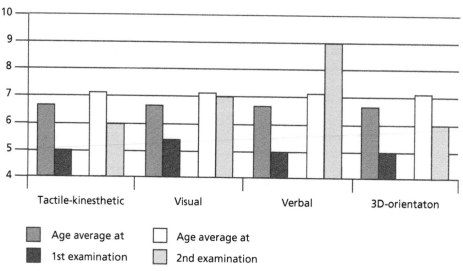

Figure 12.3   Case W.S.: performance in different tests in comparison to the age average.

horizontal position with a blockage of the right SI joint.

The head-tilt to the right was impaired and on the segmental level C_1/C_2 blocked on the right side. The radiological examination showed an offset of the atlas to the right.

We interpreted these results as an attention deficit disorder with reduced impulse control, but without hyperactivity.

As the imminent change of school seemed to be endangered, the family decided to use Ritalin therapy. The performance in school stabilized immediately and her grades improved markedly. The teachers felt that she gained self-assurance and stability.

During the last weeks of the school year, the manual therapy was applied, based on the radiological examination (i.e. C_1R). After this manipulation the SI joint regained normal mobility without direct manipulation. Simultaneously the medication was stopped.

After a week the girl said spontaneously that she did not think she would need Ritalin any more. Now she was able to function normally in school and she was able to do her homework without problems.

The mother wanted to resume the medication anyway, hoping to further improve the situation. After 4 days the course of medication was stopped as it did not result in any perceptible gains. These improvements lasted well into the new school year, and she was able to function satisfactorily in the new school with grades a bit under the class average.

This case study shows how KISS can lead to an impaired level of attention and execution typical for ADD. We have not yet found reliable tests to differentiate between cases of ADD with and without a cervical factor. It is often in combination with reduced executive capabilities that we see difficulties of coping with conflicts which may lead to behavioral disturbances and phobias, in milder cases to impaired self-confidence.

As in this case, we are in favor of examining and treating functional problems of the (cervical) spine in these children, especially after we found signs of postural asymmetry of movement restrictions, even if a pharmacotherapy seemed to have already resolved the problem at hand.

References

Biedermann H 1999 Vom KISS zum KIDD. In: Manualtherapie bei Kindern. Indikationen und Erfahrungen: ein Querschnitt. Enke, Stuttgart

Biedermann H 2001 KISS-Kinder. Enke, Stuttgart

Conners C K et al 1998 The revised Conners' Parent Rating Scale (CPRS-R): factor structure, reliability, and criterion validity. Journal of Abnormal Child Psychology 26(4):257–268

Miller G 1956 The magical number seven, plus or minus two: some limits on our capacity for processing information. Psychological Review 63:81–97

Ruf-Bächtiger L 1995 Das frühkindliche psychoorganische Syndrom: Minimale zerebrale Dysfunktion; Diagnostik und Therapie. Thieme, Stuttgart

Ruf-Bächtiger L, Baumann T 1997 Neuromotorische-neuropsychologische Untersuchung des gesunden Kindes (Course in examination methods CD-ROM). Thieme

Chapter 13

Asymmetry of the posture, locomotion apparatus and dentition in children

H. Korbmacher, L. E. Koch, B. Kahl-Nieke

Perfect symmetry of the body is uncommon in nature. In a study of children aged 9–18 years, who clinically did not reveal a facial asymmetry, Vig and Hewitt (1975) analyzed the posterior-anterior cephalograms. Astonishingly, the cephalometric analysis revealed an overall asymmetry in most children, indicating that the left side of the face was generally larger than the right.

Functional and morphological asymmetry is to some extent physiological. Pirttiniemi (1994) differentiates normal craniofacial asymmetry into normal asymmetry of a directional or fluctuating nature. Directional asymmetry can be found in the anterior/posterior, the cranio/caudal and left/right dimension. Asymmetries in the anterior/posterior and cranio/caudal dimension are embryonically rooted and thus a result of the asymmetry in the central nervous system (Zilles et al 1996). Advances in molecular genetics suggest a genetic background for laterality (Collignon et al 1996). Examples of directional asymmetry are the asymmetrical structure of the brain, a consistent laterality in internal organs and left/right handedness. Another type of asymmetry is the fluctuating asymmetry that is related to stress (Siegel and Doyle 1975). Genetically coded tissues such as the enamel of teeth are most often affected (Manning and Chamberlain 1994). One of the major etiological causes of asymmetrical orofacial findings is the side difference in muscular function. The latest scientific data shows that dental occlusion is an important factor in symmetrical development of facial structures in early life (Bishara et al 1994, Kiliaridis et al 1996a, 1996b, Raadsheer et al 1996).

How is asymmetry defined? In clinical terms, symmetry means balance whereas an imbalance of a system results in asymmetry (Pirttiniemi 1998). A similar viewpoint is described by Rude (1987) who examined 500 skulls in terms of asymmetric structures. Under normal conditions, many different factors influence the morphology of the skull. These factors can be divided into three categories such as forces driving from the vertebral column, especially the occipitocervical region (OCR), cranial factors and environmental local factors such as tongue, adenoids and perioral muscles. Under physiological circumstances, all three categories of forces form a balance of power. Under pathological conditions one group gains more influence than the others and the balance of power is destroyed. Imbalance and asymmetry occurs.

The idea of an interdisciplinary treatment is one of early prevention (Huggare 1998, Pirttiniemi et al 1990). Recent scientific data shows that apart from genetically rooted development, muscular balance and dental occlusion are the keys of a normal symmetrical development of orofacial structures. In addition to the support of the trunk muscles, head posture is the result of a complex muscle system that includes the lip muscles and the hyoidontic motor system (Aragao 1991). The postural muscles contribute to the tension and function of the orofacial and deglutition muscles. Based on this muscular interaction the logical consequence is a contribution of the muscles of the craniocervical region to facial development.

Besides the preventive character, the motivation of interdisciplinary cooperation between orthopedists and orthodontists is to optimize the treatment results and to avoid relapse. Relapse is one indicator of an incomplete diagnosis (Balters 1964, Rude 1987). Delaire (1977) interpreted a relapse of an orthodontically corrected mesial position of the lower jaw as the result of a therapeutically neglected cervical lordosis in the patient. Further

specialization in medicine led to a focus on the discipline's characteristic features and the overall understanding of the chain of events is often missed.

As an anatomically and functionally complex system, head and vertebrae have been the focus of scientific interest (Christ 1993, Gutmann 1981, Ridder 1998). Studies of this interdisciplinary issue have been carried out for more than 6 centuries. But a clear statement of the relation between orthopedic and orthodontic disorders is still missing. Most studies are based on clinical impressions and have anecdotal features. Only a few controlled studies exist so far. Some cephalometric studies have shown that anatomical features of the craniocervical junction are associated with head posture, mandibular growth and angulation of the cranial base.

In general, there seems to be an association between Angle class II – i.e. distal position of the mandible in the skull – and lordosis, as well as a high incidence of lateral crossbite in patients with scoliosis and torticollis.

ANIMAL EXPERIMENTS

The results of experiments with guinea pigs and rabbits suggest interaction between occlusal plane, craniofacial growth, head posture and cardiac function. Unilateral grinding of the occlusal plane evoked changes in the posture of the upper cervical spine as well as many reactions of the motor and autonomic nervous system. The changes observed were an abnormal mobility of the tongue, a different posture of the cervical spine, loss of hair as well as changes in the ECG in terms of an inverted T wave (Festa et al 1997). Those changes became evident one week after unilateral manipulation of the vertical plane. The evoked reactions normalized after the reconstruction of the original occlusion plane (Azuma et al 1999). These results indicate that changes in the dental occlusion interact with the masticatory muscles and head posture as well as the trigeminal system that controls heart and wellbeing. Furthermore dental occlusion is one cofactor of craniofacial growth. As Poikela et al (1995, 1997) proved, unilateral masticatory function caused asymmetric craniofacial growth in rabbits.

DIAGNOSTIC RECORDS

Not every asymmetry must be treated. Under physiological conditions the body compensates for a certain degree of asymmetry. Unfavorable environmental factors can accumulate and reduce the level of compensation. Discomfort appears and asymmetry becomes obvious (Pirttiniemi 1994).

An investigation of clinically healthy male pilots demonstrates the tolerance of the body to a certain degree of asymmetry. Although clinically the examined pilots were not asymmetrical in function and morphology and did not show any discomfort, the investigation revealed a high incidence of asymmetrical structure of the high cervical spine (OCR).

In order to treat any asymmetry correctly it is important to diagnose not only the asymmetrical structure itself, but also the cofactors that contribute to the final decompensation of asymmetry.

ORTHODONTIC RECORDS

Radiographic examination

As one basic diagnostic record in orthodontics, a lateral cephalogram is taken in order to analyze the relationship between the sagittal position of the upper and lower jaw and the direction of mandibular growth. The mandibular growth can evolve in two directions: a clockwise and a counterclockwise rotation. Different craniofacial angles can determine the quality of growth. As the vertebrae are clearly visible, orthodontists have taken these X-rays in order to investigate the spine parameters in relation to the growth of the lower

jaw. After drawing references points and planes, intersectional relations between occiput, atlas and axis were taken.

In a cervico-cephalometric examination Hirschfelder and Hirschfelder (1982b, 1991) found significant differences in craniovertical and craniocervical parameters between the registration in standardized cephalograms and a lateral cephalogram taken in a natural head position. The natural head position is more proclined than the fixed standardized position. During orthodontic diagnosis, routinely taken lateral cephalometric X-rays do not allow a reproducible realistic analysis of craniocervical and vertical parameters. In order to investigate asymmetry of the upper cervical spine, radiological examination should be based on the head position of the orthopedic registration in the neutral position (Gutmann 1981).

Clinical examination

An orthodontic disorder can be dental and/or skeletal (Kahl-Nieke 2001). Loss of space, crowding, labial or lingual inclination of the incisors, an infraposition or a supraposition, a dental midline shift and rotations all belong to dental disorders and should be corrected by movements of the teeth. A transversal mandibular shift, a more posterior or anterior position of one or both jaws as well as other vertical discrepancies are the most common skeletal problems. If there is still ongoing growth, a skeletal disorder can be corrected by guiding and influencing growth to a certain degree. If the skeletal discrepancy is too significant or there is no developmental growth remaining, orthodontists can compensate for the skeletal problem by moving teeth or correct the anomaly in combination with surgery.

In the 1890s E.H. Angle, an American orthodontic pioneer, published his 'Angle class' classification with the maxilla as a fixed skeletal structure within the skull. The correct relationship between upper and lower jaw was defined as Angle class I: a neutral position of the lower jaw and dentition in comparison to the upper jaw and dentition. The teeth occlude alternately and upper incisors are overlapping the lower ones. The pathologic Angle class II describes a more distal position of the lower teeth in comparison to Angle class I, which is measured in width of premolars (equivalent 7–8 mm). In an Angle class III the mandible and the lower teeth are positioned more mesially, in most cases in combination with an anterior crossbite.

Since 1932, following the publications on lateral cephalometric analysis by Hofrath (1931) and Broadbent (1931), the skeletal position of the jaws has been classified differently from the above-mentioned Angle classes (Fig. 13.1).

Cephalometric analysis revealed that even the maxilla alters in its position to the skull. Therefore a skeletal class I is defined as the neutral position of the jaws to each other. Based on the lateral cephalometric analysis, this neutral position can be measured by different angles. Consequently, skeletal class II is the more posterior position of the lower jaw to the maxilla. This can be due to a more forward position of the maxilla than normal and/or to a more posterior position of the lower jaw. The opposite is defined by the skeletal class III configuration (Fig. 13.2).

Under normal conditions, the incisors of the mandible and maxilla occlude with each other. This occlusal relation is described by the overjet and overbite. The overjet is defined as the distance between the lower incisors and upper ones in the sagittal plane, whereas the incisors' distance in the vertical plane is called overbite (Fig. 13.3). In addition the midlines of the upper and lower central incisors should be identical.

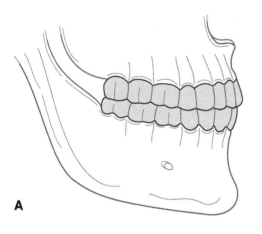

A

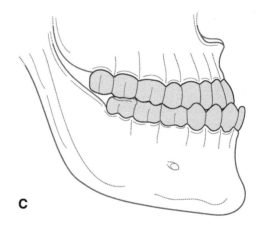

C

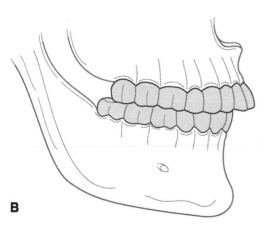

B

Figure 13.1 The relationship of the teeth as well as the jaws is defined by three different classes. In most cases dental occlusion and sagittal jaw configuration are consistent with each other. (A) demonstrates a dental and skeletal class I relation: the maxilla is in advance to the lower jaw, teeth occlude alternately by an overbite of the upper incisors to the lower ones. A skeletal and dental class II (B) occurs when the upper jaw and occlusion is in advance to the lower jaw and occlusion compared to a skeletal class I. As (C) reveals, a skeletal class III is the opposite of a class II. The lower jaw and teeth are in advance to the upper jaw and teeth.

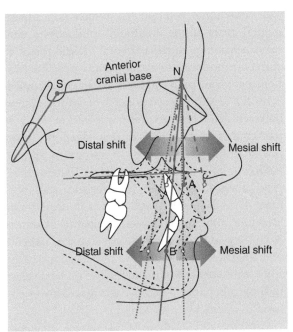

Figure 13.2   For therapeutic reasons it is important to analyze the individual skeletal position of the upper and lower jaw by a lateral cephalogram. S, sella – midpoint of the sella turcica; N, nasion – most anterior point on frontonasal suture; A, A point – position of the deepest concavity on anterior profile of the maxilla; B, B point – position of the deepest concavity on anterior profile of the mandibular symphysis. (From Kahl-Nieke 2001, with permission of Urban and Fischer.)

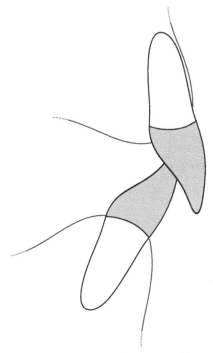

Figure 13.3   The position of the upper and lower incisors is defined by the sagittal and vertical distance between the incisors. An overjet of 2 mm is physiological. The distance in the vertical plane, the overbite, should be 2 mm as well. An increased overbite (>2 mm) is called an anterior deep bite, whereas a reduced overbite (<2 mm) is called an open bite.

In order to prove the clinical situation, extra- and intraoral pictures are taken in a standardized fixation. For better diagnosis, three-dimensional plaster models reflect the intraoral situation. A panoramic X-ray gives an overall idea of possible dental disorders. The analysis of the above-mentioned lateral cephalogram provides evidence of skeletal problems.

Examination of the soft tissues

An inspection of perioral soft tissues is essential for a good orthodontic diagnosis. The examination should start with an investigation of the posture: The head and neck muscles, the perioral and masticatory muscles as well as the muscles of the supra- and infrahyoid region all contribute

to the orthostatic posture. Furthermore, lips and nose should be investigated as they give evidence of the mode of breathing. Intraorally, the tongue position and the swallowing pattern should be observed. Habits and disorders in speech such as sigmatism (lisping) should be detected. If treatment is required, patients should be referred to a myofunctional therapist.

ORTHOPEDIC RECORDS

An orthopedic disorder can be muscular, functional or skeletal in nature. If there is a visible asymmetry in the occipitocervical region it is not a pathology by itself. Only in combination with a disturbed function may one talk of an orthopedic disorder. The functional approach is often under-estimated. But function is as real as anatomy. The neck motion can be evaluated by palpation, inspection, additional radiological records and functional analysis of the region (Biedermann 1991, Biedermann and Koch 1996, Koch and Gramann-Brunt 1999). An asymmetry in the range of lateral motion of the head in anteflexion can imply an asymmetry. A detailed description of orthopedic diagnosis is given in other chapters of this book.

REVIEW OF ORTHODONTIC DISCREPANCIES IN CHILDREN WITH ORTHOPEDIC DISORDERS

Sagittal plane

Many authors have investigated the correlation between the sagittal jaw relationship and orthopedic parameters. Although there are disagreements, there seems to be a tendency for a change in position of the upper cervical spine when the patients show a distal jaw relationship (Angle class II) (Fig. 13.4).

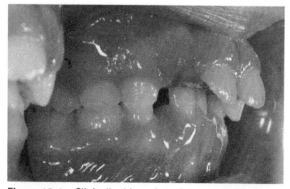

Figure 13.4 Clinically this patient shows an Angle class II relationship of 4 mm (½ width of premolars). The occlusal discrepancy results in a tooth-to-one-tooth relation which can be caused by different pathological factors: mesial movement of the upper teeth and/or distal movement of the lower teeth and/or anterior position of the maxilla and/or posterior position of the lower jaw. The skeletal causes can only be detected by a lateral cephalogram.

In functional orthopedics, which is a fundamental orthodontic treatment philosophy that takes advantage of the patients' muscle forces to correct orthodontic disorders, many possible relations between spine and jaw have been discussed. Schwarz (1926) was convinced of an interaction between head posture and jaw position. He was particularly certain that during sleep the head posture influences the mode of respiration and the pathology of orthodontic anomalies. Balters (1964) proclaimed Angle class characteristic head postures. His statement is well known in orthodontic literature, although it lacks any scientific evidence. According to Balters' clinical observation, patients with an Angle class II tend to a hyperlordosis of the spine while patients with anomalies of Angle class III show a kyphotic posture. Posture and lower jaw seem to interact.

Gresham and Smithells (1954) showed that children with a bad posture have a high percentage of Angle class II occlusion, a long-face syndrome and a significant increase in lordosis of the spine. Different working groups (Nobili and Adversi 1996, von Treuenfels 1983) revealed relations between characteristic findings, such as a hyperlordosis of the spine and Angle class II as well. In some cases a relationship between an increased overjet and a more backwardly inclined spine was detected.

Mertensmeier and Diedrich (1992) observed a correction of the concavity of the spine after orthodontic therapy. Critically, it must be taken into account that a curved spine straightens with age.

Many other studies have refuted Angle class characteristic orthopedic findings (Hirschfelder and Hirschfelder 1987, Sterzik et al 1992). Sterzik et al (1992) studied 127 lateral cephalograms of untreated children. They could not find any causal relations between sagittal position of the jaws, atlas position and head posture. Hirschfelder and Hirschfelder (1987) did not detect any correlation between specific Angle classes in children with orthopedic disorders, but observed a high incidence of postnormal occlusion (Hirschfelder and Hirschfelder 1982a).

In addition to the afore-mentioned publications Hirschfelder and Hirschfelder observed in children with disorders of the upper cervical spine a high prevalence of postnormal occlusion. About two-thirds of the children who were treated with manual therapy showed dental anomalies. A statistically significant higher prevalence of Angle class II malocclusion could not be confirmed.

Vertical plane

A similar position of the atlas is seen in patients with an anterior open bite (von Treuenfels 1984). These findings were interpreted as the cause of a reclined head posture and habitual mouth breathing (Fig. 13.5).

Transversal plane

There is still controversy as to whether children with skeletal transverse asymmetries of the dental arch tend to have specific orthopedic disorders (Fig. 13.6).

In a study of 57 children Dußler and co-workers (2002) observed no correlation between orthodontic asymmetry and any orthopedic disorder. Children with orthodontic asymmetry did not show a specific incidence of orthopedic pathologies.

On the other hand, Lippold et al (2000) recommended an interdisciplinary treatment approach in patients with midline discrepancies, since they observed a higher prevalence of orthopedic disorder in combination with midline discrepancy.

Scoliosis and torticollis

Scoliosis and torticollis are two orthopedic disorders in which many interdisciplinary approaches have been published. Except for Wachsmann (1960) all authors observed a significantly higher incidence of crossbite (26–55% prevalence) in these patients than in any control group. Prager (1980) concluded that the crossbite demonstrates the observed asymmetrical posture. Müller-Wachendorf (1961) considered the high prevalence of crossbite to be a result of the weak connective and supporting tissue and not a consequence of the scoliosis itself. Hirschfelder and Hirschfelder (1987) interpreted the results of the examination of 101 scoliotic patients as an interaction of the corporal scoliosis with the facial scoliosis. Pirttiniemi et al (1989) found a high prevalence of lateral malocclusion in patients with torticollis. The observed lateral discrepancies, i.e. dental arch asymmetry and midline deviation, were diagnosed in most cases in the upper arch (Alavi et al 1988, Lundstrom 1961).

A general agreement exists that early treatment for patients with systematic orthopedic disturbances is most effective (Lukanowa-Skopakowa 1987, Müller-Wachendorff 1961). In a longitudinal study, Pecina et al (1991) showed a positive relationship between hereditary orthodontic anomalies and idiopathic scoliosis. Since orthodontic

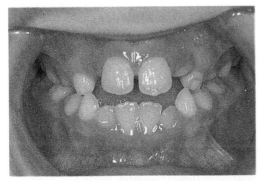

Figure 13.5 An anterior open bite caused by infraposition of upper and lower incisors to the occlusal plane.

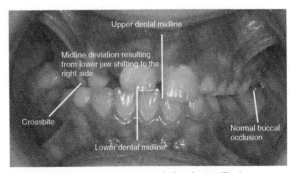

Figure 13.6 In most cases a skeletal mandibular midline shift is combined with a unilateral crossbite. As a consequence of the width discrepancy of upper and lower jaw, the lower jaw shifted to the right side with a right-sided crossbite.

disorders can be diagnosed at a younger age, the later development of scoliosis may be revealed by a close collaboration between orthopedics and orthodontics. Children with a scoliosis bigger than 10° should be examined orthodontically. Pirttiniemi et al (1989) suggested a routine orthodontic investigation of children with suspected torticollis. The aim of early orthodontic treatment is to contribute to the normalization of natural posture.

One reason supporting early surgery in children with torticollis is the attempt to prevent the development of facial asymmetries.

General orthodontic findings

For over 30 years, Solow and co-workers (Solow and Siersbaek-Nielsen 1992, Solow and Sandham 2002) have investigated the relationships between natural posture and development of the head. The posture of the upper cervical spine is related to the growth of the lower jaw (Fig. 13.7). A large cranio-

cervical angle indicates a posterior rotation of the mandible, an increased anterior facial height, reduced sagittal jaw dimensions and a steeper inclination of the lower jaw. Patients with a small craniocervical angle show a reduced lower facial height; the sagittal jaw dimensions are larger and the inclination of the mandible less steep. The only orthodontic factor that indicated an orthopedic association with the craniocervical posture was a lack of space in the anterior segment of the dental arches (Solow and Sonnesen 1998).

Solow and Tallgren (1977) explained the results of their work using the soft tissue stretching hypothesis. The soft tissue layer covering the neck and head has a restraining influence on the forward growth of the facial skeleton. An extension of the craniocervical posture leads to a caudally orientated traction on the soft tissue layer of the face. Due to the anatomy of the facial skeleton, the passive stretching of the soft tissue layer results in dorsal forces to the dentofacial structures.

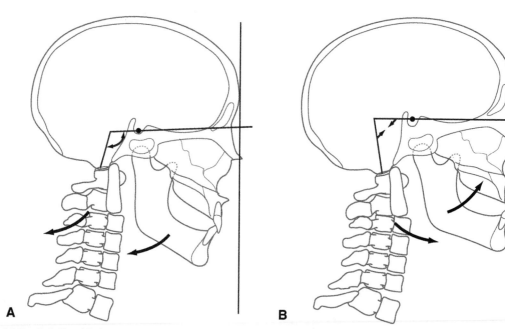

A   **B**

Figure 13.7   Relationship between craniocervical angle, rotation of the mandible, and anterior facial height (based on Solow B, Sandham A 2002 Craniocervical posture: a factor in the development and function of the dentofacial structures. European Journal of Orthodontics 24: 467–456, by permission of Oxford University Press). A: A large craniocervical angle indicates an increased posterior rotation of the mandible and anterior facial height. B: A reduced anterior facial height is most often related to a small craniocervical angle and an anterior rotation of the mandible.

The hypothesis has been confirmed by other studies. Hellsing et al (1987) demonstrated an association between lip pressure and posture of the head. With elevation of the head, the lip pressure increases. Other investigations in children with impaired nose breathing showed an increase in craniocervical angle (Solow et al 1984).

Atlas deviation

As a result of various radiological studies (Howard 1983, Sandikcioglu et al 1994), the height of the posterior arch of the atlas has been found to be correlated to different orthodontic discrepancies. In an adenoid group of 43 children aged 4–15, the posterior height of the dorsal arch of the atlas was significantly reduced (Huggare 1989). A negative correlation between the height of the dorsal arch of the atlas and the craniocervical angle was found. Furthermore in non-orthodontically treated children with an Angle class I, Huggare (1989) showed that the height of the dorsal arch could predict the growth of the lower jaw. The taller the posterior arch of the atlas the greater the tendency that growth would produce a square facial type. There seemed to be a general association between vertical development of the cervical column and face (Huggare and Houghton 1995, 1996, Kylämarkula and Huggare 1985).

Soft tissue

In children with reduced muscle tonicity, a higher prevalence of orthodontic anomalies has been investigated (Duyzings 1955, Wachsmann 1960).

Mouth breathing is thought to lead to postural changes such as a clockwise rotation of the mandible, a lowered position of the tongue, and a reclination of the head (Bahnemann 1981, Krakauer and Guilherme 2000, Rubin 1980). These postural changes may relate to characteristic morphological changes (Harvold et al 1973, von Treuenfels 1985). The appearance of a habitual mouth breather is described as 'facies adenoidea'. The term 'long face syndrome' reflects the extraoral characteristic features of a patient with habitual mouth breathing.

Similar observations have been made in patients with obstructive sleep apnea (Solow et al 1984), in children with enlarged tonsils (Behlfelt 1990, Behlfelt et al 1989), and in children with nasal allergy.

In physiotherapy, special treatment phases try to normalize the function of head and neck in order to establish an orthostatic stability of the skull with the spine. A good muscle tonicity in the orofacial region supports an undisturbed posture of the craniocervical region and furthermore of the spine (Aragao 1991, Rocabado 1987, Rocabado et al 1982, Schupp and Zernial 1997).

INTERDISCIPLINARY TREATMENT APPROACH IN CHILDREN WITH KISS SYNDROME

Since November 2001 an interdisciplinary consultation has been established at the Department of Orthodontics at the University of Hamburg. So far, 282 children aged 2–10 years (male : female = 2 : 1) have been examined at the Department of Orthodontics and at the clinic for manual therapy in children in Eckernförde. A clinical and radiological orthopedic examination was performed with particular attention to posture. The medical history of the examined children revealed at least one of the following symptoms: retarded motor patterns, retarded speech development, bad posture and vegetative illness such as headache. The evaluation of functional motion analysis as well as a radiological examination revealed in all children an anatomical and functional asymmetry of the cervical spine. After applying manual therapy, intra- and extraoral records and orofacial dysfunction were evaluated in all patients at the Department of Orthodontics. Seventy-six percent of the children showed orthodontic disorders. No correlations could be detected between the individual orthodontic records such as midline shift, sagittal jaw relationship, side of the crossbite and orthopedic pathologies. A high percentage of orofacial dysfunction was diagnosed in these children: 62%

of the children had weak orofacial muscles, and in 89% an abnormal swallowing pattern was found; 72% breathed habitually through the mouth. Although those children were undergoing treatment, myofunctional therapy had so far been neglected. Myofunctional therapy was started in two-thirds of the children and early orthodontic treatment in one-third of them. The authors concluded that the soft tissues and orofacial function seem to influence the pathology of malocclusion and orthopedic disorders. The high percentage of orthodontic treatment needed in children with orthopedic pathologies suggests an interaction of the hard tissues – jaw and spine – as well.

INTERACTIVE SYSTEM OF FUNCTIONAL BOXES

The soft tissues and orofacial function/dysfunction seem to be important factors in the pathology of malocclusion and orthopedic disorders. The combination of orthodontic disorders and orthopedic pathologies suggests that there is an interaction of the hard tissues – jaw and spine. Early orthodontic screening of children should therefore also focus on symmetric posture and function as well as on the balance of orofacial power.

To provide an explanation the following model was set up to describe the observed correlation between orofacial function and diagnostic findings: The orofacial and craniocervical region is anatomically divided into different boxes that are combined by function (Fig. 13.8). Dysfunction within one box could lead to disorder in another box. Therefore, the different boxes with different functions are combined interactively.

Some interactions have been proven so far, but the overall view has not yet been revealed.

The functional boxes are defined as follows:

- The nose with the important role of habitual nose breathing.
- The lips as the entrance to the mouth are important for nasal respiration and tongue function.

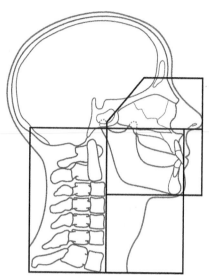

Figure 13.8 The interactive system of the functional boxes is a model to better understand the interactions of the different anatomical regions of the skull. Although each box is a system of its own, impeded function can lead to disorders within a different box. Successful treatment can only be achieved by taking the whole system into account.

Lip closure is thought to be one important condition for establishing nose breathing and somatic tongue function.

- The oral cavity with the tongue and dental occlusion. Swallowing and speech are the two important functions within this box.
- The infra- and suprahyoid muscles that contribute to an orthostatic equilibrium of the lowest part of the skull.
- The upper cervical vertebrae for the stabilization and movement of the head.

Under normal conditions, the different boxes interact in function and support each other. An equilibrium is established, and normal development is possible.

If the balance of power between the different boxes is disturbed or destroyed and bodily compensation is not possible, normal function and development is impaired. Therefore, it is very important for each medical specialty not only to examine the specific box but also to have an overall view of the whole system. Only by doing so can stable treatment results be achieved by maintaining the balance of power.

Further clinical investigation is being conducted in order to provide scientific evidence for the interaction between the different boxes.

CONCLUSION

Even though many different working groups have conducted an interdisciplinary treatment approach in children with orthopedic disorders, no clear therapeutic recommendations based on scientific evidence have been established so far.

Early treatment is recommended for children with severe orthopedic anomalies such as torticollis and scoliosis: in order to harmonize facial and postural symmetry an early bilateral treatment approach should be sought. In some cases the suspicion of an orthopedic disorder such as torticollis or scoliosis can be confirmed by orthodontic diagnosis of a crossbite.

Some authors propose a routine dental examination in cases of deviant head posture in order to start treatment at an early age. A proper treatment approach in young children should consider any condition affecting head posture and the development of the high upper cervical spine.

Radiological examination in two planes reveals skeletal deviations and clinical inspection confirms symmetry in function. A tool for clinical examination of the orofacial region can be offered by the system of functional boxes. Each medical specialty should extend the clinical view. In cases of extreme deviations the patient should be referred to the corresponding medical specialty as early as possible in order to harmonize the proper development of the orofacial and cervical region.

References

Alavi D G, BeGole E A, Schneider B J 1988 Facial and dental arch asymmetries in class II subdivision malocclusion. American Journal of Orthodontics and Dentofacial Orthopedics 93:38–46

Aragao W 1991 Aragao's function regulator, the stomatognathic system and postural changes in children. Journal of Clinical Pediatric Dentistry 15:226–231

Azuma Y, Maehara K, Tokunaga T et al 1999 Systematic effects of the occlusal destruction in guinea pigs. In Vivo 13:519–524

Bahnemann F 1981 Über das Mundatmungs-Syndrom und seine Bedeutung in der Zahn-, Mund-und Kieferheilkunde. Quintessenz 32:337–343

Balters W 1964 Die Wirbelsäule aus der Sicht des Zahnarztes. Zahnärztliche Mitteilungen 9:408–412

Behlfelt K 1990 Enlarged tonsils and the effect of tonsillectomy. Characteristics of the dentition and facial skeleton. Posture of the head, hyoid bone and tongue. Mode of breathing. Swedish Dental Journal, Supplement 72:1–35

Behlfelt K, Linder-Aronson S, McWilliam J et al 1989 Dentition in children with enlarged tonsils compared to control children. European Journal of Orthodontics 11:416–429

Biedermann H 1991 Kopfgelenk-induzierte Symmetriestörungen bei Kleinkindern. Kinderarzt 22:1475–1482

Biedermann H, Koch L 1996 Zur Differentialdiagnose des KISS-Syndroms. Manuelle Medizin 34:73–81

Bishara S E, Burkey P S, Kharouf J G 1994 Dental and facial asymmetries: a review. Angle Orthodontist 2:89–98

Broadbent B H 1931 A new technique and its application to Orthodontics. Angle Orthodontist 1:45–66

Christ B 1993 Anatomische Besonderheiten des Halses. Manuelle Medizin 31:67–68

Collignon J, Varlet I, Robertson E J 1996 Relationship between asymmetric nodal expression and the direction of embryonic turning. Nature 381:155–158

Delaire J 1977 Recidives de prognathies mandibulaires par troubles de la statique cervicale. Revue de Stomatologie et de Chirurgie Maxillofaciale 78:173–185

Dußler E, Raab P, Kunz B et al 2002 Mandibuläre Mittellinienverschiebungen und Asymmetrien des Halte-und Bewegungsapparates bei Kindern und Jugendlichen. Manuelle Medizin 40:116–119

Duyzings J A C 1955 Kieferorthopädie und Körperhaltung. Deutsche Zahnärztliche Zeitschrift 10:19–21

Festa F, Dattilio M, Vecchiet F 1997 Effects of horizontal oscillation of the mandible on the spinal column of the rat in vivo using radiographic monitoring. Orthognathodontia Italiana 6:539–550

Fischer B 1954 Asymmetries of the dentofacial complex. Angle Orthodontist 24:179–192

Gresham H, Smithells P A 1954 Cervical and mandibular posture. Dental Record 74:261–264

Gutmann G 1981 Funktionelle Pathologie und Klinik der Wirbelsäule. Vol 1: Die Halswirbelsäule. Part 1: Die funktionsanalytische Röntgendiagnostik der Halswirbel und der Kopfgelenke. Fischer, Stuttgart

Harvold E P, Vargervik K, Chierici G 1973 Primate experiments on oral sensation and dental malocclusion. American Journal of Orthodontics 63:494–508

Hellsing E, Reigo T, McWilliam J et al 1987 Cervical and lumbar lordosis and thoracic kyphosis in 8, 11 and 15-year-old children. European Journal of Orthodontics 9:129–138

Hirschfelder H, Hirschfelder U 1982a Die Halswirbelsäule im seitlichen Fernröntgenbild aus orthopädischer Sicht. Fortschritte der Kieferorthopädie 43:52–56

Hirschfelder U, Hirschfelder H 1982b Veränderungen der oberen Halswirbelsäule bei Patienten des progenen Formenkreises. Deutsche Zahnärztliche Zeitschrift 37:692–697

Hirschfelder U, Hirschfelder H 1983 Auswirkungen der Skoliose auf den Gesichtsschädel. Fortschritte der Kieferorthopädie 44:457–467

Hirschfelder U, Hirschfelder H 1987 Sagittale Kieferrelation und Wirbelsäulenhaltung: Untersuchungen zur Frage einer Abhängigkeit. Fortschritte der Kieferorthopädie 48:436–448

Hirschfelder U, Hirschfelder H 1991 Untersuchung zur Kopfhaltung im Fernröntgenseitenbild. Fortschritte der Kieferorthopädie 52:302–309

Hofrath H 1931 Die Bedeutung von Röntgenfern-und Abstandsaufnahme für die Diagnostik der Kieferanomalien. Fortschritte der Orthodontie 1:232–258

Howard J T 1983 The effects of gnathologic orthopedics on the cervical spine. International Journal of Orthodontics 21:12–19

Huggare J 1989 The first cervical vertebra as an indicator of mandibular growth. European Journal of Orthodontics 11:10–16

Huggare J 1998 Postural disorders and dentofacial morphology. Acta Odontologica Scandinavica 56:383–386

Huggare J, Houghton P 1995 Asymmetry in the human skeleton. A study on prehistoric Polynesians and Thais. European Journal of Morphology 33:3–14

Huggare J, Houghton P 1996 Associations between atlantoaxial and craniomandibular anatomy. Growth, Development, and Aging 60:21–30

Huggare J, Kylämarkula S 1985 Morphology of the first cervical vertebra in children with enlarged adenoids. European Journal of Orthodontics 7:93–96

Kahl-Nieke B 2001 Einführung in die Kieferorthopädie, 2nd edn. Urban & Fischer, Munich

Kiliaridis S, Bresin A, Holm J et al 1996a Effects of masticatory muscle function on bone mass in the mandible of the growing rat. Acta Anatomica 155:200–205

Kiliaridis S, Engstrom C, Lindskog-Stokland B et al 1996b Craniofacial bone remodelling in growing rats fed a low-calcium and vitamin-D-deficient diet and the influence of masticatory muscle function. Acta Odontologica Scandinavica 54:320–326

Koch L E, Graumann-Brunt S 1999 Kopfgelenk-induzierte Symmetriestörungen und deren Folgepathologien. Manuelle Medizin 37:67–78

Krakauer L H, Guilherme A 2000 Relationship between mouth breathing and postural alterations of children: a descriptive analysis. International Journal of Orofacial Myology 26:13–23

Kylämarkula S, Huggare J 1985 Head posture and the morphology of the first cervical vertebra. European Journal of Orthodontics 7:151–156

Lippold C, Ehmer U, van den Bos L 2000 Beziehungen zwischen kieferorthopädischen und orthopädischen Befunden. Manuelle Medizin 38:346–350

Lukanowa-Skopakowa K 1987 Zahn-Kiefer-Deformierungen und Verkrümmungen der Wirbelsäule. Fortschritte der Kieferorthopadie 48:429–435

Lundstrom A 1961 Some asymmetries of the dental arches, jaws, and skull, and their etiological significance. American Journal of Orthodontics 47:81–106

Manning J T, Chamberlain A T 1994 Fluctuating asymmetry in gorilla canines: a sensitive indicator of environmental stress. Proceedings of the Royal Society of London, Biological Sciences 255:189–193

Meno C, Saijoh Y, Fujii H et al 1996 Left-right asymmetric expression of the TGF beta-family member lefty in mouse embryos. Nature 381:151–155

Mertensmeier I, Diedrich P 1992 Der Zusammenhang von Halswirbelsäulenstellung und Gebissanomalien. Fortschritte der Kieferorthopädie 53:26–32

Müller-Wachendorff R 1961 Untersuchungen über die Häufigkeit des Auftretens von Gebißanomalien in Verbindung mit Skelettdeformierungen mit besonderer Berücksichtigung der Skoliosen. Fortschritte der Kieferorthopädie 22:399–408

Nobili A, Adversi R 1996 Relationship between posture and occlusion: a clinical and experimental investigation. Cranio 14:274–285

Pečina M, Lulic-Dukic O, Pečina-Hrnčević A 1991 Hereditary orthodontic anomalies and idiopathic scoliosis. International Orthopaedics 15:57–59

Pirttiniemi P M 1994 Associations of mandibular and facial asymmetries – a review. American Journal of Orthodontics and Dentofacial Orthopedics 106: 191–200

Pirttiniemi P 1998 Normal and increased functional asymmetries in the craniofacial area. Acta Odontologica Scandinavica 56:342–345

Pirttiniemi P, Lahtela P, Huggare J, Serlo W 1989 Head posture and dentofacial asymmetries in surgically treated muscular torticollis patients. Acta Odontologica Scandinavica 47:193–197

Pirttiniemi P, Kantomaa T, Lahtela P 1990 Relationship between craniofacial and condyle path asymmetry in unilateral crossbite patients. European Journal of Orthodontics 12:408–413

Poikela A, Kantomaa T, Tuominen M et al 1995 Effect of unilateral masticatory function on craniofacial growth in the rabbit. European Journal of Oral Sciences 103:106–111

Poikela A, Kantomaa T, Pirttiniemi P 1997 Craniofacial growth after a period of unilateral masticatory function in young rabbits. European Journal of Oral Sciences 105:331–337

Prager A 1980 Vergleichende Untersuchungen über die Häufigkeit von Zahnstellungs-und Kieferanomalien bei Patienten mit Deformitäten der Wirbelsäule. Fortschritte der Kieferorthopadie 41:163–168

Raadsheer M C, Kiliaridis S, Van Eijden T M et al 1996 Masseter muscle thickness in growing individuals and its relation to facial morphology. Archives of Oral Biology 41:323–332

Ridder P-H 1998 Kieferfunktionsstörungen und Zahnfehlstellungen mit ihren Auswirkungen auf die Körperperipherie. Manuelle Medizin 36:194–212

Rocabado M 1987 The importance of soft tissue mechanics in stability and instability of the cervical spine: a functional diagnosis for treatment planning. Cranio 5:130–138

Rocabado M, Johnston B E, Blakney M G 1982 Physical therapy and dentistry: an overview. Journal of Craniomandibular Practice 1:46–49

Rubin R M 1980 Mode of respiration and facial growth. American Journal of Orthodontics 78:504–510

Rude J 1987 Kompensationsmechanismen von Schädelasymmetrien. Fortschritte der Kieferorthopadie 48:541–546

Sandikcioglu M, Skov S, Solow B 1994 Atlas morphology in relation to craniofacial morphology and head posture. European Journal of Orthodontics 16:96–103

Schupp W, Zernial P 1997 Diagnostik und Therapie in der Kieferorthopädie unter gesamtheitlichen Aspekten. Quintessenz 48:949–963

Schwarz A M 1926 Kopfhaltung und Kiefer. Zeitschrift für Stomatologie 24:669–744

Siegel M I, Doyle W J 1975 Stress and fluctuating limb asymmetry in various species of rodents. Growth 39:363–369

Solow B, Sandham A 2002 Cranio-cervical posture: a factor in the development and function of the dentofacial structures. European Journal of Orthodontics 24:447–456

Solow B, Siersbæk-Nielsen S 1992 Cervical and craniocervical posture as predictors of craniofacial growth. American Journal of Orthodontics and Dentofacial Orthopedics 101:449–458

Solow B, Sonnesen L 1998 Head posture and malocclusions. European Journal of Orthodontics 20:685–693

Solow B, Tallgren A 1977 Dentoalveolar morphology in relation to craniocervical posture. Angle Orthodontist 47:157–164

Solow B, Siersbæk-Nielsen S, Greve E 1984 Airway adequacy, head posture and craniofacial morphology. American Journal of Orthodontics 86:214–223

Sterzik G, Graßhoff H, Lentschow B 1992 Morphologische Verknüpfungen von Eugnathien, Gebißanomalien der Klasse II/1 und Klasse III mit Veränderungen der Topographie der Halswirbelsäule im Fernröntgenseitenbild. Fortschritte der Kieferorthopadie 53:69–76

Vig P S, Hewitt A B 1975 Asymmetry of the human facial skeleton. Angle Orthodontist 45:125–129

von Treuenfels H 1983 Die Relation von Atlasposition, prognather und progener Kieferanomalie. Zeitschrift für Orthopadie 121:657–664

von Treuenfels H 1984 Kopfhaltung, Atlasposition und Atemfunktion beim offenen Biß. Fortschritte der Kieferorthopadie 45:111–121

von Treuenfels H 1985 Orofaziale Dyskinesien als Ausdruck einer gestörten Wechselbeziehung von Atmung, Verdauung und Bewegung. Fortschritte der Kieferorthopadie 46:191–206

Wachsmann K 1960 Über den Zusammenhang der Gebißanomalien mit Krümmungen der Wirbelsäule und schlaffer Körperhaltung. Fortschritte der Kieferorthopadie 21:449–453

Zilles K, Dabringhaus A, Geyer S et al 1996 Structural asymmetries in the human forebrain and the forebrain of non-human primates and rats. Neuroscience and Biobehavioral Reviews 20:593–605

GLOSSARY

analysis of lateral cephalograms the tracing of the lateral cephalogram provides information of the skeletal pattern, i.e. the quality of mandibular growth (clockwise or counter-clockwise direction) and sagittal position of the upper and lower jaw within the skull. Lateral cephalograms are taken in a standardized position: the patient is fixed by ear olives and a glabella rod. A radiograph taken in this way does not reveal a reproducible position of the head and does not demonstrate the natural head position.

Angle class I normal relationship of the molars, premolars and canines, which means that the mesiobuccal cusp of the upper molar occludes in the buccal groove of the lower molar.

Angle class II sagittal malocclusion: the lower first molar is positioned distally to the upper first molar in comparison to the Angle class I occlusion.

Angle class III sagittal malocclusion: the lower first molar is positioned mesially to the upper first molar in comparison to the Angle class I occlusion.

crossbite a deviation from the normal buccolingual relation of the teeth. A crossbite can be located frontal, lateral, bilateral and unilateral.

deep bite an increased overjet. In severe cases the lower incisors occlude traumatically with the palatal mucosa.

dental malocclusion disorder due to dental malposition. Dental malocclusion can be corrected at any age.

dental midline shift midline discrepancy due to dental deviations of the midline, i.e. an asymmetrical extraction of a tooth can lead to dental midline shift.

distal the opposite of a mesial direction.

early orthodontic treatment normal orthodontic treatment starts with the eruption of canines and premolars (late mixed dentition), which normally begins at the age of 10 years. Early orthodontic treatment may start directly after birth (i.e. in patients with cleft lip and palate), in the primary dentition or during the early mixed dentition, when incisors change and the first molars erupt. The aim of early interceptive treatment is to harmonize the development of the different jaws to each other. One indication of early orthodontic treatment is the correction of a lateral crossbite.

facies adenoidea the extraoral manifestation of patients with facies adenoidea includes narrow width dimensions, protruded incisors, incompetent lips/no lips closure. The clinical appearance has often been attributed to habitual mouth breathing.

habit a dysfunction of an unconscious nature such as a sucking habit, tongue thrust, abnormal swallowing pattern, mouth breathing, etc. Habits are physiological to a certain age in early childhood. Depending on the intensity of the dysfunction and age of the patient, a persisting habit can lead to dental and skeletal disorders.

long face syndrome excessive lower anterior facial height.

mesial describes the direction in the sagittal plane towards the frontal midline.

midline discrepancies inconsistency of upper and lower midline, which can be skeletal or dental in nature.

midline shift of the mandible skeletal discrepancy in the transversal plane.

occlusal plane defined by the buccal cusps of the upper premolars and the mesio-buccal cusps of the upper first molars.

open bite although the lateral teeth are in occlusion the incisors do not contact.

overjet distance between the upper and lower incisors in the horizontal plane.

overbite overlap of the incisors in the vertical plane.

posterior-anterior cephalogram gives an assessment of the skeletal situation in the transversal and vertical plane.

protrusion a proclined inclination of the incisors.

retrusion a retruded inclination of the incisors.

sagittal jaw position position of the upper/lower jaw within the skull. It is of therapeutic interest to know the cause of a skeletal deviation in order to treat efficiently: i.e. a skeletal class III can be caused by a pathological mesial position of the lower jaw and/or by a distal position of the upper jaw.

sigmatism disturbances in the articulation of 's'.

skeletal anomaly three-dimensional deviations of the position of the upper and lower jaw which should be treated skeletally. During growth, skeletal anomalies can be corrected to a certain extent orthopedically by the orthodontist. In adolescence, skeletal problems can be corrected surgically or by dental compensation.

skeletal class I normal balanced relationship between upper and lower jaw which can be assessed by analysis of the lateral cephalogram in terms of an angle or the distance between a defined landmark at the maxilla and mandible.

skeletal class II increased (positive) sagittal distance between maxilla and mandible.

skeletal class III decreased (negative) sagittal distance between maxilla and mandible. In severe cases the landmark of the mandible is ahead of the landmark of the maxilla. Consequences of this skeletal discrepancy are a decrease in the overjet and a concave profile.

The different levels: practical aspects of manual therapy in children

Chapter 14

Practicalities of manual therapy in children
Interaction with parents and children, tricks and tips for diagnosis and follow-up

H. Biedermann

COMMUNICATION PROBLEMS

A lot of things happen before we see a child and the family for the first time. The most important step is to draw the family's attention to the fact that manual therapy may have something to offer in resolving their particular problem.

The professionals we interact with can be divided in two broad groups. The larger group comprises the 'classic' pediatricians whose worldview is that of an internist, i.e. predominantly patho-morphologically oriented. The smaller group is made up of neuropediatricians, physiotherapists and other caregivers who – through their professional experience – are already in contact with the possibilities of functional pathology.

These two groups have big problems communicating with each other. They may know about the other's language, but even then understanding does not come naturally.

Most of the pediatricians we collaborate with are social pediatricians and neuropediatricians, doctors trained in rehabilitation and care of disabled children. Because they use physiotherapy extensively in their planning, they have at least a notion of the possibilities such an approach can offer. The functional approach is not new to them.

In most cases the first patients referred to us are those with clear 'mechanical' problems, i.e. a postural asymmetry or muscular imbalance. After the first contact, these colleagues are as a rule very astonished that other – in their eyes non-related – problems have been resolved, too. Chapter 10, by Kühnen, provides a few such case histories.

The communication with physiotherapists is easier. They know first-hand how much interaction there is between the muscular system and the autonomic system, to name but two, and they are aware of the power of the functional approach. At least in Germany they depend on referrals from medical doctors, and they cannot refer patients directly, at least not officially. In reality there often is such a trusting relationship between the mothers and the physiotherapists that they have more influence than is apparent at first sight.

However, it cannot hurt to explain one's point of view as clearly as possible, which is one reason why we have drawn up several leaflets for parents concerning the main indications for manual therapy in children.

LEAFLET FOR KISS CHILDREN

We send the following leaflet to parents in preparation for the first visit.

You will bring your baby to us for treatment in the next week, most probably after a conversation with your pediatrician or physiotherapist. To complement the information you received there we would like to give you some explanation regarding our diagnosis and treatment.

During more than twenty years of treating children and babies we have discovered how problems of fixed posture and unbalanced symmetry can be improved by an adapted therapy of the spinal column at the neck. My friend and teacher Gutmann started this in the 1950s and we have been able to systematize this since. Meanwhile we have treated more than 25 000 infants under the age of two.

Based on this extensive experience we came to some general conclusions.

The most important problem regarding the spine and the neck is the *KISS syndrome*, Kinematic Imbalances due to Suboccipital Strain. The main symptoms we encounter in these cases are:

- wry neck
- fixed and bent trunk
- asymmetry of the face
- flattened back of the head
- asymmetrical use of arms and legs.

Often these problems coincide with sleeping disorders, difficulties of breastfeeding on one side, colic or incessant crying.

We do not know beforehand how much we can help in individual cases by treating the upper part of the spine, but in two-thirds of our patients, one treatment is sufficient to achieve a thorough improvement or at least a more solid base for further physiotherapy, simplifying future treatments.

Comparing our young patients to the general statistics available we found some risk factors: a difficult birth with the use of vacuum extractors or forceps, prolonged labor and/or breech position of the unborn increase the probability of KISS. We see twins much more frequently, too. If one of your children has already had successful treatment for KISS the likelihood of similar problems is much greater if the newborn is of the same sex.

All these observations are based on statistical analysis, which means that we have to examine every individual case separately, albeit with a bigger chance of finding the corresponding results.

Radiographs:
To examine the baby thoroughly a radiograph of the cervical spine is essential. Without this we cannot come to a firm decision as to whether your baby needs treatment or not. During the first year, one plate is sufficient in most cases; if ever we need more plates we shall explain the reasons to you. In children who are older than 2 years, we

need two plates, one from the side and one frontal picture.

As technology of films has improved considerably during the last decades the amount of radiation needed for a plate is about 10–20% of what was necessary in the 1970s and 1980s. Digital equipment has reduced this further. Compared to a plate of the lungs and thorax the dose used for the neck is negligible. Having said that I want to accentuate that we do not order these plates thoughtlessly. We think that the information obtainable from them more than warrants the necessary exposure.

If ever you have any more questions don't hesitate to ask us.

The treatment:

As we found out in analyzing our treatments the success rate is much higher when we can make sure that the babies were not treated elsewhere in the 2 weeks preceding your first visit. Accidents immediately prior to this date, or an acute infection with fever, are not a good base for examination and treatment, either. In this case do not hesitate to phone us, and we can postpone your date. It is better for the child to wait a few days and be seen in the best possible circumstances.

Based on the evaluation of the radiographs, your report and the examination of the baby, we come to a decision about the best treatment. In most cases this will consist of a manipulation of one or several levels of the spinal column. The exact technique used in an individual case depends on a lot of factors, e.g. the age and mood of the baby. We shall ask your permission to treat beforehand, as the best way to proceed is to move on smoothly from examination to the treatment – not least to spare the mother's additional stress. Most parents are not aware of the moment of manipulation and are a bit astonished (and relieved) to get the baby back so soon.

Nobody should be so arrogant to exclude any risk 100%, but to our knowledge there have never been any serious complications in manual therapy of babies. Incidences in the treatment of adults

concern, in almost every case, improper techniques, repeated manipulations and superficial examination prior to treatment.

What do the parents tell us?

Most parents mention some (but not all) of the following items in their case history:

- fixed posture of the head to one side or to the back
- insufficient control of the head
- fixed retroflexion of the head with arms pulled back ('parachutist')
- fixed posture while sleeping, with head bent back
- difficulties getting the child to sleep
- often waking up at night, crying
- asymmetry of the movements and use of arms and legs
- asymmetry of the posture of the trunk
- uneven maturation of the hip joints
- pes adductus (i.e. a bent and curved foot)
- highly irritable neck; the baby does not want to be touched there
- 'head banging' – the baby bangs its head against the sides of the bed
- asymmetry of the facial features
- flattened and asymmetrical back of the head
- asymmetrical position of the ears
- colic
- incessant crying.

These complaints can have a lot of different causes, but when they are found in combination – and when there is a prompt improvement after our therapy – it seems fair to say that problems of the cervical spine were at least partly responsible.

Some remarks about further development:

Three to four weeks after our treatment your child should be examined by a proficient specialist at home, be it the pediatrician or a physiotherapist. These colleagues determine if and what further treatment is necessary. If they decide that you ought to come back to us for a check-up (which is the case in about 15%) we would like to see your child 6–8 weeks after the first visit.

We strongly advise some rest for the cervical spine after our treatment. Therefore we would like to ask you to stop any physiotherapy during that time. We also would like you to refrain from any sport or exercise which might put stress on the neck, i.e. a header or head dive, etc. After these 3 weeks it is much easier to judge if and what kind of additional treatment is necessary. About a third of the babies will need additional help, mostly physiotherapy.

Manual therapy and physiotherapy can and should be combined. A baby who is successfully treated with manual therapy profits more from physiotherapy or speech therapy and the professional attention of these specialists helps to control the outcome of our efforts, too. Any rush in adding as much as possible therapeutically worsens the result, and the necessary patience is something which has to be learnt conscientiously.

Parents who have seen the sometimes dramatic improvement due to manual therapy tend to be overly concerned afterwards. We do not have to exaggerate; in almost every case there are no special precautions necessary after manual therapy. It suffices to avoid direct irritation of the neck during these 2–3 weeks.

If the child catches a cold, a temporary relapse into the old postural pattern is possible. If this lasts only a few days, no further measures are necessary. If it lasts for more than a week it might be fitting to consult us or another specialist, e.g. your physiotherapist at home. If in doubt, do not hesitate to contact us by phone or email.

Our experience has shown that a routine check-up at the age of 3 is very useful. We often find minor dysfunctions which were not apparent earlier but could cause more trouble if left alone too long.

The next check-up is usefully scheduled around the first school year. This marks the transition from the free-wheeling baby period to the more sedentary lifestyle of a schoolchild. Any functional problem of the musculoskeletal system tends to be aggravated by this reduction of exercise and these disorders often manifest themselves in a way that does not help to see the connection with a biomechanical base of the situation.

Babies with a family where scoliosis or other orthopedic problems occur should be screened more thoroughly than other children, be it at home by their pediatrician or at a specialist clinic.

LEAFLET FOR KIDD CHILDREN, i.e. schoolchildren

Today you came for the first time with your child to be examined and treated. Most probably you have already talked with your pediatrician and/or physiotherapist about it. To complement their information we would like to give you some information about the kind of therapy we provide and its possibilities (and limits). This leaflet should help you to formulate further questions.

During the last decades we have learned to look at many problems of schoolchildren from the viewpoint of spinal disorder. Think, for example, of headaches: most have their main origin in disorders of the spine. The prime candidates for such an examination of the spine are problems of posture and maladroit movements.

One example may help in understanding how these problems can go much further than that.

A child cannot move its head freely – and often this problem started very early on. The constraints of neck mobility have to be compensated further down, i.e. at the thoracic level. An untrained observer might not notice much about the restrictions of the neck mobility due to this compensation mechanism, but the eye–hand coordination depends on it as much as the equilibrium and the ability to orient oneself in a given space.

This malfunctioning confronts the child with many difficulties when the causal connection with the spinal apparatus is not obvious at first sight:

- Early on (in the months after birth) we can find a fixed posture, colic, incessant crying and a non-standard motor development.

- Later on these children often have problems learning to bicycle or walking on stilts.
- Lack of confidence in their own perception often leads to fear of heights and being afraid of unknown situations.
- Bad coordination results in clumsiness – they are regarded as fools (and sometimes these children cultivate a clown image to conceal their inabilities).
- With poor spatial orientation comes a hearing impairment, especially in filtering out background noises and concentrating on one person. These children seem to lack concentration when, in fact, they are just tired of having to concentrate too much.
- With such a difficult base for their perception these children become as frustrated as we adults would be in such a situation; they are easily annoyed and irritable. They acquire a reputation of being impatient, aggressive and that 'they never listen'.
- Too slow, too timid, too clumsy – many of these children withdraw and avoid situations where they fear not being up to the task. Those around them often reinforce this attitude through their refusal to play with them, or to help them over minor problems – and a vicious circle sets in.

The broad spectrum of the situation described here makes it evident that it fits many cases. Almost every child has a phase where one or more of these items fit in, certainly those children with the label 'hyperactive'. But this little cascade of events shows, too, how minor problems of motor coordination can get built up till they reach serious proportions and influence the entire life of such a child and its family.

When does it make sense to think of a problem of the vertebral spine as being at the root of these disorders? Basically always when coordination problems, headaches and postural imbalances are involved. If one finds an impairment of function in these children, a test manipulation should be made to decide if and how much the spine is part of the problem. It is not for nothing that the word 'posture' has a double meaning. . .

Our therapy aims at restoring the function of the entire spine. The most important areas are the junctions of the spine with the head and the pelvis, i.e. the suboccipital region and the iliosacral joints. Beginning here the entire spinal apparatus is examined and if necessary treated.

At the first session we normally find quite a few of these blockages all over the spine. Most of them vanish after the 'big' problems are taken care of. Once the upper cervical spine moves freely again most blockages in lower regions of the cervical spine and the thorax subside spontaneously, so we do not have to treat every blockage we find on the way.

Once the functioning of the spine is restored, we strongly advise allowing the body enough time to reorganize its motor patterns. Years ago we realized that the results of our treatment were *better* when the manipulation was not immediately followed by another therapy. So we advise that children be given 2–3 weeks to adapt, before further evaluation of the situation by the physiotherapist who knows the condition of the patient. In some cases we propose modifications to the exercises applied, but mostly we leave these decisions to the pediatricians and physiotherapists who already know the child. Equally important is to avoid unnecessary stress to the neck, i.e. somersaults or headers. During the week after manipulation we would advise you to refrain from sport completely, as the skills might be temporarily diminished and a certain amount of roughness is almost unavoidable in any sport.

In quite a few cases children complain about aching muscles and headaches. Some mention that 'my head seems to sit differently on my shoulders' or 'my neck feels lighter than before'. Such comments show how far the reorganization of the motor system goes. The best strategy is to wait and leave the child alone. Some analgesics may be necessary, but in most cases a bit of sympathy and a warm compress is sufficient.

The best interval between the treatment and the check-up seems to be 6–8 weeks. It helps to have some time after the treatment to enable you to judge the effects on your child.

The opinion of the (nursery-) school teachers, coaches and physiotherapists is very important to us. Try to get their opinion before you come back for the check-up. Based on your report and the examination we shall discuss the developments and what was achieved. Then we can see what other measures have to be taken – if any. In quite a few cases it suffices to monitor the development of the child rather loosely, i.e. once or twice a year. If ever something happens that worries you, these check-ups can be brought forward.

The following questionnaire [see Figs 14.1–14.3] is based on a well-established protocol. The questions are necessarily vague, but we shall ask you to fill out such a questionnaire every time you come back. This has proved very useful for the follow-up.

THE MAN DRAWING TEST

To assess the actual situation of a schoolchild, a lot of different tests are on offer. Most of them require quite some time and the aid of a qualified helper. Most children coming to see us have already done one of these tests. We do not want to confront them with yet another of these questionnaires as such an enquiry reflects on the child's self-perception, too.

On one hand we have at our disposal enough information to come to a qualified judgment of the child's sensorimotor and intellectual development – at least in most cases. On the other hand these data are not comparable and to assess the effects of our therapy we would have to repeat the same questionnaires or ask the specialists who did the first tests to repeat them. This is in most cases not practicable.

To minimize the impact of such a standard test on children and to keep the necessary time within the constraints of a consultation, we opted for a mixed approach. We ask the parents to fill in the questionnaire shown in Figures 14.1–14.3 – which can be done very quickly – and ask the children to do a drawing containing a house, a tree and a person.

Some examples of the 'before and after' are shown in Figures 14.4 and 14.5, and needless to say, not all of the drawings depict these amazing improvements. The combination of the two types

Observation	Grading the activity Tick the appropriate box (how often)			
	Not at all (0)	A little bit (1)	Rather often (2)	Always (3)
Restless				
Impulsive				
Disturbs other children				
Short attention span, does not finish the work				
Constant fidgeting				
Inattentive, easily divertible				
Cannot wait, easily disappointed				
Cries quickly				
Mood changes quickly and drastically				
Prone to fits of rage				
Starts a lot and does not finish the work				

Figure 14.1 Parents' questionnaire. Based on Conners Parent Rating Scale (Sorensen et al 1982).

Observation	Grading the activity			
	0	1	2	3
Restless		X	X	
Impulsive		X	X	
Disturbs other children		X	X	
Short attention span, does not finish his work			X	
Constant fidgeting		X		X
Inattentive, easily divertible				X
Cannot wait, quickly disappointed	X			X
Cries quickly	X	X		
Mood changes quickly and drastically	X		X	
Prone to fits of rage	X	X		

Figure 14.2   Completed parents' questionnaire – example 1 (Daniel, 9 years). White crosses: parents' comments before treatment. Black crosses: parents' comments after treatment.

Observation	Grading the activity			
	0	1	2	3
Restless		X		X
Impulsive		X		
Disturbs other children	X	X		
Short attention span, does not finish his work	X		X	
Constant fidgeting			X	X
Inattentive, easily divertible			X	
Cannot wait, quickly disappointed		X		X
Cries quickly	X	X		
Mood changes quickly and drastically	X			
Prone to fits of rage	X			

Figure 14.3   Completed parents' questionnaire – example 2 (Simon, 9 years). White crosses: parents' comments before treatment. Black crosses: parents' comments after treatment.

of information gives us nevertheless some insight into the direction of the development since the first visit. Quite often the parents tell us that 'nothing really changed' and the comparison of the list and the drawing says something different. In putting the first and second drawing or questionnaire next to each other we can use them to discuss with the parents if their initial comment holds true. We have to keep in mind that some of these developments are rather slow and that it is difficult for the parents to be aware of such a gradual improvement, as they are in contact with their children every day. Quite frequently these improvements are more easily seen by an aunt who visits the family only every few months than by the mother or father.

We started asking for these drawings about 4 years ago and in doing so we realized that some details have to be standardized, too. The children have to have a good table to sit at, we have to ask the parents to refrain from helping and it is probably better not to use colors. On one hand one learns a lot from the use of colors, e.g. if the child is able to limit the coloring to borders. On the other hand this additional dimension distracts from the 'hard' information – both arguments have their merits and we have not yet made any definite decisions about this.

LEAFLET ON POSTURAL PROBLEMS

Dear parents,
We all know the situation depicted here [see Figs 14.6 and 14.7] – and we all know that it does not help a lot to tell the child to 'sit straight'. Twenty to twenty-five seconds later the old posture is back. Unconscious support of the head during school lessons is another well-known problem. Many children in such circumstances start to fidget

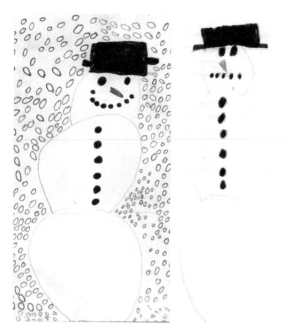

Figure 14.4   The snowman: these two drawings were sent by a mother with the comment: 'My son always drew persons or trees not straight. I got so used to it that I did not notice it any more. A few days after the treatment he suddenly was able to draw straight! So I asked him to make a second drawing of a snowman, which I include here.'

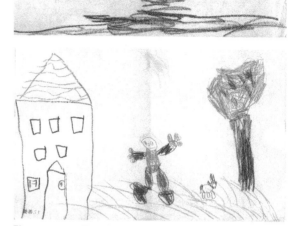

Figure 14.5   Two drawings: these two drawings were made 5 weeks apart by a 6-year-old boy.

and wriggle on their chairs. Before we label them as 'hyperactive' it might help to think about how much sitting still we ask of them at a time when mother nature wants them to move around freely.

The support for the head shown here is in itself not bad; the child tries to minimize the stress on the passive support structures of the head and we have to be alert to this. A child in such a position has to push up to improve its situation.

A lot of money is spent on seats, but often the desk is overlooked. You can do a little experiment yourself: look at somebody who reads a book or a newspaper which is flat in front of him at a table and you can watch how the back of the neck suffers. Once the book is tilted and in a slightly sloping position the reader immediately sits straighter. This stress of the support structures is even stronger in people who have soft ligaments – as all children do. In quite a few of our young patients we found 'special constructions' at the neck vertebrae which complicate the situation even further. As long as this posture is only assumed for a few moments it does not matter too much. But in doing homework, children have to sit like that for lengthy periods of time – and concentrate on the task at hand, which aggravates the situation further. This stress is not felt as pain by most of the younger children; they tend to complain about headache or tiredness and less about neck pain.

During lessons such a tilt desk is not so very important, as the attention shifts from the blackboard and the teacher to the exercise book. Only during tests should we see to it that the surface is tilted, too.

Many parents want to do well and buy desks for their children which can be tilted entirely. In most cases, this is a waste of money. Homework is done in the living-room, the kitchen or the terrace, but

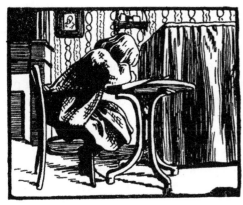

Figure 14.6 Illustration in postural problems leaflet (from a children's book published in 1886).

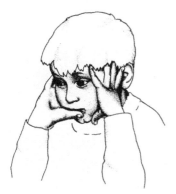

Figure 14.7 Illustration in postural problems leaflet.

seldom at the – expensive – tilt desk. Even if the desk is used, most children refuse to tilt it as everything slides down when they do so.

Our proposal is therefore to supply a removable tilt top which can be carried to where the work is done. Children accept it as soon as they realize how much better they can get on with their homework when such a desktop is used. An angle of 20° seems to be optimal.

Working with computers:

Nowadays, most children start working with computers in primary school. Whereas the posture while working at a computer is in principle better than at a typewriter, there are quite a few aspects which can be annoying, from reflections on the screen or a flickering screen to a jamming keyboard. The height of the support for the keyboard is often too high, which forces children to lift their shoulders and overload the neck muscles. If the children work with material alongside the screen we should take care that these papers or books are positioned correctly. If a book is put next to the keyboard and the gaze shifts back and forth, the head has to do a diagonal movement which only the more robust can handle. Again, this is not that important if the session lasts only a few minutes. Once children are in front of a PC for more than 10 minutes these considerations should be taken into account.

It is especially important to sit right in front of the screen. This demand seems superfluous – till you actually watch your children. You'll be surprised what you find...

AN ONGOING PROCESS

The leaflets reproduced above are some of the material we use to communicate with families, but it is certainly not everything. The selection presented here is to give an idea of how to avoid some of the pitfalls in communication which – if not taken care of – may complicate the interaction needlessly, thus endangering the intended outcome of the treatment.

The way we interact with families and doctors has changed considerably during recent years. Due to the thousands of children who profited from our treatment we enjoy an amount of goodwill (from the doctors) and positive expectations (from the families) inconceivable some years ago. Some of the leaflets we gave out in the 1980s and 1990s would be far too timid nowadays, and the questions asked then ('My GP at home told me there were cases of paraplegia after manual therapy in children') do not come up any more, thankfully. As Gandhi once said, 'First they ignore you, then they laugh at you, then they fight you, then you win'. Let us say we are past stage three, but not yet at stage four. This reflects in the way one has to interact professionally. The question is no longer: 'Does this work at all?' but more if and when manual therapy is best applied.

And, naturally enough, quite a few of those who ridiculed the potential of manual therapy initially switch their position somewhat astonishingly and tell their patients that there is no need to see a specialist as they are able to do that little bit of pushing and cracking themselves.

Luckily, parents are quite picky about what and who gets close to their children, so to protect them from these self-appointed specialists is the lesser problem. The bigger problem seems to be to convince these parents not to do too much.

The majority of patients think the quality of an operation depends only on the skill of the surgeon – and the outcome of manual therapy on the talents of the specialist. In both cases, the 'before' and 'after' are almost as important as the treatment itself. And in both cases, it helps to give the individual who underwent the treatment time to react and not start any additional therapy too early.

So we do like to stress the point that children should not be given additional treatment immediately after having undergone manual therapy. In order to make parents comprehend that this is neither out of disregard for the other healing professions nor to make our contribution more important than it is, we have to tackle this sensitive subject on a case-by-case basis – so no leaflet for this (important) subject.

To find a balance between these competing urges – of the parents (to do whatever it takes to help their children) and the manual therapist (who knows that quite frequently less is more) – needs a lot of tact and sensitivity. These qualities are as elusive as they are essential to achieve a good therapeutic result, and whatever advice one can give is only a small and ephemeral detail in a big picture. So this quote from Antoine de St Exupéry may be appropriate to close this chapter: 'Perfection is achieved, not when there is nothing more to add, but when there is nothing left to take away'.

References

Sorensen J L, Hargreaves W A, Friedlander S 1982 Child global rating scales: selecting a measure of client functioning in a large mental health system. Evaluation Program Planning 5(4):337–347.

Chapter 15

Manual therapy of the sacroiliac joints and pelvic girdle in children

Freddy Huguenin

CHAPTER CONTENTS

INTRODUCTION

To understand the biomechanics of the pelvic girdle one must understand its dysfunctions and determine the axes of treatment. The functional anatomy includes actual sacroiliac articulations, axial sacroiliac articulation and the pubic bones which constitute the elements of the pelvic girdle. Therapeutic actions, always limited to the physiological articular interaction, will respond to a precise palpatory diagnosis based on examination of the areas of sacroiliac and pubic irritation.

ANATOMICAL REMINDERS

Contours of the cartilaginous surfaces of the sacroiliac articulation. The contour of cartilage in vivo has the following features (Fig. 15.1):

- *On the iliac side:* depression of upper and lower limbs, depression of the middle anterior pole.
- *On the sacral side:* elevations corresponding to the depressions of the iliac side.

The consequence of these articular poles – which bring about an interlocking of cartilage – is that only sliding movements are possible. A reduced range of rotation is only possible at the price of a light opening of articulation.

Figure 15.1 Elevations and depressions on the articular surface of the sacroiliac joint, according to H. Weisl. 1, Elevations of the sacral surface. 2, Depressions of the iliac surface (adapted with permission from Weisl H 1954 The articular surfaces of the sacroiliac joint and their relation to the movement of the sacrum. Acta Anatomica (S. Karger AG, Basel) 22:1-14).

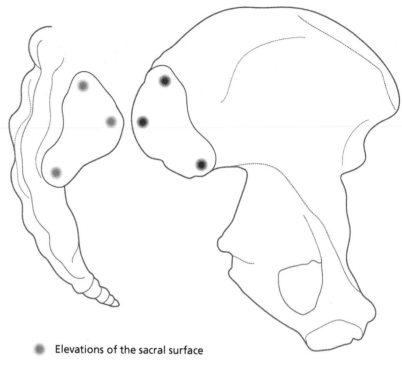

● Elevations of the sacral surface

● Depressions of the iliac surface

Figure 15.2 Axial sacroiliac joint according to Bakland. S, sacral cavity; P, prominence (*pyramide iliaque*) (adapted from Bakland O, Hansen J.H 1984 The axial sacroiliac joint. Anatomica Clinica 6: 29-36).

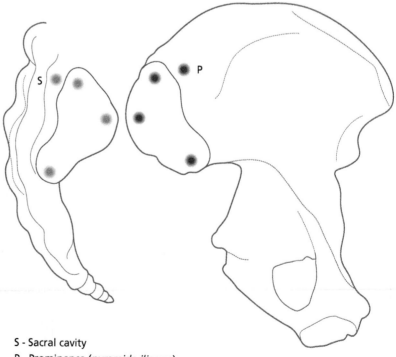

S - Sacral cavity
P - Prominence (*pyramide iliaque*)

Axial sacroiliac joint. The sacroiliac articulations are certainly among the most complex articulations of the locomotive system. Their classic anatomical description most often ignores the axial sacroiliac articulation, the 'Nebengelenk-fläche am Kreuz-und Hüftbein' (accessory joints at the sacrum and ilium) of the German literature (Luschka 1858). Without going into too much detail we can look back to 1753 to find the description by Albinus of an articular surface of the sacrum corresponding to a tubercle of the iliac bone. In 1864 Luschka described articular surfaces in sockets on the sacral side raised on the iliac side which can be considered as a transversarius accessorius process of the second sacral vertebra. Petersen in 1905, Derry in 1911, Jazuta in 1929, Seligmann in 1935, Trotter in 1940 and 1964, Hadley in 1952 and 1973, and Bakland in 1984, gave detailed descriptions of the axial sacroiliac articulation. Bakland and I even tried to understand the role that it could play in the biomechanics of the pelvic girdle.

The iliac prominence (*pyramide iliaque* in French), described a long time ago by anatomists (Testut and Jacob 1893, Rouvière 1932), is articulated with a sacral cavity, encrusted with cartilage,

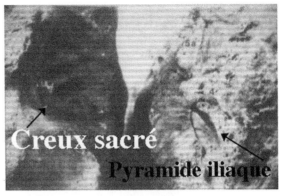

Figure 15.4   Sacral cavity (*creux sacré*) and iliac prominence (*pyramide iliaque*) (from Rouvière 1932).

without an articular capsule (Figs 15.2–15.4). This axial sacroiliac articulation has limited mobility (Fig. 15.5). Its ligament (the axial ligament) goes from the iliac pyramid to the first joint tubercle (Fig. 15.6).

The pubic bones.   The pubic bones are part of the articular system of the pelvic girdle. They have all the characteristics of an articulation and are

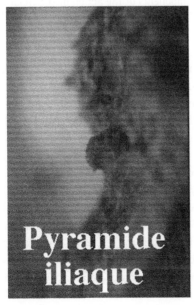

Figure 15.3   The iliac prominence (*pyramide iliaque*) (from Rouvière 1932).

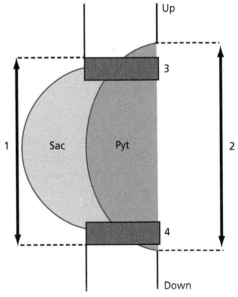

Figure 15.5   Limitations of mobility of the sacroiliac joint (redrawn from O. Bakland's drawing, kindly authorized by the author). 1, Depth of sacral cavity; 2, height of prominence; 3, cephalic joint play; 4 caudal joint play.

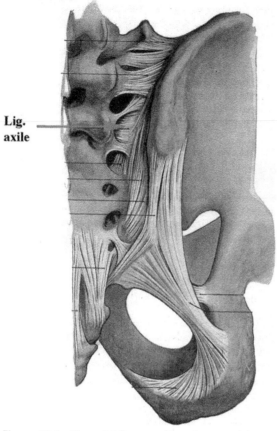

Lig.
axile

Figure 15.6 The axial ligament (from Testut and Jacob 1893).

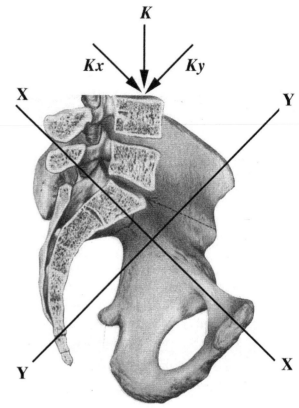

Figure 15.7 Stresses. K, weight of the body; X–X, plane of the pelvic ring; Y–Y, plane perpendicular to X–X; K_x and K_y, components of the action of the weight of the body on the pelvis (from Testut and Jacob 1893).

made up of ligaments, which correspond to frena of movement.

Ligaments. The entire sacroiliac and pubic bones ligament system responds to constraints described by Pauwels (1948), in the standing position as well as in monopodal support (Figs 15.7–15.9).

ANALYSIS OF ARTICULAR STRESS

Stresses at the sacroiliac level are compressions in their lower part and openings in the upper part thereby bringing about the conditions of a sliding rotation at each monopodal support. (Fig. 15.8). At the level of the pubic bones, the stresses are three-fold: shearing, compression and ventralization (Figs 15.8 and 15.9).

These observations according to Pauwells (1948) match clinical findings: if one of these components is blocked, the conditions of functional pathology are met. The treatment must aim at correcting these impaired movements according to the laws of mobility of the pelvic girdle. The sacroiliac joint must therefore be considered as a four-pole articulation (Fig. 15.2). The actual sacroiliac articulation is limited to sliding movements. The axial sacroiliac articulation limits the movements of flexion and extension of the sacrum and iliac wings and allows for minimum rotation. Articulation of the pubic bones is involved in all movements of the iliac wings in relation to one another.

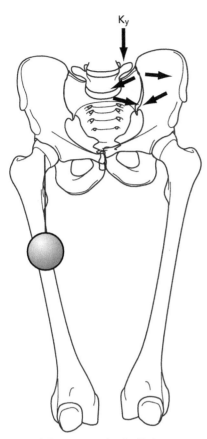

Figure 15.8 Joint stresses in the Y plane.

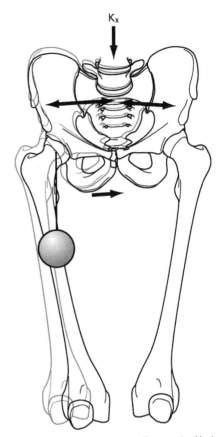

Figure 15.9 Joint stresses according to the X plane.

AXES OF MOBILITY OF THE PELVIC GIRDLE

In order to understand diagnostic maneuvers and manipulations of the pelvic girdle, it was necessary to experiment with the axes of mobility. This is what Lavignolle et al did, firstly on cadavers, then in vivo (Lavignolle et al 1983). The results of their research exactly match clinical work and agree with the methods of treatment proposed here. The determination of working axes, bending the right thigh at 60° and extending the left thigh at 15°, has to be perfomed before measuring the ranges of rotation (Fig. 15.10).

Experiments on humans show the following results.

Bending the thigh (nutation of the corresponding iliac wing, Fig. 15.11) at a rotation of 12°: the axis passes in front of the left ischio-pubic leg, under the right sciatic indentation, behind the right iliac wing.

Extending the thigh (counter-nutation of the corresponding iliac wing, Fig. 15.12): at a rotation of 2°, the axis of extension passes in front of the right ischio-pubic leg, over the left ischio-pubic leg, behind the ilium, and at the level of the cotyloid brow of the left acetabular socket.

Mobility of the iliac wings in relation to one another (Fig. 15.13): the relative rotation of the iliac wings is 10°. The left-right iliac wing axis passes across the left obturator hole, behind the two ischio-pelvic legs, and at the level of the cotyloid brow of the right acetabular socket.

Crossing of the working axes (Fig. 15.14): all the axes cross one another at the level of the pubic bones at a point that Lavignolle calls the instanta-

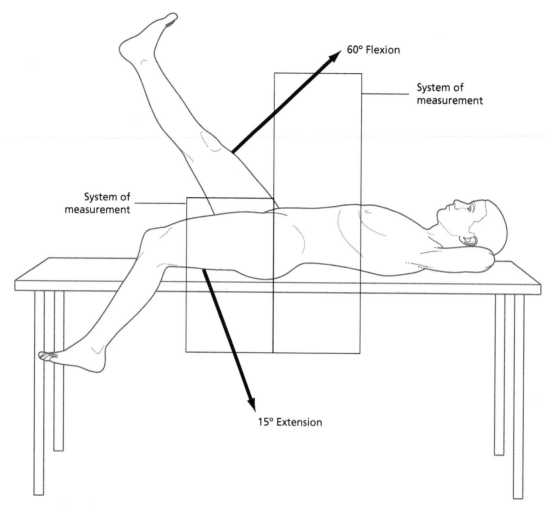

Figure 15.10 Experimental data retrieval of Lavignolle et al (1983).

neous center of rotation in the sagittal plane. The axes of rotation have a quasi-constant position in relation to each other.

Previous rotations of the pubic quadrilaterals (Fig. 15.15): Lavignolle et al (1983) found a movement of anterior rotation of the pelvic quadrilateral of about 6 mm from the side with the bend, 4 mm from the side with the extension. The result between the two iliac wings is 2 mm from the right pubic quadrilateral (Fig. 15.15). These rotations are physiological when they are reversible during movements. They become significant with respect to functional pathology when they persist

and become painful. This fact led to our palpation examination of the pubic quadrilaterals, since a locking always appears as the support of a part of the quadrilateral that was previously moved.

POINTS OF DIAGNOSIS

At the sacroiliac level (Fig. 15.16) direct palpation is not possible. On the contrary, during a dysfunction the multifidus muscle (spinal crossing) which joins the sacrum at L_5 and L_4 presents a tendinosis which corresponds to one of the poles of the dys-

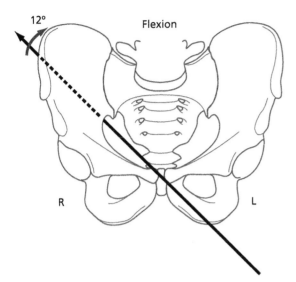

Figure 15.11 Bending the thigh: a rotation of 12°. The bending axis passes in front of the left ischio-pubic leg, under the right sciatic indentation, behind the right iliac wing.

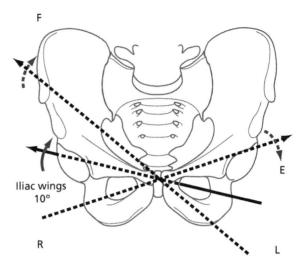

Figure 15.13 Mobility of the iliac wings in relation to one another: the relative rotation of the iliac wings is 10°. The left-right iliac wing axis passes across the left obturator hole, behind the two ischio-pelvic legs, and at the level of the cotyloid brow of the right acetabular socket. F, flexion; E, extension.

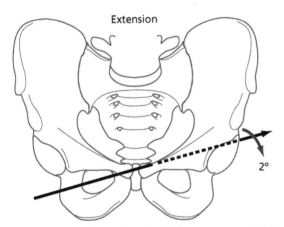

Figure 15.12 Extending the thigh: a rotation of 2°. The axis of extension passes in front of the right ischio-pubic leg, over the left ischio-pubic leg, behind the ilium, at the level of the cotyloid brow of the left acetabular socket.

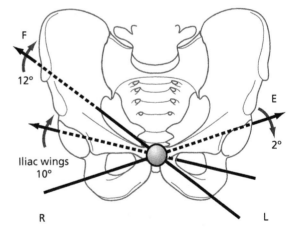

Instantaneous centre of rotation in sagittal plane

Figure 15.14 Crossing of the working axes: instantaneous center of rotation.

functional sacroiliac. These points, described by Max Sutter (1973, 1975), are situated on the backside of the sacrum, exactly on the intersecting line of the insertions into the aponeurosis of the large buttock with the insertions into the multifidus muscle. It is probable that insertions into the sacro-tuberale ligament are also sensitive to palpation on the free edge of the sacrum and on the posterior superior iliac spine.

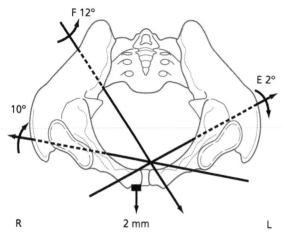

Figure 15.15 Previous rotations of the pubic quadrilaterals. The result between the two iliac wings is a prominence of 2 mm from the right pubic quadrilateral (right 6 mm – left 4 mm).

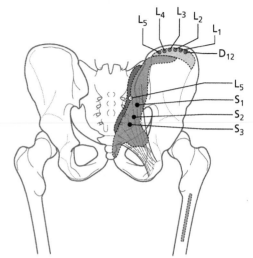

Aponeurosis:
- ▨ Multifidus
- ▨ Gluteus maximus
- ▨ Gluteus medius
- ▨ Sacrotuberale ligament

- ● Areas of sacroiliac irritations zone
- ○ L_5 Irritation zone
- ● Tendinosis in the middle buttock

Figure 15.16 Areas of sacroiliac irritation of the L_5, tendinosis of the middle buttock corresponding to the dysfunctions from L_5 to T_{12} (D_{12}). m, multifidus muscle; G, gluteus maximus; M, gluteus medius; S, sacrotuberale ligament.

These palpation points designated S_1, S_2, and S_3 are what we call the areas of irritation. It is also interesting to note that painful points on insertions into the average buttock can move thoracic-lumbar dysfunctions from T_{12} to L_5 (Fig. 15.16).

At the pubic quadrilateral level (Fig. 15.17) the palpation is done on the internal edge of the right and left quadrilateral which, in functional pathologies, is backward, anterior, irritating the transversal anterior ligament system which is felt by the patient as a needle prick for a pressure of 100 grams. These points of palpation named P_1, P_2 and P_3 are what we call areas of irritation. It must be noted that a stretching 'block' is expressed by P_1, that of bending by P_3, and that a conflict between the two iliac wings is a P_2.

CLINICAL CASES

Boy of 14 months: While learning to stand and walk, this boy fell regularly, either forward or backward. During a clinical examination, he was diagnosed with an atlanto-occipital dysfunction of the pelvic girdle (S_1 to the left, P_1 to the right).

Treatment of the pelvic girdle and of the atlanto-occipital dysfunction immediately allowed the child to keep his balance. Only one treatment was necessary.

Eight-year-old boy: His behavior did not lead us to suspect any anomaly. But when the child tried to maintain his balance on a wooden fence and to walk on it, he rapidly lost his balance. A clinical examination revealed a dysfunction of the pelvic girdle. The treatment according to the pubic bones of P_3 corrected functionality and the child could walk the 10 meters of the fence without losing his balance.

Girl of 2 months: Since birth she had not been able to use her arm, which remained inert alongside her body. Neurological examinations revealed nothing in particular. The clinical examination revealed a

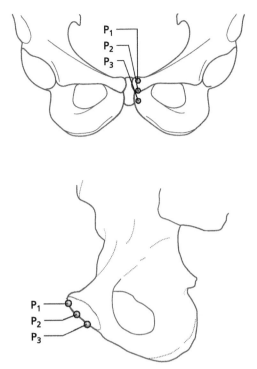

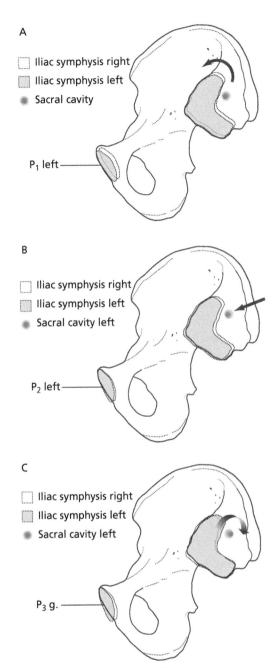

A

☐ Iliac symphysis right
▨ Iliac symphysis left
✳ Sacral cavity

P₁ left——

B

☐ Iliac symphysis right
▨ Iliac symphysis left
✳ Sacral cavity left

P₂ left——

C

☐ Iliac symphysis right
▨ Iliac symphysis left
✳ Sacral cavity left

P₃ g. ——

Figure 15.17 Areas of irritation of the pubic bones on the pubic quadrilateral.

functional pathology of the atlanto-occipital joint and of the pelvic girdle. Immediately after treatment of both dysfunctions, the baby raised her arms for her mother to lift her up.

TREATMENT OF THE JOINTS OF THE PELVIC GIRDLE

Figure 15.18 shows the constitution of the zones of irritation of the symphysis, movement of the iliac wing, the symphysis and sacroiliac axial according to Huguenin (1991). The symphysis is practically always involved in sacroiliac dysfunction.

The therapies use the right (healthy) iliac wing as a lever for mobilization in the direction opposite to the pathology. The actual treatment of the pelvic girdle is based on the knowledge of the functional axes (Fig. 15.19). This also includes sus-

Figure 15.18 Constitution of the zones of irritation of the symphysis, movement of the left iliac wing, the symphysis and sacroiliac axial according to Huguenin (1991). The arrow indicates the movement of dysfunction of the left iliac wing of which the symphysis carries the zone of irritation. A: Anterior seesaw (P₁). B: Distortion between the iliac wings (P₂). C: Posterior seesaw (P₃). The therapies use the right healthy iliac wing as a lever for mobilization in the direction opposite to the pathology.

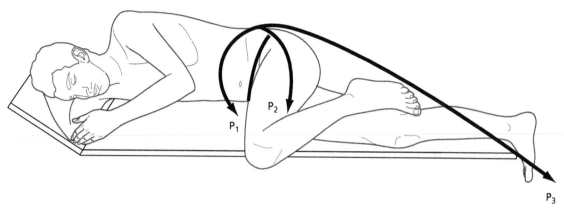

Figure 15.19 Direction of the movements to make the healthy iliac wing restore the congruence of the pubic bones in accordance with the diagnosis of P_1, P_2 or P_3.

pected dysfunctions caused by palpable myogeloses (painful hardening of muscles due to hypoxia) on the iliac crest for any syndrome lasting more than 3 weeks.

Treating children (newborn to puberty) or pregnant women has to take into account the special anatomical situation of these patient groups. Different treatments are done according to diagnosis of the pubic bones, which always decides the direction of the treatment. Clinical findings show us that treating the pubic bones always corrects a sacroiliac dysfunction.

DIRECT TREATMENT OF THE SYMPHYSIS

The patient lies on his back. He must be very relaxed. Holding points of fixation and treatment must be done gently.

- Treatment of the right P_1 (Fig. 15.20A and B). The stationary hand holds the booster iliac wing of the area of irritation (in the example: the therapist's left hand) while the right hand presses on the pectineal (pecten ossis pubis) line, causing a rocking motion in the caudal direction (arrow), thus bringing the left P_1 in congruence with the ventralized right P_1. Mobilization limit is greatly reduced to 2°.

- Treatment of the left P_3 (Fig. 15.21A and B). The stationary hand, the right hand in the example, is pressing on the pectineal line of the side of the area of irritation. The treating left hand presses on the upper edge of the opposite iliac wing, at the level of the antero-upper iliac spine, and causes a lateral opening movement and a dorsal rotation of the right iliac wing (arrow). Mobilization limit is 12°.

- Treatment of the left P_2 (Fig. 15.22A and B). The right hand is stationary, in the example by maintaining the iliac wing below the antero-upper iliac spine. At the same time, it causes a lateral distraction by supporting the thenar, allowing the pubic bones to open. The left hand does the pushing and manipulation in the dorsal direction and in the direction of the P_2 rotation (arrow). Mobilization limit is 10°.

All these treatments are done by a more or less limited sliding of the healthy iliac wing on the booster iliac wing of the area of irritation.

Especially after verticalization – i.e. after the first birthday – the proper functioning of the pelvic girdle assumes an increasing importance for the development of mobility and orientation of the growing infant. The techniques described here complement the treatment of the craniocervical area, the other pole of the vertebral spine.

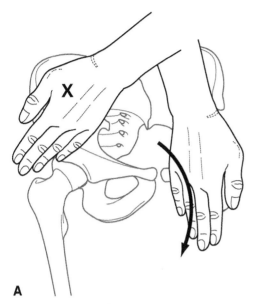

A

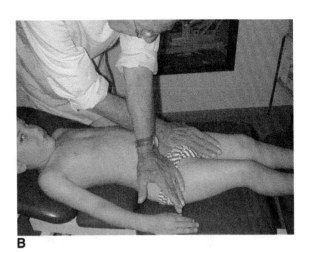

B

Figure 15.20   (A and B) Treatment of the right P₁.

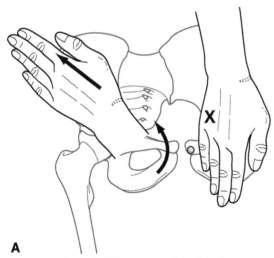

A

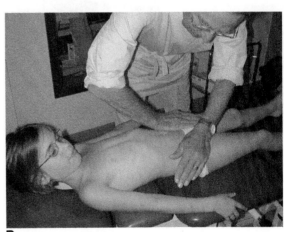

B

Figure 15.21   (A and B) Treatment of the left P₃.

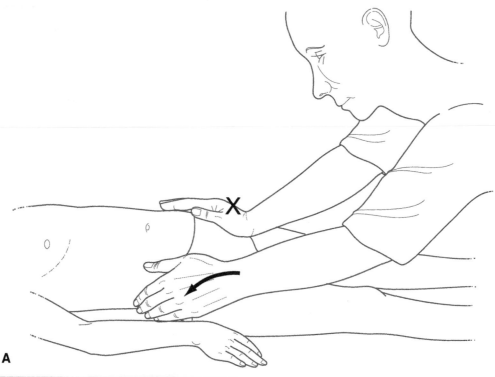

A

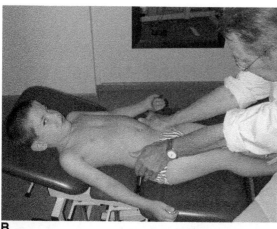

B

Figure 15.22   A and B: Treatment of the left P_2.

References

Bakland O, Hansen JH 1984 The axial sacro-iliac joint. Anatomica Clinica 6:29-36

Huguenin F 1991 Médecine orthopédique, Diagnostic. Masson, Paris

Lavignolle B, Vital J M, Senegas J et al 1983 An approach to the functional anatomy of the sacroiliac joints in vivo. Anatomica Clinica 5:169–176

Luschka H 1858 Die Halbgelenke des menschlichen Körpers. G Reimer, Berlin

Pauwels F 1948 Contribution à l'explication de la sollicitation du bassin et particulièrement de ses articulations. Zeitschrift für Anatomie und Entwicklungsgeschichte 114:167–180

Rouvière H 1932 Anatomie humaine descriptive et topographique. Masson, Paris

Sutter M 1973 Beitrag zur Kenntnis des spondylogenen pseudoradikulären Syndroms L1. Manuelle Medizin 11:43–46

Sutter M 1975 Wesen, Klinik und Bedeutung spondylogener Reflexsyndrome. Schweizerische Rundschau für Medizin 64(42):1351–1357

Testut L, Jacob O 1893 Traité d'anatomie topographique. Doin, Paris

Chapter 16

Manual therapy of the thoracic spine in children

H. Mohr, H. Biedermann

Manual therapy in infants and small children is challenging and exciting for a number of reasons, not least the much clearer picture one gets of the influence of functional disorders beyond their immediate vicinity. In newborns it is safe to declare the occipitocervical (OC) junction by far the most important part of the vertebral spine with a potential for functional disorder vastly greater that its size. No other part of the vertebral spine plays a significant part in neuromotor development at that stage.

The region coming into focus next is the iliosacral junction with its influence on the functioning of the abdominal muscles and autonomous regulation (see Chapter 15). The thoracic spine manifests its role much later – and more discreetly. We see impaired function in the thoracic region as soon as there are coordinated movements, i.e. 4–6 weeks after birth, and we can release these blockages during the examination.

Studying the normal development of newborn babies, it seems very probable that any such impairment of the function of the thoracic spine would resolve spontaneously, too, albeit after some time.

Infants and elementary school pupils seldom present specific thoracic complaints. However, during early puberty, there is often a tendency towards interscapular pain, poor sitting posture, thoracic kyphosis and a poorly developed equilibrium when sitting, with a resultant insufficient sitting posture. The kyphotic sitting posture often develops as a result of KISS II; in such cases, the positional reflexes and the extension functions of the spinal column have not developed efficiently. The complex interaction between this biomechanical level and the input via the autonomous regulatory network is still poorly understood. Suffice it to say that the pseudo-dorsalgia caused by gastric irritation (Kunert 1963) plays as important a role in adolescents as it does in adults.

So the thoracic spine plays a part in the pathogenetic context of functional disorders, but not as a prime mover. The dysfunctions situated on the thoracic level have in many cases a strong tendency to disappear after the underlying structural problem is taken care of. But this process can be speeded up by treating those local problems simultaneously.

Inefficient breathing in the upper thorax is often the inevitable result of a kyphotic sitting posture. Asymmetry, caused by KISS I, is in itself often the cause of asymmetrical breathing patterns, which develop as a result of asymmetrical motion of the ribs. The literature refers to osteoarthritis of the first rib in 20-year-olds (Nathan et al 1964). This phenomenon is only conceivable as the result of a faulty use of these structures over the years, e.g. due to asymmetry as a consequence of KISS I. Similarly the vertebral osteochondrosis (Scheuermann's disease) is in our view connected to a previous KISS II symptomatology. As with KISS, these developments have to be seen in the context of a genetic predisposition. More often than not we find the same posture in father and son, and for good measure the cousin displays the same stance as well. The complex interaction between the genetic base and individual development leaves enough room for therapeutic maneuvers, and knowing about a predisposition does not mean there is no point in the therapist taking any action.

In young children, internal organ pathology has far less influence on the structures and functions of the thorax when compared to what is often observed in adults (Kunert 1963). Instead, the result is usually poor posture and restricted breathing motion. In pediatrics, little attention is paid to these complex functional disorders of the thoracic region because the child seldom presents with orthopedic complaints and if noticed at all, these complaints are more likely to be seen in the setting of internal disorders.

During the evaluation of the case history we often discover that children with poor posture and inadequate motor functions have a previous history of KISS I and/or KISS II. As the child grows older, both the insufficient posture and the complaints arising from the autonomic nervous system (ANS) increase, with headache and fatigue being the most marked. As the thoracic spine lies in the intersection between the biomechanical spinal irritations and ANS disturbances originating from the epigastric zone, it serves as a stage for referred pain from other areas. These external irritations can be the cause of thoracic joint dysfunctions which in turn lock the entire process into a feedback loop.

INTERDEPENDENCE OF FUNCTION AND MORPHOLOGY

Functionally, the thoracic spine is the stable intermediary between the cervical and the lumbar levels. The cervical spine, the craniocervical junction, the lumbar spine and the pelvis are those areas where there is three-dimensional movement within broad frameworks of motion.

During the first few months, a C-scoliosis can often be observed in the unburdened horizontal state. In the case of KISS I, the tonic neck reflexes direct the entire spinal column, including the pelvis and hip joints, into such an asymmetry. The resulting pelvic distortion and oblique transverse pelvic inclination is frequently the cause of an asymmetrical base for verticalization and walking. This can cause the C-scoliosis to increase during initial verticalization (Meyer 1991).

Scrutinizing the course of the reflex-induced C-scoliosis in the non-weight-bearing state and the resultant compensatory S-scoliosis in the verticalization phase requires the attention of the manual therapist in order to employ adequate therapy in the earliest possible stage: i.e., before the beginning of the child's third year. Due to the limited three-dimensional movements of the spine during the first 2 years of life the shapes of the joint structures and the vertebrae come to be defined by these asymmetrical functions.

At a later stage, the morphology of the vertebral joints largely defines the adverse functions. In other words, the scoliotic posture in the cradle is triggered by reflex patterns defined at the OC junction, and later the morphology maintains the asymmetry. The initially functional pathology determines the morphological fate – later the acquired morphology determines the function. The pathogenetic potential of such an asymmetry might only become apparent when other, non-related factors come into play, i.e. an asthmatic crisis in the case of a thoracic functional disorder or an irritation of the autonomic nervous system via epigastric problems – often of psychosomatic origin.

In the case of KISS I a lateral flexion of C_0–C_1 and C_2–C_3 can usually be found. This lateral flexion is then adopted by the cervical spine, often even by the whole spine.

During the testing of the neck reflexes, this lateral flexion of the cervical spine will remain more or less fixed. In the case of this specific lateral flexion, the sternocleidomastoid muscle causes a heterolateral rotation of atlas and occiput in order to neutralize this lateroflexion and keep the head horizontal. Neurologically, the left asymmetric tonic neck reflex (ATNR) will be more active, if not dominant, so that extension in the arm and leg is often observed. The homolateral side of the trunk will have more muscle tone.

With lateral flexion of the whole spine to the right, the quadrate lumbar muscle will actively maintain the lateral flexion of the lumbar spine to the right. Simultaneously, the right quadrate lumbar muscle will fix the inferior ribs on the right in expiration. Because of its insertions on the iliac bone, the quadratus lumborum will exert a cranially directed force on the pelvis.

A left convex C-scoliotic posture is the logical consequence of this. The lumbar scoliosis causes an oblique inclination of the transverse pelvic line, with the left side positioned lower.

Influenced by the left ATNR component, extension in the left leg will be stronger. This extension of the stronger left leg will then be utilized during verticalization. The left leg will thus become the 'privileged' weight-bearing leg and this will cause the sacrum to tilt.

The pelvic distortion becomes more pronounced, as a result of a dorsal tilt of the iliac bone, and the left leg becomes relatively shorter (Cramer 1956). The left leg becomes the main weight-bearer as it is relatively shorter, but also because it has a higher muscular tone under the influence of the persisting left ATNR component.

The existing left convex lumbar scoliosis – until now purely functional – is then maintained and will eventually become fixed.

The left psoas muscle reflectorily neutralizes the physiological left rotation of the lumbar vertebrae (Michele 1962). Due to its constant state of contraction, the left psoas muscle will become shorter and hypertonic, resulting in a slight fixation of the femur in external rotation within the hip joint. The whole left leg is then prematurely and constantly burdened, and optimal function is hardly possible.

During examination of the left side, the following details are observed in a situation like the one mentioned above:

- valgus of the foot and even extreme pes planus with further shortening of the leg (occasionally a slight valgus of the knee can be observed)
- limited hip function (internal rotation/extension and hypertonic psoas muscle)
- left sacroiliac joint blocked
- contra-nutation in the right sacroiliac joint
- poor equilibrium while standing on the left leg, due to disturbed sensory function of the joints
- limited function of C_2–C_3 on the right side
- elevated state of the first four ribs on the right, with limited function.

The functional asymmetry of KISS in the cervical spine and below has, as a consequence, asymmetry of the pelvis and lumbar spine. Neumann remarked that this process of scoliosis must be neutralized far in advance of the third year of age, because at approximately that time the ossification of vertebral structures is complete (Neumann 1960). He proposed manual therapy as the appropriate treatment in these cases, while problems which arise after the third year of age more often than not should be treated by orthopedics. In relation to KISS, orthopedics is not the up-to-date treatment option; nor are any other modes of remedial exercising or postural correction advisable before the basic problem – a functional disorder of the upper cervical spine – is taken care of.

Diagnosis within the framework of the KISS syndrome consists of the sort of subtle diagnosis that is characteristic of manual medicine, namely acknowledging and distinguishing reversible limited functions of joints. It is with this four-dimensional framework (i.e. taking into consideration the timeline) that we can bring some structure to the otherwise confusing symptoms and come to a viable diagnosis. This implies that manual therapy in very young children should be applied during the first year of life, in order to prevent a morphological fixation and future orthopedic problems.

To balance the head and bring it into a horizontal position, the cervical C-scoliosis has to be compensated elsewhere by a counterswing, resulting in an S-scoliosis. This process starts at the beginning of verticalization (Meyer 1994). The thorax and the thoracic spine have an important role in this process because of the length of this part of the spine and also because of its adaptability. The cervically initiated asymmetry and the consequent occurrence of lumbar asymmetry due to pelvic distortion must be negotiated in the thoracic region in the compensatory search for equilibrium.

ANATOMICAL CONSIDERATIONS

The cervical spine has extensive three-dimensional mobility, partly in order to facilitate spatial orientation and motion. The rotations are especially important, and the rotation of the head is the most important component for rapid spatial orientation. The lumbar spine, on the other hand, is typically defined by another type of three-dimensional function, combining extensive stability with motion and only slight mobility in each segment. These are also the key movements contributing to lateral flexion.

In a biomechanical sense, the thorax constitutes the 'stable' center of the body. Many movements take place relative to the thorax, and this region buffers and stifles both lumbar and cervical motion. Integrated into a web of the more than 170 joint and cartilage connections, it has only limited mobility compared with the cervical and lumbar regions. But for this very reason the motion patterns are extremely complex, and even more so at the thoracic level. The biomechanics of this area are thus more difficult to describe than those of the cervical or lumbar spine, which have a far bigger range of movements.

Within their physiological barriers, the cervical and lumbar vertebrae function in three-dimensional freedom. Due to the connections of the ribs and the sternum, the dorsal vertebra is restricted in its movements with obvious restriction in its range of movements. The thinness of the dorsal intervertebral disks does not allow for much intersegmental motion, thus providing a stable environment for the vital organs, such as the heart and the lungs, and solid points of attachment for the respiratory diaphragm, as well as for the shoulder girdle.

A good example for this role as a stable base for the adjoining structures is its function for the shoulder girdle, for breathing, and for regulating blood pressure, and also as an intermediary between the cervical and lumbar spine.

The upper thoracic spine acts as a transition area between the free movement of the cervical spine and the stability of the middle and lower dorsal segments.

In a functional sense, the fourth dorsal vertebra is considered to be the base of the cervical spine. For this reason, T_4 (D_4) is often nicknamed the 'sacrum of the cervical spine'. T_4 is actually the least mobile of all vertebrae.

The articular connection of the ribs lends additional stability to the thoracic region. Figure 16.1A shows the first rib, completely bridging the intervertebral space T_1/T_2. Figure 16.1B, depicting the fourth rib, displays a slightly different biomechanical picture. Here the articulation is confined to one vertebral level.

The rib cage and its 12 vertebrae can be subdivided into four functional groups:

- T_1–T_3: cervicothoracic transition
- T_4: stable base for the cervical spine; least mobile vertebra of the spinal column
- T_4–T_{10} forms the kyphosis, of which D_8 is the most dorsally situated
- T_{11}–T_{12}: lower end of the thoracic cage.

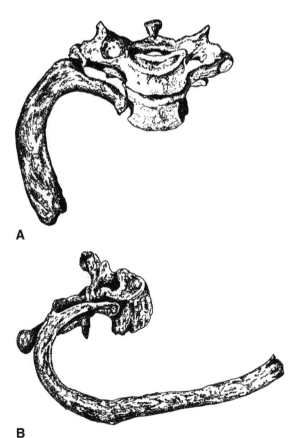

A

B

Figure 16.1   The costovertebral joints.

The dorsal (thoracic) vertebrae have oblique joint facets in a transverse plane. These joints, by nature of their position and shape, have a minor weight-bearing function. The joint capsule is strong yet elastic, and is provided with a stabilizing padding, which penetrates the joint from the dorsal portion of the capsule. The corpora have a considerable (static) weight-bearing task, especially in the case of a kyphotic posture and during sitting.

Due to the position of its facets, T_{12} usually functions as a transitional vertebra to the lumbar spine, and its inferior facets display a more lumbar alignment. The thoracic intervertebral disks become thicker and wider as we move downwards.

The thoracic disks are less vulnerable than the lumbar disks for a number of reasons: intervertebral mobility is strongly limited by the ribs; the disks are relatively thin; and the rotational axes of the vertebrae are situated within the disks. Furthermore, the thin segmental nerve root exits through a large intervertebral foramen, above the level of the disk. As a result, disk–nerve root problems are scarce in the thoracic level.

There are numerous joint connections in this area: intervertebral, costovertebral, costotransverse, costosternal, intercostal, sternoclavicular joints and the intersternal connection (manubrium corpus). Due to this complexity, a considerable range of distortions is possible. This allows for the breathing movements, and the constantly changing postures and positions that occur in daily life, and many types of sports.

Within this complexity of joints, minor dysfunctions frequently occur, together with limited function and segmental pain points. In respect to KISS–KIDD children we can objectify this at a very early stage, namely by the asymmetrical sitting posture, caused by a previous or persisting torticollis. Even the slightest torticollis (with ATNR component) causes asymmetrical regulation of movements in the lower portion of the trunk. In these cases, asymmetrical rib functions are evident. The long levers of the blocked ribs consequently have a limiting influence on the intervertebral joint functions.

ANATOMICAL AND FUNCTIONAL ASPECTS OF THE RIBS

The ribs articulate with the dorsal corpora and disks at the following attachments (Fig. 16.1):

- first rib head attaches to the corpus of T_1
- the second rib head attaches to the edges of the corpora of T_1, T_2 and the intervertebral disk
- this pattern is repeated for the third through to the tenth ribs; and at the same time, the rib articulates with the transverse process of the vertebra of its own level
- the second through to the tenth ribs form double-chambered synovial joints.

The superior ribs suspend from the concave transverse processes by their costal tubercles, which allows for a considerable range of rotation. This is necessary for the raising of the thorax during inspiration. The seventh through to the tenth ribs 'rest', as it were, on the transverse processes, allowing for more sliding motion.

The ventral attachment of the ribs varies widely. Whereas the first rib articulates with the manubrium sterni only, the ventral fixation of the second rib is more complex, being attached to the transition area between manubrium and corpus sterni – an unstable connection. The middle part of the thoracic spine connects rather uneventfully to the corpus sterni via the cartilaginous part of the rib. The lowest ribs have increasing degrees of freedom, costae 8 through to 10 connected to the cartilage of costa 7 and the last two (costae 11/12) without any anterior attachments to the sternum.

The costotransverse joint is a joint with a sliding motion, whereas there is more of a rotation within the costovertebral joints. The rib has the effect of a long lever on the costotransverse joint and a short lever (collum costae) on the costovertebral joint.

Between the two 'sensory' and three-dimensionally mobile areas of the spinal column (the cervical and lumbar region) we view the thoracic area as a biomechanical 'transmission station' from the lumbar level up to the craniocervical level and vice versa. The thorax with its relative stiffness lacks muscles like the sternocleidomastoid and the psoas major. The psoas major moves the rib cage three-dimensionally, just like the sternocleidomastoid, which moves the head three-dimensionally in space.

The middle portion of the spine, from which the thorax is suspended, is largely dependent upon a well-functioning lumbar spine to maintain equilibrium, integrating influences from the cervical and lumbar area. The thoracic spine constantly bears the weight of the head, arms, thorax and the mass of the internal thoracic organs, hence the necessity for stability. This stability, in conjunction with little mobility, renders the thoracic spine susceptible to static and dynamic overload and muscular dystonia. This is the case when foot, hip and/or pelvic function are functionally disturbed.

BREATHING

Because of the orientation of the costovertebral and costotransverse joints, the superior ribs induce a sagittal plane for a thoracic enlargement. Within rib joints 6–10 there is a movement like that of a bucket-handle: i.e., a transverse enlargement of the thorax occurs. The position of the thorax in the sagittal plane is of great importance for the rib functions: in the case of a thoracic kyphosis we observe a limited breathing movement, mainly due to decreased function of the costotransverse joints ('sterno-symphysal overload' – Brügger 1977). Breathing (Fig. 16.2) requires uninhibited thorax dynamics, which depends upon optimal functioning of the vertebral and rib joints (Bergsmann and Eder 1982, Eder and Tilscher 1985). Free and synchronous breathing in both halves of the thorax (symmetrical function) is the basis of economical breathing. One dysfunction within this complex neurophysiological chain can unsettle the whole pattern. Because of the vulnerability of

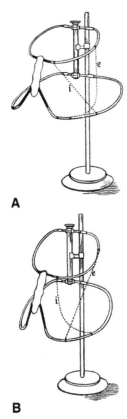

A

B

Figure 16.2 Breathing mechanism (Fick 1911). This classical model shows inspiration (A) and expiration (B). The strings are symbolic representations of the intercostal muscles.

the joints of the thorax (poor posture), breathing can rapidly become impaired.

Craniocervical problems as in KISS will provoke muscular reactions in the upper thoracic structures, for example: torticollis with an opisthotonic component. Even in early childhood, this can lead to asymmetry of the ribs, in conjunction with blocked joints, especially in ribs 1–4. The total thoracic balance of function can become deregulated at a very early age.

The respiratory movement of the thorax is a complex event involving the nerves, the muscles and the joints, in which the base tone of the scalenus and intercostal muscles plays an important part. The scalenus muscles help in the process of moving the first and – to a lesser extent – the second ribs. On inspiration the muscle tone increases and on expiration this tone decreases. However, it has been shown that the intercostal muscles also have a constant base activity without any rhythmical increase or decrease in the base tone. As a result of this base activity, the ribs remain at a constant distance from each other, both on inspiration and on expiration, a function which passive connective tissue membranes could not perform as they would overstretch on inspiration.

The scalenus functions require good mobility of the upper ribs and thoracic vertebrae, but are also dependent on the optimal functioning of the occiput and upper cervical spine complex. Functional restrictions or a fixed position of the upper four rib joints when breathing in can easily lead to an insufficient respiration pattern. This is because restrictions in the upper cervical spine interfere with proprioception and with the base functions of the respiratory muscles, which in turn drive the base functions of the respiratory process. This illustrates the functional connection between the craniocervical junction and the upper thoracic region.

Whereas the scalenus muscles make it possible for the thorax to expand in cranial, sagittal and lateral directions, the diaphragm initially enables this in the lower part of the thorax at a later stage of the respiratory movement. At rest, the diaphragm takes care of the majority of the respiratory functions, amounting to approximately 70%. At this point the scalenus muscles are not being exerted.

In order to move the sternum cranially, the thoracic spinal column needs to perform a stretching function. As a consequence, the erector trunci thoracalis, in particular, has an important part to play in respiration. On inspiration, the upper thoracic spinal column is extended and on expiration it is inflected. This involves small movements among the vertebrae themselves, which are nonetheless important as these movements make it possible for the 'rigid' thorax to remain the ever-mobile part of the body. The influences on the thoracic region from the movements of the lumbar spinal column and from within the upper extremities and the neck require a great deal of coordination on the part of the thoracic structures.

The anatomy of the sympathetic nervous system, which originates almost entirely from between C_8 and T_2, is important; Hansen and Schliack (1962) have clearly shown the ortho-sympathetic influences. As a result, thoracic functional disturbances lead to irritation and muscular hypertonus of the shoulder girdle and the cervical area (cervicogenic tension headache), while pain in the abdomen and the lower part of the body is often related to lower thoracic functional restrictions. Children with an insufficient sitting posture can gradually develop these types of symptoms, too.

As in craniocervical problems in small children, the question is only rarely one of orthopedic abnormalities on the thoracic front, and if this is the case, these can always be diagnosed using radiology. Thoracic functional disorders in the form of bad posture and restrictions of movement are easy to diagnose and can be linked to growth processes and related neck pains and headaches. Lumbar symptoms and pelvic problems also play their part in thoracic functional disorders, and all of this means that observation, inspection and functional examination by means of palpation should be carried out with great care.

PROBLEMS OF RESPIRATORY BIOMECHANICS

As a result of a prolonged opisthotonic position in the craniocervical region (KISS II), the growing child will have to compensate for the fixed dorsal inflection position of the head by means of increased thoracic kyphosis when lifting the head. This is because the somewhat upturned head position is compensated for by a more pronounced thoracic kyphosis, thus allowing the child to look horizontally. If there is a case of dorsal inflection obstruction in the C_0–C_1 motion segment, then it will not be possible for the baby's lifting reactions to take place optimally, in part

because C_2–C_3 will be functionally restricted as a result of the functional restrictions in C_0–C_1. This restriction in the lifting function of the occiput will have its own influence on the extensor functions of the thoracic spinal column. So, in the biomechanical sense, as well as in the neuromotor sense, the extensor function of the thoracic spinal column can become insufficient and deteriorate into thoracic kyphosis, also referred to as the sternal stress position.

Thoracic kyphosis entails a forced expiration position of the ribs, and as a result of the anterior position of the head, the cervicothoracic region is constantly overburdened because the ribs have to facilitate inspiration. This is why a loss of function can be observed in the upper thoracic area of the intervertebral disks as well as in the rib joints, as a result of which the scalenus muscles become hypertonic and shortened by the extra burden. This is referred to as T_4 syndrome, also described as 'serratus anterior syndrome'.

As a result of the fixed expiration position of the thorax, particularly in the sitting position, the diaphragm will not be able to function properly either, which means the already heavily burdened and hypertonic scalenus muscles will be taxed even further to aid upper thoracic respiration. In addition to the constantly stressed scalenus musculature, the cervicothoracic junction is also heavily burdened by the anterior position of the head which, although it actually weighs 4 kilograms, exerts a force of between 15 and 20 kilograms at that point as a result of the lever effect.

The cervicothoracic junction is thus constantly overburdened and the consequence is that the schoolchild sitting in kyphosis is continually breathing superficially and insufficiently. The kyphotic expiration position is the position of a weary and depressed person, a position which is not right for anyone, and even less so for a young child. The present-day television and computer culture is a constant negative factor, which induces a kyphotic sitting position: the 'laissez-faire' position. It seems obvious that such a position, if maintained long enough, favors the development of a juvenile kyphosis with the classic Schmorl's nodes (Schmorl and Junghanns 1968).

Inspiration is an active muscular event, while expiration is mainly passive, in particular because of the elasticity of the rib cartilage, which means that little effort is involved in bringing about the expiration position. The kyphotic sitting position is a permanent expiration position for the schoolchild; in this fixed position further expiration is either not at all possible or extremely restricted.

Because of the fixed expiration position of the thorax, physiological inspiration is almost impossible, in particular because the weak abdominal wall cannot use the stomach as a fixed point, which means that there is no support point for the transversus thoracis of the diaphragm. As a result, proper abdominal respiration is almost impossible, which is why caudolateral thorax expansion cannot take place. Because abdominal inspiration is insufficient, subconscious use will be made of upper thoracic respiration.

The functional restriction of the first ribs results in the cranial thorax being incapable of expanding laterally, and the upper thorax in particular (together with the scalenus and sternocleidomastoid muscles) will be heavily taxed. These comparatively small muscles will then have to lift the entire thorax, just at the time when it is fixed in an expiration position.

If this situation persists for too long, both expiration and inspiration will become superficial, with small inadequate thorax and rib movements, while the child will have to produce extra muscular effort in order to achieve proper ventilation.

Therapeutic manipulation measures and specific remedial therapy are definitely indicated in this case. If a history of KISS can be found, treating small and growing children with therapeutic manipulation (combined with remedial therapy and posture advice) is usually an adequate solution. It is just this combination of unblocking a restricted range of movements (as a base) and re-education of the postural and breathing automatisms which achieve a lasting result. Neither of the two measures alone will bring therapeutic success.

We often see that with a KISS I child the asymmetrical posture in the craniocervical junction is the cause of increasing asymmetrical steering in the motor apparatus covering the entire spinal column, and pelvic and hip joints, and can even lead to asymmetrical functioning of the feet. The left–right imbalance then expresses itself in C-scoliosis and one-sided pes planus (flat-foot), a restricted functioning of the hip and a unilaterally blocked sacroiliac joint. In the process of standing up, this asymmetry will translate itself in thoracic terms into compensating S-scoliosis, a left/right asymmetry in the rib positions and asymmetry in the vertebral and rib functions. It is well known that with thoracic functional disorders, an asymmetry in the ANS balance can also arise, opening a further negative feedback loop.

FUNCTIONAL CONSEQUENCES OF KISS II IN THE THORACIC REGION

The anteversion of the head following KISS II causes a load increase on the segments T_1–T_4, combining hypertonic scalenus muscles and hypertonic dorsal (postural) muscles. This postural anterior positioning of the skull, as well as a previously experienced KISS II phase, are the causes of poor extension of the thoracic spine and a reflexive hypotonia of the muscles of the cervicothoracic area. As a result of KISS II, the righting reflexes of the head and extension of the thoracic spine will be laborious and even lagging. This is how the foundation of a kyphotic posture is determined early on. Pathological afferent joint impulses cause insufficient efferent postural regulation – and this is revealed in the thoracic area.

An accentuated and fixed dorsal kyphosis is in effect a posture in a permanent state of expiration, resulting in a further burdening of the already hypertonic scalene muscles (auxiliary breathing muscles) during inspiration, which creates problems in the upper thoracic area. Lumbar problems influence the lower thoracic structures (psoas, respiratory diaphragm, the quadrate lumbar muscles and the erector spinae). In the whole thoracic area there is a close interdependence between internal organs and their accompanying thoracic segments (Kunert 1963).

There is a broad consensus that thoracic problems in children are much less evident than in adults. However, a clear KISS/KIDD history, poor posture, and a history of sensorimotor problems with poor results in school, attention deficiency, autonomic instability (such as headache and fatigue), justify an extensive examination of the child and, in most cases, subsequent treatment with manual therapy. In most of these cases the disorders found on the thoracic level are secondary to the problems originating at the cranial or caudal junction of the spine, but their neglect can lead to long-lasting problems of posture and function, too.

The biomechanical complexity and vulnerability of the thoracic area, and frequently an enduring hyperactivity of the autonomous nervous system, are often reasons for the child's descent into a vicious circle of vertebrogenic and autonomous nervous functional disorders, thus keeping the child in an unbalanced state. These complexities have as one reason an initial KISS situation, developing slowly, but surely. Many pediatricians claim that colic and torticollis neonatorum will recover spontaneously, but it seems probable that these form the basis for later problems (Biedermann 2000).

Thanks to the improved documentation of children's development (see Chapter 10) we are now much better able to relate biomechanical functions of the elementary schoolchild to the earlier occurrence of KISS symptoms during infancy. Whereas the craniocervical area is the most important cause of KISS syndrome, in the case of KIDD the thoracic spine plays important roles both autonomically and biomechanically. Therefore, the examination and treatment of the thoracic spine in schoolchildren with their perplexing complaints is more than justified.

Thoracic problems in adults present pronounced patterns of complaints which have been discussed in numerous publications. In children, this symptomatology is less pronounced and usually scarcely – if at all – present. These symptoms include:

- pronounced limited arm, shoulder and neck functions in the case of upper thoracic functional limitations (Janda 1968, Lewit 1985)
- neurovascular compression syndromes in various forms
- pseudo-anginous complaints
- nocturnal tightness in the chest and stifling of breathing
- distinct costosternal complaints.

SOME CLINICAL PICTURES

The developments outlined above are encountered in various clinical contexts which are not necessarily orthopedic. More often these problems of a dysfunctioning thoracic spine and rib cage are hidden behind internal or pulmonary disorders. In this regard the transition between the situation in children and in grown-ups is fluent, and most of what we encounter and treat on the level of the thoracic spine follows the same rules found in all relevant textbooks.

This collection of commonly encountered problems is intended to shed some light on the thoracic pathology without intending to present a full outline. But it should show that one special aspect of functional problems of the thoracic region lies in the chronic character of these ailments. Even those problems (such as an acute blockage of a rib joint), where we can help immediately, have a strong tendency to recur, and thus need more than just a manipulation.

It goes without saying that in all cases of thoracic dysfunction we have to consider the OC and lumbosacral junction, too, as most of the problems gain their chronicity from extra-thoracic influences.

Acute thoracic vertebral blockage

This is brought about by sudden, uncoordinated movements (e.g. sport), whereby it is possible to observe movement restrictions and hypertonic musculature. It can be treated by careful manipulation or mobilization. In children, it is sometimes difficult to elucidate the trauma component as the onset of the discomfort may be delayed. Whereas in adults we often find a more ventrally situated area of referred pain (the classic 'pseudo-stenocardia') the localization of the children's pain stays mostly close to the spinal midline. These problems fall into the category of trivial manual therapy (see Chapter 22) and are often treated on the fly, i.e. they do not last long enough to necessitate a dedicated visit to the specialist. But we find them often while screening for other problems and would advise treating them accordingly.

Mechanical dyspnea syndrome

Mechanical dyspnea syndrome is frequently the result of a (traumatic) blockage of one or more thoracic vertebrae and the costovertebral joints in the vicinity. Symptoms include one-sided thoracic pain, occasional intercostal pain, and pain while lifting, coughing and straining. The relevant costotransverse joint is sore when pressed. There is a feeling of breathlessness and the affected rib is usually in the inspiration position. Therapy involves manipulating the rib joint carefully, and then mobilizing the rib back to the inspiration position. These blockages are more important in children with internal breathing problems like asthma or obstructive bronchitis, as they tend to worsen an already precarious situation, certainly if combined with a kyphotic posture.

The main difference to the situation in adults is that we still have a chance to influence the individual's postural pattern before the growth process is terminated, albeit to a lesser degree after the beginning of the teenage years. It is imperative to combine the elimination of the acute problems with a re-education of the postural balance. This asks for quite some diplomatic skills, as motivating an adolescent to do exercises is a far from easy task.

Sternal stress syndrome (Brügger) as a result of a kyphotic posture

Symptoms include interscapular pain and a pressing, heavy, sometimes breathless feeling retrosternally. The sternum is literally constantly overburdened by the pressure of the ribs on the sternocostal connections, while the carrying function of the thoracic vertebrae is transferred to the costosternal connections. The sternoclavicular and the five upper costosternal connections are painful when pressure is applied.

A child does not usually complain about the pain there, but this is exactly why palpation provides objectivity in this situation. When the child is sitting up straight, these points are less sensitive to pressure than in the kyphotic sitting position.

It is quite possible that this sternal stress syndrome is at least partly caused by KISS II in the beginning of the sensorimotor development. The sternal stress position in turn, because of the anterior position of the head, maintains this dorsal inflection of the occiput and the child gets into a vicious cycle of biomechanical and neurovegetative imbalance. The therapy in cases with late KISS II (after the second birthday) must then encompass treatment of the whole spinal column, supplemented with muscle-strengthening exercises and advice on posture.

The remnants of the Galant reflex (a deep abdominal reflex in which contraction of the abdominal muscles occurs on tapping the anterior superior iliac spine) can be observed in a newborn infant until the fifth month after birth, and may continue to persist in a growing child to such an extent that hypersensitivity of the skin of the thoracolumbar area can be observed during the examination. This segmental hypersensitivity can be caused by thoracolumbar kyphosis, as described by Brügger (1977) (possible KISS II).

If (as a result of KISS I) an asymmetrical position of the pelvis is caused, resulting in a pelvic contortion, then on the anterior rotation side the shortened quadrate lumbar muscle can maintain the pelvic contortion as well as the expiration position of the ribs on that side of the body. If the child remains in such a scoliotic sitting position for years, then this may well have an adverse effect on the vital functions of the diaphragm and the caudal rib movements; for children who remain in this scoliotic sitting position for hours on end at school, chronic problems will eventually develop. Phrenic respiration being insufficient, the cranial part of the thorax is called on to perform an extra effort. As the child often already has an insufficient sitting posture and hypertonic scalenus muscle, the vital capacity of the lungs as well as the child's overall vitality will deteriorate significantly.

Restoring the lumbothoracic kyphosis to lordosis is of essential importance and requires, again, a lot of tact and sensitivity in proposing the therapy. When one looks at a family as a connected whole, one realizes how the children are often only an exaggerated version of the parents' behavioral and cultural patterns. To motivate a young adolescent to do sports without including the parents renders this endeavor much less efficient.

Tietze syndrome

This is actually a segmental equivalent of the sternal stress syndrome. This usually involves the costotransversal joints on one side only. As a result of a rotational blockage of T_2, T_3 or T_4, the ventrally rotated processus transversus will exert pressure on the rib and this pressure will be passed on to the costosternal connection. Furthermore, the costosternal connection of the second rib is the most unstable connection on the junction between corpus and manubrium sterni. The sternal connections are swollen and painful to pressure in this situation and there is also intercostal pressure pain. It is therefore understandable that careful palpation of a possible rotation position of the vertebra in question must be carried out, and that specific remedial therapy must be given. The vertebra must be rotated back into the neutral position in order to take the pressure off the costosternal connection.

Many thoracic symptoms are accompanied by cervical problems but arthrogenous functional restrictions in the C_0–C_3 area also have their restricting influence on ribs 1 and 2 as a result of the scalenus musculature. Over time, a child (KISS II) with a kyphotic sitting posture and anterior position of the head builds up functional restric-

tions from C_0–C_3 up to T_6–T_7. Mumenthaler and Schliack see one of the causes of these problems in the subscapular musculature (Mumenthaler 1980, Schliak 1955), while Lewit (1985) believes the cause is mainly to be found in the costotransverse joints. Maigne (1968) is of the opinion that the interscapular pain is caused in the segment C_6–C_7. If there is also a question of a history of KISS I, then these functional restrictions will also develop in asymmetrical patterns.

In adults the shortening of the scalenus group is often caused by temporomandibular problems. This has to be taken into account in older adolescents, certainly if orthodontic appliances have been employed recently. The intimate interdependence between orthodontics and the functional situation of the cervicothoracic junction is grossly underestimated (see Chapter 13).

Idiopathic kyphosis (Scheuermann's disease)

When one tries to see the postural development of children in a long-term perspective, the links between the kyphotic posture of a teenager and an initial KISS symptomatology become evident. A quantitative analysis is almost impossible to achieve as we do not always have a detailed and reliable database of the first years. One clear indicator can be found in the photo album of the first years: time and again one sees the same postural details at a very early stage.

Again it has to be stressed that the interactions between the genetic predisposition and the individual's development are far from simple, but at least we have to try to influence this in as positive a way as possible. The therapy is basically one of re-education and motivation for sports and movement. It is almost too trivial to mention it, but it is important to take into account the family context when advising for specific schedules. In one family there is a sports tradition and it is perfectly possible to encourage father and son to go swimming together on a regular basis; in another family the daughter can be encouraged to follow a girlfriend to her ballet lessons. If it seems that sport is not too popular with the family in question, there are always other options: singing in a choir does wonders for the posture and the breathing technique necessary to partake in a choir motivates some children to improve their posture much better than an unloved sports lesson.

Functional problems of the thoracic spine due to scoliosis and/or cerebral palsy

Very often the major reason for recurring functional problems on the thoracic level lies in a neurological or morphological pathology which will not subside. A cerebral palsy is almost always accompanied by an asymmetrical posture and thus an asymmetry of the thoracic spine. This leads to side differences in the movement range of the ribs

and in consequence to an asymmetrical breathing pattern. The effects of an idiopathic scoliosis are very similar on the thoracic level.

In both cases, it is highly advisable to alleviate the symptoms of the problem at the root of the pathology by treating the – secondary – functional impairments on the level of the intercostal or costovertebral joints. In children the situation is more dynamic than in adults, so one can assume that a regular unblocking of these functional impairments helps the developing body to at least become less fixed in its asymmetry than would be the case otherwise. Manual therapy is part of a palette of adjuvant measures and has to be integrated into a total concept encompassing, for example, physiotherapy and sports therapy, patient exercises and other activities.

Here, as always, we should try to work as efficiently as possible. As a rule, manipulations can be spaced 2–3 months apart even in cases where the chronicity of the underlying problems necessitates repeated interventions.

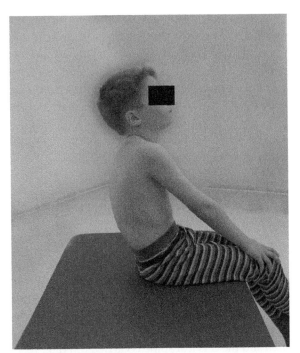

Figure 16.3 Thoracic muscular hypotonia combined with a hyperlordosis and muscular hypertension in the suboccipital region. These children have a disproportionately high incidence of KISS II in the early phase of their development.

INTEGRATION OF THORACIC EXAMINATION AND TREATMENT

As mentioned earlier, children will seldom complain directly of spinal pain. It is thus up to the therapist to find the causal connections between the often rather general symptoms and their spinal functional component. It is often appropriate to treat the child's thoracic spinal column if the examination detects restricted movements in these areas. If on top of that we see in the case history that the child has suffered from KISS syndrome in the past or is currently suffering from KIDD, an insufficient posture, or an autonomic imbalance accompanied by headaches, the link between these general complaints and the functional impairment on the thoracic level is plausible enough to justify treatment.

Few small children will put their physical problems into words; at most, after treatment they may sometimes say, 'That feeling has gone.' The KISS–KIDD symptoms recognized by the parents are therefore more significant than whatever few words the child may be able to utter. The case history taken by the therapist often confirms the suspicions of the parents, while the physical/functional examination should provide further details. In the clinical situation the therapist must take into account the child's candor, their preparedness to 'wait and see' and their vulnerability. Often the tolerance of children for long-term burdens is grossly underestimated. It is only after this stress is lifted that they perceive the difference.

When the child and therapist meet each other, there must be mutual trust, and the therapist then explains the aim of the therapy clearly and simply to the child. Many doctors are of the opinion that it is unnecessary to treat a KISS–KIDD child because the child does not really complain and it therefore seems as though therapeutic manipulation is not necessary. However, when objective examination of such a child takes place, functional restrictions can be found from the OC junction to the hip joints.

The therapist should first take a case history, and should then inspect the child, undertake palpation, perform a segmental functional examination and test the muscles.

The case history focuses on signs indicating a KISS/KIDD problem. It may entail autonomic imbalance, organ problems, cold or sweaty hands and feet, headaches, tense neck muscles, stomach pains and vague pains in the lower back, postural insufficiency, trauma, clumsiness at sports and games. As always the final diagnosis depends at least as much on listening carefully to the stories told by the parents and the child than on the clinical findings. Without the guidance of the preceding interview we would lose our orientation in the jungle of conspicuous details of the clinical examination.

But before the active examination starts we observe the child, observe how it walks into the room or how it behaves on the parent's lap.

- What is the child's sitting posture in the waiting room?

- How does the child sit down (kyphosis, asymmetry, etc.)?
- How is the head held, in a straight posture or tilted anterior or posterior?
- Is there a lateroflexion of the cervical spine (possible minimal torticollis and upper position of the homolateral ribs)?
- Does the child have cold hands (autonomic imbalance)?
- What is the respiratory pattern like at rest (upper thoracic)?
- Is there rapid upper thoracic respiration (stress)?
- Is the upper thoracic respiration asymmetrical?
- Is respiration superficial?
- Is there an emphasis on respiration (associated with depression)?
- Are the arms rotated inwards?

The child should be examined while standing up and assessed in relation to the lumbar spine and the cervical spine, unilateral lifting of the shoulder, kyphosis–lordosis posture, scoliosis (assess pelvic position) scapulae alatae, shortened pectoral muscles and the position of the feet (rotated outwards/inwards, symmetrically or only on one side). These observations are part of the overall examination and have to be checked against the local functional capabilities of – for example – the thoracic spine.

DETAILS OF THE THORACIC EXAMINATION

The complexity of the anatomy and its functions makes it difficult to decide whether the problems have been caused by vertebral or by rib problems, although it is usually a combination of the two. Within the framework of the overall functional diagnosis, examination of the lumbosacral area and the cervical spine is carried out (Fig. 16.4). As a result of palpation and functional examination of the thoracic spine, many problems often come to light involving the restricted inflection function of the thoracic spine, and painful areas in

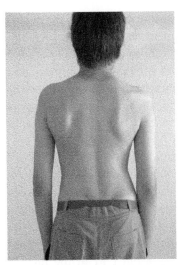

Figure 16.4   What the back can tell you. Just by looking at this teenager we get information about the lumbar asymmetry and an impression of a fairly good muscular balance of the thoracic area. The shoulder blades are well attached to the thorax and the postural muscles provide compensation for the basal asymmetry.

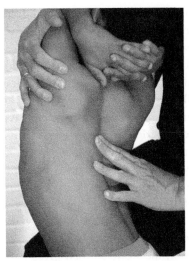

Figure 16.5   Classic examination of segmental mobility, considering the intervertebral and the costovertebral aspect.

the paravertebral structures of the thoracic spine.

Most of the examination pertaining to the thoracic spine is integrated into the general check-up, but some details may be worth mentioning separately. When examining the child in an upright position we have to leave time enough for the child to attain a stable (or unstable) posture. Often during the first seconds an almost normal posture can be achieved and it is only after 5–10 seconds that the problems come to the surface. After this neutral stance we ask the child to stand on one leg, bend forward, etc. (see Chapter 10). The examination of the thorax is just *one* part of this assessment.

After having examined the child in a standing position we continue to check segmentally, first in a sitting position, then lying down. Again the first moment is reserved for an examination of the child's spontaneous posture. If we encounter a suspicious detail, for example an asymmetry which does not fit into the overall picture, we can always ask the child to stand up and sit down again. One should refrain from commenting about the posture to the parents present, as the child will

immediately adjust its posture to such a remark. The next step might be to ask the child to breathe in deeply, thus getting an impression of the breathing type while sitting (as compared to the thorax movement in a standing position).

After the non-touch phase comes the segmental examination (Fig. 16.5), first in neutral position, then moving the trunk in flexion/extension and checking the segmental movements individually. Several tests are at our disposal:

- palpation per segment of the painful areas: cervical-thoracic and thoracic-lumbar junctions
- muscular painful areas (localized pain/radiating pain)
- is there a twitch response?
- painful areas in the costotransversal, paravertebral and interspinal region
- costosternal connections: superficial/deep palpation of the tissue resistance
- intercostal musculature: trigger points, excitability, passive extension.

Lying down on the back gives an impression of the posture uninfluenced by gravity, and it is often surprising to see that the asymmetry while standing is maintained even then. The next item that is relevant for the evaluation of the thoracic function is the palpation sensitivity of the upper abdominal area. Children with signs of gastritis typically complain about pain in the middle of the back – much like adults. If we confine our therapeutic efforts to the manipulation of the segments in question our success will be temporary at best.

Departing from the mid-back pain we proceed to the epigastric irritation, which may have its origin in a difficult situation at school or in the family – how we deal with this is a different question and one we cannot discuss here. But one has to be aware of the basic fact that the thorax acts very frequently as a resonance board for problems originating well outside its confines.

Lying on the stomach then gives access to the detailed examination of the resistance of the skin and subcutaneous tissues, complementing what we found during the examination while standing. The most important detail accessible in this position is the turgor of the skin and the subcutaneous tissues. The comparison of the findings in sitting and lying positions can sometimes shed light on the role of gravity in local dysfunctions and helps to differentiate between a more biomechanical or a primarily reflective origin of a zone of thoracic sensibility (Illi 1949).

THERAPY

The most important aspect to keep in mind when comparing manual therapy of the thoracic spine to that of the cervical spine is that the thoracic spine is much more fault-tolerant than the cervical spine. Whereas any therapeutic maneuver at the cervical level – and even more so at the OC junction – should be planned and executed with the utmost reserve, the limits on a trial-and-error approach are much less strict here. Due to its restrained movements the thoracic spine is in general well protected against mechanical overload, but less so against tilt and blockages. Most of the problems originating at the thoracic level can be resolved with fairly simple techniques. Even these 'trivial' manipulations (see Chapter 22) profit

from an exact application of the necessary forces. Any treatment on the thoracic level has to be preceded by a thorough examination of the pivotal areas of the spine, and even more so in children than in adults. But as mentioned above, the chronicity of the underlying problems determines the outcome of the local treatment on the thoracic level.

This should take place in relation to the cervical (KISS/KIDD) problems and that is why thoracic therapy occurs within the framework of a full treatment. Indeed, the complexity of such thoracic problems means that treatment should be as broad as possible. Not only do complex biomechanics play a big part in the literally palpable problems; the ortho-sympathetic deregulation (which may have been going on for many years) also plays a significant role in the pathology or 'unwell-being' of the child. In addition to the biomechanical disorders, there are also often ANS disturbances, which are frequently assumed to be innocent.

For specific manipulation techniques, readers should refer to the 'classic' textbooks about manual therapy. Here we mention those treatment techniques that are most useful and most effective for children.

Soft tissue techniques

Soft tissue techniques are situated in the intersection between manual therapy and 'normal' physiotherapy/massage. These techniques come in various guises, be it connective tissue massage (Kohlrausch 1955), periosteal massage (Vogler 1955) or the more 'modern' osteopathic techniques (Greeman 1996, Scott-Conner and Ward 2003). The former two methods date back to the first half of the twentieth century and – especially in central and eastern Europe – many similar methods were taught. The basic techniques are absolutely identical to those applied to adults and the only difference is that in children one has to use even less force than in grown-ups.

Mobilization techniques for ribs and vertebrae

In a growing child, forceful manipulation should be avoided. Because of overall physiological mobility it is easy to diagnose segmental functional restrictions and as a result it should be possible to operate purely in segments.

Treatment techniques of the thoracic area are quite similar to the maneuvers used in adults. Figure 16.6A shows a mobilization of the second and third rib, Figure 16.6B a dorsal manipulation of T_4/T_5. Much less force is needed than in adults.

In relation to the cervical spinal column the cervicothoracic area belongs with the cervical spinal column. The three-dimensional cervical functions run through up to T_4, which in functional terms is the basis for the cervical spinal column and is the least mobile of the spinal vertebrae. In the case of cervical problems the cervicothoracic junction must also be treated. The most obvious therapy methods for the upper thoracic area are mobilization of the upper four ribs and the intervertebral joints; mobilization of the first and second ribs can be carried out in either the sitting or the lying position.

After the rib joints have been mobilized on the dorsal side, they can then be mobilized to the expiration position via the sternum and the anterior ribs, that is to say via the long lever. This technique is most effective during expiration, so the child should be asked to breathe out slowly.

The lower costovertebral joints are best dealt with by using springy and oscillating treatment techniques in the ventral position, so that the therapy hand is positioned on the angulus costae and the heterolateral processus transversus is kept in a fixed position. This technique can be used either on just one rib or on several ribs at once. As before, it is important to proceed gently, quietly and in a focused manner. It is also possible to carry out the mobilization in a gentle manner as the child breathes out. Manipulation techniques, as described for adults, should not be used in the treatment of children.

Mobilization of the intervertebral joints can take place in two directions. In the sagittal area, while the child's hands are on his or her neck, dorsal inflection mobilization can be carried out, so that the underlying vertebra is kept in a fixed position. This technique can be applied up to T_{10}.

A logical progression of this technique is three-dimensional mobilization in dorsal inflection carried out while the child is sitting down. In the sitting position the thoracic spinal column is able to move as freely as possible in the space. While carrying out this technique the child stays seated on the chair with his or her feet on the ground; in other words, the child is not brought out of balance (Fig. 16.7).

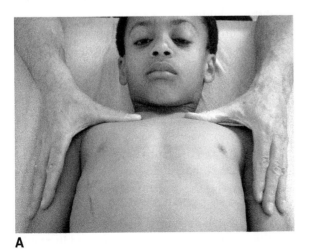

A

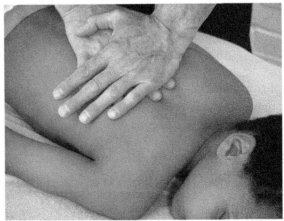

B

Figure 16.6   A: Mobilization of the second and third rib. B: Dorsal manipulation of T_4/T_5.

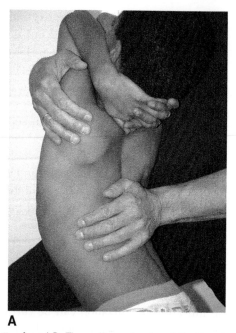 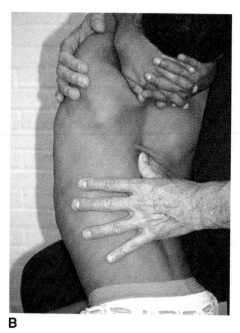

A   **B**

Figure 16.7   A and B: Three-dimensional mobilization. In using this technique the therapist has a lot of freedom to choose the most effective position in order to achieve the manipulation with the least discomfort possible. The position shown in part A is better suited for the costovertebral joints.

When treating a child with a thoracic kyphotic sitting position accompanied by insufficient respiration, mobilization of T_7–T_9 is very important, as this is physiologically the highest part of the thoracic kyphosis. This is very common in children with a medical history of KISS II.

Embedding manual therapy of the thoracic spine in a broader approach

Both children and parents need to pay attention to the most important part of the therapy: conscious posture correction and mobilizing, and muscle-strengthening exercises for the back. The most important point, however, is to ensure that they are aware of the relevant posture correction. At home, as well as at school, measures should be taken to promote a correct sitting posture (for example, a tilting desk table is very effective). These corrective measures will have a positive influence on posture stress and the autonomic imbalance, and such auto-corrections should

become automatic for the child. Postural stress is a source of thoracic pain, while sitting is a static stress. Although children do not often complain about pain, it is in the thoracic region in particular that the pain threshold is often lowered, and this frequently becomes clear when using provocations in painful areas: this is all the more reason to treat these children.

In treating the thoracic region of the spinal organ we are busy with an area which displays much less spectacular pathologies than the two pivotal regions of the spine, but one which needs attention, too. Here – more so than in the other areas – manual treatment of the functional disorders has to go hand in hand with rehabilitation, re-education and preventive measures.

So, although the thoracic area is not of primary importance in the functional pathology of the spine, nevertheless if this inconspicuous but basic part of the whole therapy is taken care of, the quality of our therapy will improve and its results last longer.

References

Bergsmann O, Eder M 1982 Funktionelle Pathologie und Klinik der Brustwirbelsäule. Fischer, Stuttgart

Biedermann H 2000 Primary and secondary cranial asymmetry in KISS-children. In: von Piekartz H, Bryden L (eds) Craniofacial dysfunction and pain. Manual therapy, assessment and management. Butterworth & Heinemann, London, p 46–62

Brügger A 1977 Die Erkrankungen des Bewegungsapparates und seines Nervensystems. Fischer, Stuttgart

Cramer A 1956 Zur Funktion der Ilio-Lumbo-Sacralverbindung. Erfahrungsheilk 5:264–270

Eder M, Tilscher H 1985 Schmerzyndrome der Wirbelsäule. Hippokrates, Stuttgart

Fick R 1911 Handbuch der Anatomie und Mechanik der Gelenke. Fischer, Jena

Greeman P 1996 Principles of manual medicine. Lippincott Williams & Wilkins, Philadelphia

Hansen K, Schliak H 1962 Segmentale Innervation. Thieme, Stuttgart

Illi F 1949 Soigner le dos de l'enfant – c'est prévenir le 'rhumatisme' chez l'adulte. Geneva

Janda V 1968 Die Bedeutung muskulärer Fehlhaltung als pathogenetischer Faktor vertebragener Störungen. Archives of Physical Therapy 20:113–116

Kohlrausch W 1955 Reflexzonenmassage in Muskulatur und Bindegewebe. Hippokrates, Stuttgart, p 133

Kunert W 1963 Wirbelsäule und Innere Medizin. Enke, Stuttgart, p 281

Lewit K 1985 Manipulative therapy in rehabilitation of the motor system. Butterworths, London

Maigne R 1968 Douleurs d'origine vértebrale et traitments par Manipulations. Expension Scientifique, Paris

Meyer T 1991 Methodiek van Manuele Therapie. Rotterdam, p 37

Meyer T 1994 Das KISS-Syndrom. (Kommentar). Manuelle Medizin 31:30

Michele A A 1962 Iliopsoas. Charles C Thomas, Springfield, IL

Mumenthaler M 1980 Der Schulter-Arm-Schmerz. Huber, Bern

Nathan H, Weinberg H, Robin G C, Aviad I 1964 The costovertebral joints: anatomico-clinical observations in arthritis. Arthritis and Rheumatism 7:228

Neumann C 1960 Sulla Genesi della Scoliosi nell' et. . . evolutiva. Giornale Sanita 21:451–452

Schliak H 1955 Zur Segmentdiagnostik der Muskulatur. Nervenarzt 26:471

Schmorl G, Junghanns H 1968 Die gesunde und die kranke Wirbelsäule im Röntgenbild und Klinik. Thieme, Stuttgart

Scott-Conner C, Ward R 2003 Foundations for osteopathic medicine. Lippincott Williams & Wilkins, Philadelphia

Vogler P 1955 Periostbehandlung. Thieme, Leipzig, p 174

Chapter **17**

Examination and treatment of the cervical spine in children

H. Biedermann

The young physician starts life
with 20 drugs for each disease,
and the old physician ends life
with one drug for 20 diseases

Sir William Osler

Every goldsmith, software engineer or surgeon is
– depending on their observational skills – sooner
or later confronted with the same baffling fact: of
the multitude of procedures his teacher considered essential only a very few are used in everyday practice. 'You need 10% of the code for 90% of
the end-user's needs' is a standard quotation in
software engineering – only to continue a second
later with '. . . and the other 90% of the code for the
last 10% of the user's needs'.

We shall try to be as encyclopedic as required
– but not to the point where every possible technique is covered. Some will be left out and my
only excuse is to rely on the reader's creativity
and encourage everybody to seek their own
way.

PRECAUTIONS

The principle *nil nocere* is as much the basis of
planning of the procedure as in any other context.
The extensive literature of complications after
manual therapy offers a few clues on how to
proceed:

- optimize the fixation prior to manipulation
- do not use reclination and/or rotation unless absolutely necessary
- leave enough time to react and reach a new equilibrium
- manipulate as fast as possible, i.e. with an impulse of minimal duration
- use the minimal energy sufficient to achieve the therapeutic effect.

These are the purely technical considerations applicable to all manual therapy. But especially in children and the newborn, three further important points have to be added:

- win the confidence of the parents first
- try to the best of your abilities to establish a positive communication with the young patient
- immobilize the child reliably in the moment of treatment.

All this sounds quite obvious, but putting it into practice is quite a different matter. Winning the parents' confidence starts well before the first visit to the consulting room and could be classified under 'marketing' – it is something that can be taught to a great extent. How to interact with the young patients, on the other hand, is much more difficult to 'teach' and even more complex to learn. An innate ability to win the confidence of small children helps.

I have seen quite a few colleagues whose body language signaled very clearly that to win this basic confidence was not their most obvious talent. It is not impossible to treat children who do not like you – but it is a *lot* more difficult than with that magic connection as a base.

Not that the children where there was a good contact at the beginning of the examination would not complain and be angry after the manipulation; it is their unalienable right to be furious. Certainly those children who suffer from a neurological condition which necessitates fairly regular treatments every few months do develop a love/hate relationship with the therapist: intellectually they realize that their condition improves after the

treatment, but viscerally they hate the moment of manipulation – as much as some adults, by the way.

So we have to make our intervention as smooth and agreeable as possible without deceiving the child. I never tell them 'this won't hurt' – if it does, they are rightly annoyed by my blatant lie. So it is better to say 'this might be a bit unpleasant for a moment' – and do it quickly. Disrespect hurts children much more than a short moment of pain.

The smaller the child, the more it is essential to package examination and therapy in a play and cuddle situation. If you tell the observing parents 'now I shall do the manipulation' you can be sure that their immediate apprehension is as quickly transmitted to the child and results in a sharp heightening of its muscular tonus. Therefore it is advisable to inform the parents beforehand that examination and treatment are performed together – or you create a *fait accompli* – whatever seems appropriate for the parents concerned. Most parents do not mind being a bit surprised to get the child back before they were able to observe an intervention, but there are others where it is better to inform them beforehand. I find it difficult to give a clear classification; to make this distinction well is part of one's professional intuition.

A successful treatment comprises three basic steps:

- identifying the problem
- defining the therapeutic steps
- applying the treatment itself.

As very often when a specialist is involved in the final outcome, at least one initial step depends on the insight and initiative of a non-specialist: we can only help those who come to us. Realizing this motivates us to use the utmost effort to ensure the best possible information is provided to those involved with children, in order to enable them to think of the possibilities manual therapy can offer for an existing problem in a child under their care.

We did a – quite cursory – check of our patient database of the year 2000 to see how many children were referred to us with a clear indication for manual therapy. As it turned out there was roughly a split into three groups:

About 28% were referred to us by general practitioners or pediatricians with a diagnosis and/or query referring to a functional problem of the vertebral spine ('vertebrogenic headache', 'KISS', 'dorsalgia', etc.).

A second group of 41% of the children were sent by physiotherapists who treated these children and realized after some of their own treatments that those children would profit from a specific manual intervention.

The last group of patients basically came because the parents saw the effects of manual therapy in another child first and thus got the idea of trying this kind of therapy here too (22%), or because friends and relatives proposed it (9%).

However brilliant our therapeutic procedures may be, to prove their worth we first need the children to be present with us and the consent of the parents to treat them. Here, too, a little 'marketing effort' may be helpful. So we try to provide kindergarten personnel, teachers and others involved with children with information about how manual therapy can help them with some of their problems. But the best – and most convincing – argument comes from non-professional sources, i.e. the stories other parents tell.

Realizing this, we might use our waiting room as a therapeutic tool. When we surmise that parents coming for the first time may be very sceptical about our approach we give them some extra time in the waiting room; almost inevitably they get involved in a discussion with parents who come for the check-up and who (we hope) dispel anxieties much more efficiently than we could ever do it ourselves . . .

LESS IS MORE

Another problem of our approach in manual therapy stems from the long delay between the treatment and the ensuing amelioration (see Fig. 17.1).

In about two-thirds of cases the effect of the treatment shows in the first 48 hours after the manipulation, but the other third of the successfully treated children need between 2 and 4 weeks to display a change for the better, sometimes only after an initial rebound. This is especially frequent in schoolchildren. We tell parents explicitly that they might encounter an even more 'difficult' child in the first days after our treatment and that this aggravation of an already tiring situation has to be weathered by the family. It is tempting to try to combine several other modes of treatment to alleviate this phase – for example by using psychopharmaceuticals.

As far as our experiences indicate, this approach is ineffective. It seems better to allow enough time for the results of the manual therapy to take effect; they tend to be more profound and stable when the organism is given the chance to re-adjust its functions to the post-manipulation situation without further stimuli.

Again, this proposition is based on the observations of the outcome of our patients. In the beginning we routinely advised the parents to resume other therapies and treatments immediately after our intervention. This was in most cases physiotherapy and we took care to motivate the parents to continue with the exercises at home the next day and see the therapist soon afterwards. In a few cases our advice was not followed, sometimes because the family went on holiday, sometimes because other problems were more pressing and prevented the mother from exercising with the child. In even fewer cases this 'non-compliance' was reported back to us, as it takes some courage and trust of the parents to tell this. In these few cases the result of our treatment was mostly much *better* than in children who followed the prescribed procedure.

By asking some parents to stop additional treatment in the weeks following our intervention we saw a trend in the data proving this counterintuitive observation.

Our standard procedure for patients undergoing manual therapy is thus to ask for a period of

2–3 weeks after manual therapy before other treatments are resumed and/or the effect of our treatment is evaluated. In a small minority of patients it might be advisable to shorten this interval, most often in patients with a very low general muscular tonus. In these cases the possibilities of manual therapy are generally more limited, one extreme being patients with trisomy 21 (Down syndrome).

THE 'TWIN-PEAK' PHENOMENON OF MANUAL THERAPY FOR CHILDREN

Figure 17.1 shows a diagram analyzing interviews with parents of 264 babies treated at our practice. Two reaction peaks are clearly visible. The first peak is testable by the classic procedures advocated by evidenced-based medicine, but between the treatment and the second peak lie more than 14 days and it is often difficult to convince parents to refrain from additional therapies during that time. In the example in Chapter 21 showing the documentation of movement patterns it was clear that the effect of a single manipulation lasted well over 6 months, and that during that time an adaptation to this new situation took place. Such a long-term effect can be documented by a multitude of follow-up studies, but it is very difficult to verify this in a rigorous protocol, as it is almost impossible to take all the other contributing factors into account.

The main lesson one should draw from these data is to give the patients time to respond to a manipulation. This is true for all age groups but is especially important in children. *We do not aim at the mechanical level when we treat children, so the improved mobility or the reduced pain level is just a means to another end, which is in most cases a better sensorimotor equilibrium.* The timing of a therapy is as important as the technique used.

TREATMENT TECHNIQUES

Some of the basics will be presented here, but with the caveat that this chapter does not claim to be more than an aide-mémoire. Those of us used to reading books about manual therapy are accustomed to the chapters about treatment techniques showing the therapist and the patient in more or less close contact, where the latter undergoes (in the strict sense of the word) the manipulations exercised by the former. One is reminded of a cookbook: if you know how to do it, such a demonstration might help to freshen up one's memory, but for a novice it makes frustrating reading. Having said that, we shall anyway try to illustrate some of the techniques used here, but it must be emphasized that these pictures are not intended as a replacement for practical demonstrations.

The standard position

The majority of children can be treated in a relaxed and neutral position as shown in Figure 17.3.

The therapist sits on the examination bench and the child lies on his or her back in front of the therapist. This position is the most relaxed for children and it permits the parents to hold the child. There is always a trade-off between over-immobilization and annoying the child: the more persons partake in the task, the more irate the child tends to be. For the beginner it is certainly the better option to ask the parents to help with holding the child. We

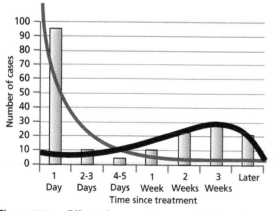

Figure 17.1 Effect of manual therapy relative to the time of the manipulation (Biedermann 1999).

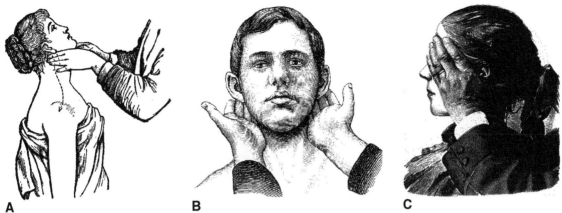

Figure 17.2 A few oldies. These pictures are taken from books published between 1860 and 1910. A: Techniques of 'massage' (Livre d'or de la santé, Paris, 1864). B: 'Kneading the nerves' (Bum 1906). C: 'Enhancing circulation' (Naegeli 1875). The idea behind the therapy has changed, but the *modus operandi* is much the same.

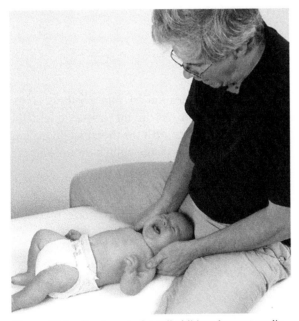

Figure 17.3 Treatment of small children is most easily achieved as shown.

use this option very rarely and prefer to wait a little bit till the child relaxes his muscular tonus for a moment. This procedure is not only more elegant, but it gives you better control over the reaction of the child to the manipulation and it is – last but not least – less stressful for the child to be confronted with only one adult. Finally it exculpates the parent in the eyes of the child, and makes it easier to comfort the little one after everything is achieved.

Sitting positions

Another possibility is to have the child sit on your lap. Depending on the direction of the manipulation, there are two basic varieties and the positioning of therapist and child is comparable to the situation during examination (Fig. 17.4).

Figure 17.4 shows the position for those children who need a lateral impulse, in this case from the left. This position allows a very tight control of the child's movements and we use this option often in children with ADD-like symptoms. These children are especially sensitive to close contact and even more so to an examination of the cervical spine. They oppose this very intensely and to be able to even examine them, one has to be prepared to use some coercion. It is essential to make sure beforehand that the parents understand the necessity for such a procedure and to go through with the examination and treatment in one go. As soon as one stops on the way, the child quite rightly assumes that there is an exploitable dissent between parents and therapist and will use this to the maximum.

In those cases where you cannot be sure that the parents agree, you will have to forego any attempt to use a quick and efficient therapy. It is not

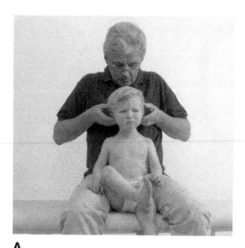

A

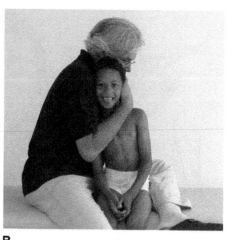

B

Figure 17.4 A: Treatment of C1 in sitting position. Sometimes children refuse to lie down and it is easier to accommodate this wish. B: A more 'controlled' approach. This position gives a maximum of control and is useful in situations where the child does not want to be treated. For further explanation see text.

advisable to proceed against the will of the parents, even if you are sure that it would be for the best of the child. In some cases such a problem arises only with one of them and it is sometimes possible to resolve this by asking the more nervous partner to leave the room temporarily. In quite a few cases this calms down the atmosphere considerably, as the child loses his audience. Very often children, being much more sensitive to such non-verbal acts of communication, relax once the nervous parent has left the room, and a treatment considered impossible can go ahead.

Figure 17.5 shows how we treat children in a sagittal direction: the child sits on the therapist's knees and faces the therapist directly. The two foreheads have contact and the two hands of the therapist are firmly positioned behind the transverse process of the atlas.

This procedure can be modified so that the patient sits on the bench and the therapist kneels in front of the patient or sits opposite him on a stool. Sitting is more gentlemanly, and kneeling is more flexible, as one can adapt one's height more easily.

A slight modification of this position is the 'hugging' position. As in the last example the child sits face to face with the therapist on his lap. The therapist embraces the child's thorax and has

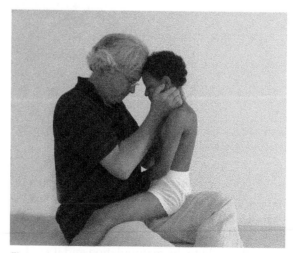

Figure 17.5 Sagittal manipulation of C_1/C_2. This position gives the therapist good control and through the skin contact with the forehead, a precise way of gauging the necessary pre-tensioning.

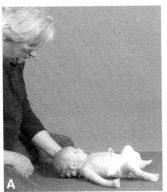
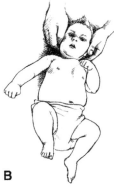

Figure 17.6 The 'classic' treatment position for infants and smaller children. A: The positioning of the baby. At the same time this makes it possible to test the mobility of the suboccipital region very exactly. B: The treatment.

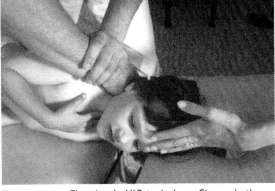

Figure 17.7 The classic HIO technique. Shown is the treatment of C2. The mother's hand supports the forehead of the child, thus giving additional reassurance.

good control of the sometimes quite incompliant young patient.

Standing positions

This position lends itself to the treatment of the lower cervical spine and the cervicodorsal region.

It is very similar to the classic techniques for grown-ups and the precise application depends on close cooperation between therapist and patient. These techniques are thus applicable mostly in older children – if they are willing to take part in the effort.

Lying position

Most babies will be treated lying on their back with the head oriented towards the therapist. Figure 17.6 shows an example. Which posture one prefers depends on the width of the examination bench and the flexibility of the hip joints of the therapist.

CONCLUSION

One could classify the treatment positions nonconventionally as those for cooperative children and those for uncooperative ones. Looking back at over 20 years of dealing with infants and children it is obvious that the techniques used did develop in response to the constant dilemma of wanting to be as soft and kind as possible on one hand and having to be in command, anyway.

However we label our treatment, the basics stay the same: transfer of a mechanical impulse of variable energy from the hand of the therapist to the spine of the child. We can call this chiropractics, manual therapy, atlas therapy, osteopathy and the like; basically this is it and the few examples shown here are intended to give but an impression of the enormous variability of the techniques applicable. To end this chapter we show a 'classic' HIO ('hole in one', Palmer 1934), a technique suitable only with older children who cooperate (Fig. 17.7).

References

Biedermann H 1999 KISS-Kinder: eine katamnestische Untersuchung. In: Biedermann H (ed) Manualtherapie bei Kindern. Enke, Stuttgart, p. 27–42

Bum A 1906 Handbuch der Massage und Heilgymnastik. Urban & Schwarzenberg, Berlin

Naegeli O 1875 Nervenleiden und Nervenschmerzen. Basel

Palmer B J 1934 The subluxation specific – the adjustment specific. Chiropractic Fountain Head, Davenport, IA

SECTION 4

Radiology in manual therapy in children

Chapter 18

Functional radiology of the cervical spine in children

H. Biedermann

THE STARTING POINT

Defending the merits of classic radiological plates in manual therapy poses its challenges nowadays. On the one hand, there are those who pretend that taking these plates is a completely superfluous exercise. Statistics are quoted which show that examination of these plates does not improve the detection of contraindications – so why bother?

On the other hand, the 'modern' radiologists point out that magnetic resonance imaging (MRI) is the state-of-the-art procedure for a detailed investigation of this anatomically complex region. If radiological examination is necessary, why not the most thorough one? Waibel's essay (see Chapter 20) covers the more morphologically oriented radiology while this chapter deals with the functional interpretation of the radiographs (for additional information see Swischuck's monograph [Swischuck 2002]).

Once in a while one finds papers about radiological findings in the cervical spine related to functional disorders (Hartwig 1964), but they are few. Lewit and Gutmann stressed the importance of plates of the cervical spine as the basis of functional examination at any age (Gutmann 1953, Lewit et al 1992).

In the following pages we shall concentrate on the cervical region of the vertebral spine, as it is the most complex and also the functionally most important in children. The analysis of the pelvic girdle and the lumbar spine – important as it is for evaluation of the development of the hip joints – plays a much less prominent role in manual therapy in children. There are cases where an X-ray picture of the lumbar spine and the pelvic girdle is essential, but for the overwhelming majority of cases it is the cervical spine and its functional analysis that is the most rewarding. It poses the biggest problems, too, as its signs are subtle and have to be evaluated with care.

Last but not least, the radiograph of the cervical spine is one of the most difficult plates to take at any age – and with babies (generally uncooperative partners) this task does not get easier. In Chapter 19, we shall try to be of help in this difficult task.

HOW WE USE RADIOLOGICAL INFORMATION

The most commonly held idea about the use of X-ray plates is to look for *morphological* changes. In these cases one needs to define a standard, and anything deviating from that standard is considered more or less pathological.

I am not in a position to judge the validity of this assertion in all circumstances. For the purposes of orthopedic surgery – and even more so in dealing with problems related to the vertebral spine – it is safe to say that whatever non-standard facts can be extracted from a radiological picture (X-ray, CT scan, MRI, etc.), they have to be compared with and validated by the clinical examination.

Publications abound which reiterate the well-known (but often ignored) fact that there is no such thing as a radiological diagnosis of, for example, a discus hernia (Hollingworth et al 1998, Murrie et al 2003, Penning et al 1986, Wood et al 1995) – a clinically relevant hernia, one has to add to avoid useless squabbling. The radiological findings as such need the causal connection with the clinical picture to be validated and only then should they be accepted as a basis for clinical decisions (van der Donk et al 1991).

Nowadays we are able to see with ever better quality the patho-morphology of a given region.

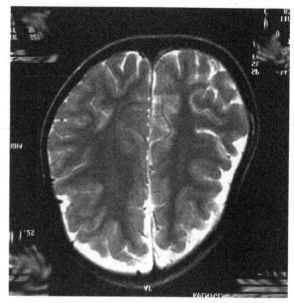

Figure 18.1 Cranial asymmetry in an MRI. This cut shows the occipital flattening of a typical KISS II case. These distinctive asymmetries allow a prima-vista diagnosis of cranial asymmetry which has to be examined for other possible causal factors. In the overwhelming majority of cases, a functional background (i.e. KISS II) is the most probable reason.

But there is no straight and short path from this initial finding to a valid decision about what to do with the patient.

Humans are visual; 'One picture is better than a thousand words'. But once in a while pictures are overloaded with a significance, when they can only constitute a basic framework for further evaluation based on the case history and the clinical evaluation, as is quite often the case in the morphological radiology of the vertebral spine.

One school of thought among those active in manual therapy takes the obvious and radical consequence to disregard X-ray analysis completely. This argument is facilitated by the fact that many of those applying manual therapy to the vertebral spine often do not have ready access to radiographs, as is the case for most physiotherapists. Departing from the just cause of putting the findings of radiological examinations into perspective, they extend this argument beyond its breaking point and disregard X-rays altogether, thus losing a valuable source of information.

THE FUNCTIONAL ANALYSIS

This chapter aims at restoring the balance between over-confidence and total neglect: on one hand those who do not bother to take radiographs at all, and on the other hand those for whom only an MRI or a CT scan suffices. In order to get to the middle ground we shall first introduce a conceptual frame for radiological data extraction: the *functional analysis*.

This functional view is not completely alien to radiologists, in fact it is the basis for some of the newer research tools such as positron emission tomography (PET) scans which are used to analyze the momentous changes in the metabolic rates of different brain regions. So far, so good – but the idea that an 'ordinary' X-ray picture of the cervical spine can give us more than strictly morphological data has not yet reached the medical mainstream.

But it is precisely the functional level which yields the most relevant data in dealing with vertebrogenic problems. The functional analysis is in no way a contradiction to a morphological approach, as we shall see in several examples here. At the end of this chapter it should be comprehensible that the evaluation of the functional implication acts – quite contrarily – as a catalyst to deepen insight into minor (and otherwise easily overlooked) patho-morphological details.

In following the leads provided by the functional approach of the X-ray analysis, our attention is often attracted to minor details which would have been easily overlooked without it. It is the interaction between morphological and biomechanical levels which influences the function – and for the brain this (impaired) function is all that counts (Lewit 1994).

In young adults, and even more so in older persons, this fabric of interaction can be very complex and difficult to decipher. Luckily the situation is much less complicated in dealing with children and babies. Whereas the latter show a complex pattern of inborn and acquired features, the main morphological problems in newborns are congenital malformations and/or the anatomical variants found in this evolutionarily volatile region.

A second aspect of the functional analysis of the X-ray pictures of small children is the dominance of functional over morphological details. In adults it is the morphology that determines the function: an arthritic joint facet diminishes the local range of mobility; an asymmetry of a vertebra induces an asymmetrical posture.

In the small child – and even more so during the first year – it is more often the (mal-) function which determines the way the morphology will differentiate. We see more and more examples where a timely intervention mobilizes the functional situation and the imminent morphological pathology could be averted (see Fig. 8.13). The functionally fixed posture results in a morphological response. This is *one* major reason why the functional analysis of the X-ray pictures is of such paramount importance in dealing with our young patients.

The search for an optimal treatment of a baby's functional problems is much easier if we are able to read the signs correctly. And the problems involved are not confined to postural or kinetic phenomena only. The validity of this approach can only be determined by the improved quality of our interventions based on functional radiological analysis. It can be demonstrated that our therapy is more effective when using the functional analysis of standard X-ray pictures of the cervical spine, thus reaching the therapeutic goal with fewer treatments.

Minor anatomical deviations are too elusive to be clinically recorded. So it is not possible to find out before, either in the medical history or in the course of the palpatory findings, where it would make sense to take a radiograph and where not. It is impossible to define 'risk groups' who then should have a radiographic examination, or to exclude groups of patients where, if a patient were to be manipulated, a prior radiographic examination would be unnecessary. Not even block vertebrae can be made out during a palpatory examination. (In an experiment during a training course, several patients were examined by proven experts and the findings compared. Neither of the two patients with block vertebrae was identified [Lewit 1980, personal communication].)

THE PROJECTIONS MOST USED IN THE CERVICAL SPINE

Any radiograph taken for diagnostic purposes has to be justified by the information eventually gained through it. Most authors of books on manual therapy put the emphasis on the contraindications of manipulation as the main justification for a standard X-ray picture of the cervical spine. This is undoubtedly correct and important – but it is certainly not the whole picture. Standard radiographs are not a very convincing tool in searching for tumors or neurodegenerative diseases, which are the most important contraindications for manual therapy in infancy and early childhood. Osseous malformations are easier to spot on conventional radiographs. At least as important is the role of the functional examination of the radiograph in order to fine-tune one's manipulation technique and to improve the precision of the diagnosis – and make statements about the long-term prognosis, too.

Since we routinely take radiographs to examine and treat small children we look for indicators which might allow us to screen for those children where a radiography is not necessary. If there was a clinical marker which gave a reasonably accurate gauge to exclude those children where a radiograph is unnecessary, we could save some costs and ionizing radiation. Regrettably no such criteria have been found yet. This is why we advise taking a radiograph of the cervical spine of *every* child who undergoes a manipulation, regardless of the technique used. In newborns, one plate of the cervical spine in an anteroposterior (a.p.) projection does suffice as a standard; whenever this plate shows signs of a morphological problem, it has to

be determined if the sagittal projection might enhance the information or if it is necessary to use costlier procedures such as CT or MRI to obtain a sufficiently precise diagnosis.

From month 18 on we routinely take lateral plates, too. At that point in time the child is used to the upright position and the tonus of the neck muscles is sufficiently developed to allow for an upright positioning of the child, thus enabling a projection which shows the occipitocervical (OC) junction and the lower cervical spine uneclipsed by the occiput and the shoulders. When using the lateral projection in smaller children, there is a big chance that a morphological analysis is made impossible by the hyperlordosis of the cervical spine and the overlapping of the osseous structures on the plate.

ADDITIONAL PROJECTIONS

In our monograph on the functional radiology of the cervical spine (Gutmann 1981), quite some space was given to projections that are hardly used any more today. The ready availability of CT scans or MRI makes it possible to gain a much deeper insight in the complicated topographical situation of the upper cervical spine. Nevertheless it is sometimes important to be able to gain additional information on the spot, be it only to prepare a more precise question for the additional examination required or to decide immediately if such an expensive and time-consuming examination is necessary at all.

In (small) children these cases are very rare; whenever an atypical case history requires additional diagnostics we first refer these children to a specialist for further neuropediatric investigation. If our radiographs show signs that do not offer a clear diagnostic solution, the children in question are sent to a specialist. In most cases, MRIs are the method of choice for further investigation.

In referring patients, it is important to include a concise explanation of their problem, as the OC junction is a kind of no-man's land for radiologists, too. In examining the cervical spine the first focus of attention for an average radiologist is more often than not the intervertebral disks. If one asks for a CT scan of the cervical spine it is not uncommon to get a detailed examination of the disks C_3–C_6 but the OC junction is at best depicted cursorily. If one asks for an MRI of the skull, the examination stops at the foramen magnum. Detailed instructions about what has to be depicted is therefore essential; sometimes a phone call is the best way to convey this information, which might otherwise be lost between the two classic fields *intracranial* or *cervical spine*.

These examples are not meant to be exhaustive of the problems encountered at the OC junction but are intended to give a healthy fright lest one overlooks something important in taking a too cavalier attitude towards an unclear situation.

Let us be candid: there are quite a few cases where the solution is not 100% clear and where we proceed, anyway, in order to use the outcome of the manipulation to judge the validity of our initial diagnosis. But even in those cases where an initial improvement made this diagnosis look correct, one has to be aware that a reappearance of the initial problems – certainly without plausible reasons (e.g. trauma) – has to alert us to other, much less frequent, but more serious possibilities.

Two case histories illustrate this point: in both cases the initial picture was unclear or indicative of a functional problem with the 'appropriate' trauma present. In the first case the child improved after the first treatment only to relapse 4 weeks later (Gutmann 1987). After the second relapse, a CT scan revealed a tumor as the structural cause of the dizziness and headaches. The second case came to a specialist in manual therapy after several trial treatments with such an atypical clinical picture that he referred the child immediately to a neuropediatrician (Koch 1999). These cases admittedly represent only a tiny minority, but their mention should help to dispel any illusion that we operate in a risk-free area. Low-risk it is – until now no serious complication following manual therapy in children has ever been reported, and the one case study dealt with Vojta

physiotherapy (a physiotherapeutic system widely used in central Europe for the treatment of neurological disorders in children; Vojta 1992) and a baby with signs of circulatory problems (Jacobi et al 2001). The case reported by Jacobi et al (2001) is in fact very instructive, as the complications arose only after repeated treatments involving pronounced rotation and/or extension of the head.

The relational analysis of the four parts of the OC junction is in some ways simpler in small children than in adults. The osseous structures visible on the plates are much less developed, thus rendering attempts to determine, for example, a rotational component almost useless. The main information to be gained is about the symmetry in the frontal plane and proper alignment in the sagittal plane. These two – essential – items are difficult enough to achieve in our small patients.

THE A.P. VIEW

The approach in analyzing this projection is quite comparable to the one in adults.

Initially we have to make sure that the skull is in a neutral position (see Fig. 18.5). If the septum nasi, protuberantia occipitalis externa and the middle of the incisors are on one vertical line we can be reasonably sure that the head is in a neutral position.

The open mouth is essential to allow an unobstructed view of the suboccipital area. Before the age of 5–6, it is almost impossible to get children to open the mouth voluntarily. This leaves two strategies: we can try to wait for the moment when the crying child opens the mouth wide to intimidate us or we force the mouth open, using a cork or the finger of one parent.

We have to admit that the picture thus obtained does not fulfill the ideal of a spontaneous individual posture which would be ideal to judge the radiograph functionally. On the other hand, we have to take into account that the pathology we are looking for is in most cases so relevant that the

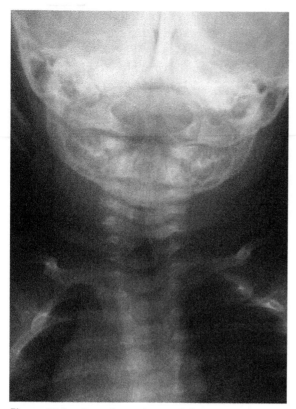

Figure 18.2 A good a.p. picture of the suboccipital region of a 3-month-old.

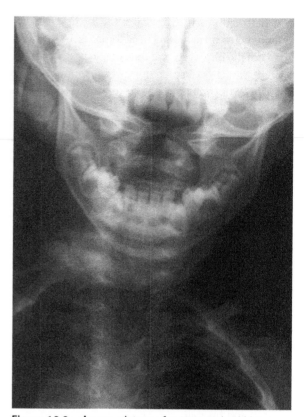

Figure 18.3 An a.p. picture of a 15-month-old boy, showing a dysplastic joint C_1–C_2 on the right side.

interference of the parent's intervention is secondary and the picture can be analyzed, anyway, albeit with the necessary reservations.

The biggest changes occur in the first 12–18 months, as a comparison between Figures 18.2, 18.3, 18.4 and 18.5 shows. One main difference is the size and orientation of the articular cartilage of the atlanto-occipital joint.

We were able to show in an analysis of our radiological data how the frontal angle changes from 153° for the first 3 months to 145° at the first birthday and 126° at the age of 10 (see Fig. 18.4). The sagittal angle changes from 36° for a newborn to 28° for an adult (Ingelmark 1947).

These differences may explain two phenomena we see only in infants:

The movement pattern in side-bending. Figure 18.6A shows the normal situation in adults

(Jirout 1990, Kapandji 1974). In a lateroflexion of the head the atlas is forced by the inclination of the joints C_0/C_1 and C_1/C_2 to shift towards the concave side. Examining the movement patterns with the head and neck in side-bending position, Jirout found this movement in 64% of cases and called it the 'typical' pattern. In one-third of cases the atlanto-occipital relation did not change and only in 3% of cases C_1 shifted to the concave side of the movement (Jirout 1990). The lateral shift forces the axis into a rotation which moves the processus spinosus C_2 to the convex side. This movement pattern looks obvious considering the anatomy of the OC region and it was verified experimentally time and again. In small children, on the other hand, we consistently found the opposite pattern, i.e. that C_1 moves to the convex side of the head (Fig. 18.7A). This is only possible

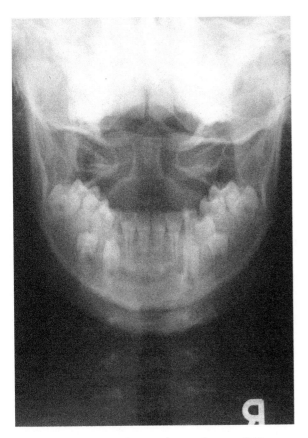

Figure 18.4   An a.p. picture taken at the age of 10 years.

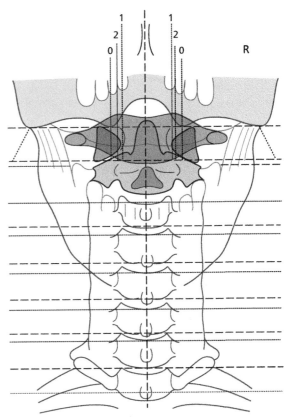

Figure 18.5   Schematic view of the upper cervical spine a.p., in an adult (reproduced with permission from Gutmann 1983). The comparison with the three examples shown in Figures 18.2 to 18.4 explains the differences between the situation in an adult and that in infants. The cartilaginous layer is much thicker in the first months and the condylar angle flatter. The basic points of reference are the same: septum nasi and the middle of the mandible as the markers for symmetry of the head and posture; the two triangles of the massae laterales of C_1 and the stump of dens axis which develops only later in life.

because the much flatter frontal condylar angle enables C_1 to move like this.

The second observation is connected to this. It is remarkable that infants suffer much more often from a reflective fixation of the head in retroflexion (KISS II) and we wondered if there was an anatomical reason for this phenomenon. Studying the literature we found the above-mentioned changes in the sagittal condylar angle. Taking them into account it seems plausible that this steeper angle favors the retroflexion fixations we often see in small children, as a more parallel orientation of the joints makes it easier to slide smoothly in the sagittal direction.

The orientation of the condylar angle in the sagittal direction is not visible on conventional radiographs of the cervical spine. The only projection where we would be able to measure this angle is the axial projection, today almost completely abandoned and replaced by MRI or CT scan.

These two biomechanical characteristics of the newborn lead to distinctive patterns of pathological function. In particular, the much steeper sagittal condylar angle is almost certainly the cause of the KISS II postural fixation. It would be very interesting to examine this angle in children with

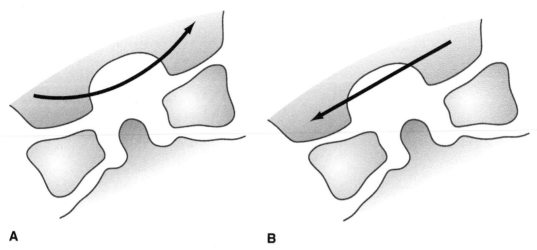

A   **B**

Figure 18.6 Movement pattern in lateroflexion of the head (reproduced with permission from Jirout 1990). A: The normal movement in adults and bigger children. The atlas moves under the occiput towards the concave side of the head, following the wedge-shaped massa lateralis. B: This movement pattern is only to be found in a small minority of adults (Jirout (1990) found ± 2%). Here the atlas moves to the 'upper' side, i.e. the convex side. In small children before verticalization, this is the norm. In our material we found more than 86% with this movement pattern.

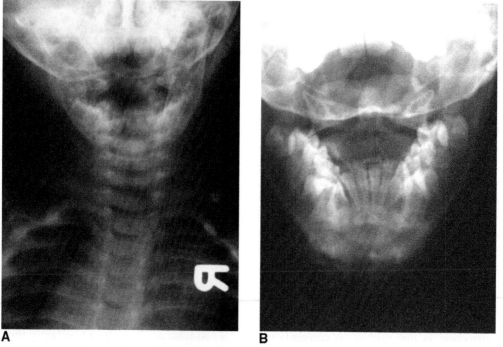

A   **B**

Figure 18.7 Two examples. A: a 7-month-old girl showing a displacement of C_1 to the convexity. B: This child is older (10^1/$_2$-year-old girl) and the movement pattern corresponds to the 'adult' variant: C_1 moves to the concavity.

KISS II and compare it to the standard value for the same age group.

DETAILS IN THE A.P. PROJECTION

When we first started analyzing the plates, the main emphasis was on the functional aspect, i.e. to get reasonably clear information about the relative situation of the main structures C_0–C_3. This is easier in children than in adults, at least regarding the rotational component which cannot be determined except in very distinctive cases. Also for practical considerations the translational component is the most relevant. In combination with the clinical picture this gives us a reasonably safe base to determine the direction and the level of the manipulation.

Beyond this 'utilitarian' aspect, the functional analysis reveals quite a lot about the qualitative aspect of the problem at hand. A minimal asymmetry in the suboccipital region exerts a much less stringent influence on the technique used later for treatment than a massive displacement.

The term 'subluxation' seems unfortunate and was rightly abandoned in recent years, but that leaves us without a simple and striking expression to distinguish between these two possibilities.

The offset between atlas and axis is most visible at the gap between the respective massa lateralis atlantis and the dens, but in order to judge the situation correctly we have at least to make sure that the axis is in a reasonably unrotated position.

The first and most reliable fixtures for the examination of the symmetry of the suboccipital region are the condyles, as we were able to show with statistical analysis of many plates (Gutmann 1981). Therefore it is indispensable to be able to locate these on the a.p. plate. In almost every case it makes more sense to judge the position of C_2 relative to the occiput. The relative position of C_1 and C_2 is secondary and only relevant for the treatment if we can be reasonably sure that C_0/C_1 are in a neutral position.

The second and very interesting aspect of this functional analysis is that it directed our attention

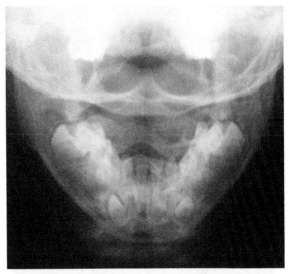

Figure 18.8   A rather common combination of dysplastic joints C_0–C_1 and a persistence of the medial gap between the two ossification centers of axis. These should be fused at this age (5-year-old boy). The lateral projection showed a dysplastic corpus axis, too.

to minor and often overlooked morphological aspects of the upper cervical spine (Fig. 18.9). Minor variations in the orientation of the joints, details of the implantation of the dens in the corpus axis and asymmetries of the condyles get their relevance from our knowledge about the irritability of the biomechanical equilibrium in this area.

Interesting, too, is the fact that we see many more of these 'irregularities' in small children than in adults. During the growth process many of these minor variants are compensated for by compensatory measures and are much more difficult to find later on.

On the other hand, we saw that initially quite pronounced morphological problems were markedly reduced after a timely intervention. This is especially true for asymmetries, which are almost always permanent in older adolescents and adults and which can quite often be reduced or made to disappear in smaller children.

One aspect should not be forgotten, too: some cases of asymmetry have their origin beyond the suboccipital region. Therefore we strongly advise including the upper cervical spine in the a.p.

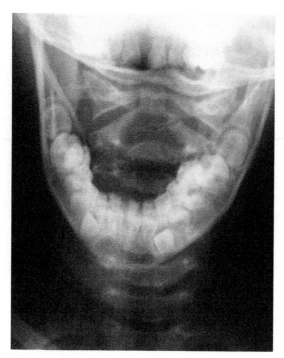

Figure 18.9 Persistence of the apophysis between dens and axis (5-year-old girl). The suboccipital region is very variable. Most block vertebrae are found in the segment C_2–C_3, for example, and other variants are quite common here, too. We can safely assume that this apophysis will be closed in a few years. This finding has no clinical significance besides the fact that it alerts us to look for additional morphological irregularities.

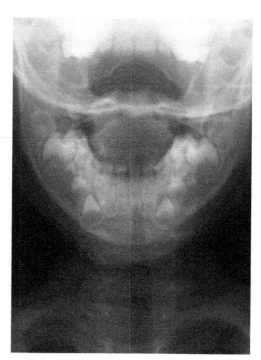

Figure 18.10 Dysplastic joint C_1–C_2: This 4-year-old boy has a fixed lateroflexion of the head. Initial therapy by another specialist did not lead to a marked improvement. Our radiograph showed a 'hump' at the medial part of the joint facet of C_2 in the C_1–C_2 level and a marked asymmetry of C_1 against the occiput. This is a clear sign of a morphologically dominated situation. There is a good chance of getting to an almost normal situation in the long run, but this will need repeated interventions over several years (normally every 6 to 9 months).

projection, often cut off in a misguided attempt at radiation protection. Most hemivertebrae or other segmentation anomalies responsible for a scoliosis of the cervical spine are located in segments C_6–T_3 (Swischuk 2002) and are easily visible – if this area is not shielded by radiation protection.

If one can be more precise about the likely outcome of a therapy, the parents will be more patient and keep faith even when – as predicted – success does not come quickly.

THE LATERAL PROJECTION

Many things said above for the a.p. projection hold true for the lateral plates of the cervical spine, too.

Again there is an intricate interdependence between the functional and the morphological aspects, giving the latter's analysis the necessary impetus. If one does not take into account the relevance of minor changes in the morphology of C_0–C_3 for the functional situation, these small details lose any interest. Figures 18.11, 18.12 and 18.13 show some examples.

The main interest under functional considerations is focused on the transitional area between clivus and dens. This region contains an extraordinary density of structures central to survival. In humans, this region has to cope with much more mobility than in quadrupeds. This makes the compromise between mobility of the head and protection of all these delicate structures very demanding.

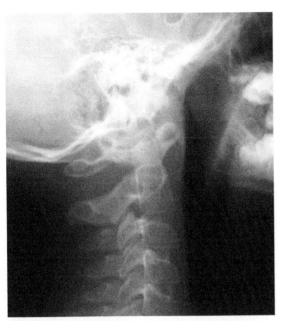

Figure 18.11   Hypoplastic posterior arch of C_1 in combination with hyperplasia of the anterior arch in a 10-year-old boy. These two phenomena are often combined. This arouses suspicion about the symmetry of the lumbosacral area. Very often these children need orthodontic treatment, too.

In infants there is additionally a relative insufficiency of muscular protection in this area. The head contains a full third of the weight of a newborn, whereas the muscular connection between the skull and the trunk is not at all proportional to this, let alone that the coordination of the postural muscles is not yet developed. Primitive reflexes help the fetus to cope with the stresses of the birth channel. Later on – and especially in the transition period between the predominance of the primitive reflexes and the more complex patterns the infant acquires during the first year – this already frail balance is further weakened and the structures of the brainstem suffer more translational and bending stress than later in life.

One of the protective measures to shield these parts of the central nervous system at this point in time is the repair potential of the infant's brain (Valk et al 1991). Another one is the different biomechanical pattern in the suboccipital area (see

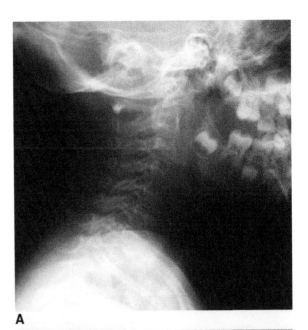

A

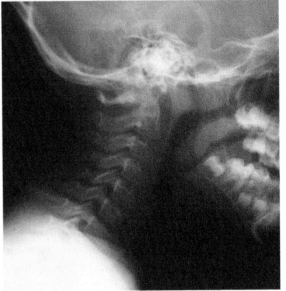

B

Figure 18.12   Disappearance of initial rotation after manual therapy. This 5-year-old girl was unable to keep her head straight on the first picture. The shoulders are in a neutral position, the head is somewhat turned and the maximum of the enforced rotation occurs at the level C_2–C_3. On the second plate, taken 3 months later, the cervical spine is in a neutral position and the slightly dysplastic dorsal arc of C_1 clearly visible.

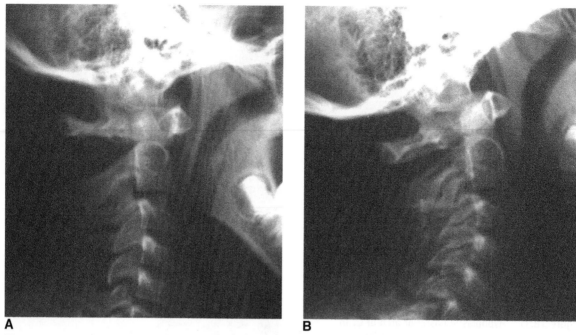

Figure 18.13 Normalization of atlanto-dental joint angle. This 7-year-old boy came with complaints of headaches after school. The first picture shows the typical cleft in the cranial portion of the atlanto-dental joint. At the follow-up the joint facets were almost parallel again. Besides the manipulation we advised the use of a tilting work surface (see Chapter 14).

below). The best protection for the pathways crossing this region is an optimal functioning of all parts involved. This is why minor variants in the anatomy of this vulnerable area can have a big influence on function.

In the early years we started out from the assumption that these alterations (a dens recurvatus, for example) develop spontaneously and the best we can do is to take preventive measures to prevent overload. Once we had examined these children and found the accompanying functional disorders we treated these, anyway.

Figures 18.12 and 18.13 show two examples of children with 'non-standard' biomorphology of the suboccipital area and at the check-up we found, to our surprise, that the initial bend in the articular surface of the dens had disappeared almost completely. The amount of dominance of function over morphology surprised even us 'professional optimists'. These examples are an excellent motivation to keep following up these

children – once a year is almost always sufficient. With such a minimum of intervention we can help them to overcome their genetic predisposition and develop this crucial biomechanical area as optimally as possible.

Fused vertebrae are not as uncommon as one might think. The incidence varies according to the different levels, but the fusion between C_2 and C_3 is the most common (Fried 1963). This is also the biomechanically most relevant level, as the fusion lengthens the lever of axis in anteflexion.

Another interesting detail worth looking for is the closure of the dorsal arc of the atlas, something much more easily checked on the lateral projection (Fig. 18.11). In itself this non-fusion of the dorsal arc does not signify a lot, but – as we try to explain later – it should alert us to the fact that these individuals have a much higher chance of developing a lumbosacral asymmetry, too. As there is normally no need to take plates of the lumbar spine in small children the consequence of this finding is primarily to make us check the static situation even more thoroughly than normal.

Quite frequently a 'stepping' phenomenon is seen in children, even more so when they display signs of a generalized hypermobility. On lateral plates of the cervical spine of these children, one can see a horizontal displacement between all levels of the visible vertebrae (Kamieth 1983). As long as this shift is generalized and harmonious, it is not a sign of pathology, but nevertheless a clue indicating that excessive and prolonged anteflexion of the head should be avoided, e.g. somersaults.

Isolated hypermobility is, in almost every case, post-traumatic and as such attributable to some well-defined event in the past. This is rarely a problem during childhood.

Rotation of one or more components of the upper cervical spine has to be analyzed as well as possible in order to locate the main stress level, which in most cases coincides with the level where a manipulation delivers the best results. Figure 18.12 shows an example of a rotation beginning at C_2/C_3 and of the normalization of the clinical signs some months after treatment.

RADIOLOGICAL DOCUMENTATION OF THE EFFECT OF MANUAL THERAPY

It is well known that in adults the relational situation between the different parts of the cervical spine does not change after treatment (Gutmann 1975, Lewit 1985). In almost every case the clinical improvement cannot be aligned with a change in the radiographs, the only exception being cases of acute trauma. In children, this is different. More often than not we can see quite marked differences between the first picture and the follow-up. It is not the rule to take a second picture if the clinical improvement is satisfactory. In Figure 18.12 the second plate was taken to obtain a clearer view on a suspected dysplasia. In most cases, new plates are only taken if a trauma occurred in the meantime.

THE OC REGION IN THE NEWBORN

At birth, many of the features of an adult's X-ray picture of this region are not yet fully developed (Fig. 18.14):

- apophyses open
- dens axis not ossified
- much thicker cartilaginous material between the bones in the joint areas
- everything is softer, less accentuated, e.g. the angle of the C_0/C_1 joint is almost horizontal.

This situation is less easily interpreted radiologically, as many of the necessary markers to determine rotation or translation cannot be fixed as precisely as they can in adults. But this 'softness' of the situation reflects only the undetermined state of the biomechanical components.

Differentiation of, for example, the rotational position of the cervical vertebrae is less precise than in adults, but for most practical purposes

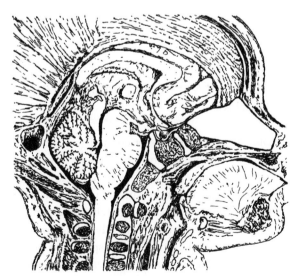

Figure 18.14   The suboccipital region in the newborn (adapted from von Lanz and Wachsmuth 1955).

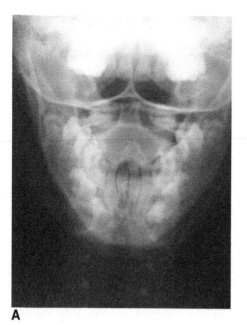
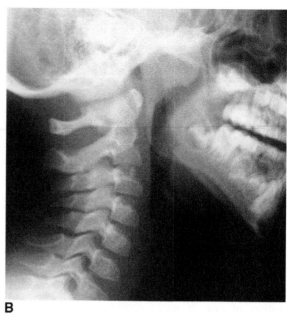

A   **B**

Figure 18.15   Flat joint plane C_0–C_1. This is a very subtle sign and both projections have to be analyzed together. In the a.p. view a flat condylar angle C_0–C_1 is combined with a marked asymmetry between the two joint components. The lateral view shows a line where the joint C_0–C_1 should form an angle of 140–150°, which means that the joint plane is almost horizontal. This portends the reappearance of functional problems after therapy.

much less relevant for the treatment, too. The cushioning influence of the extended per-articular cartilaginous strata prevents the 'hard' blockages we find in adults. This is one of the reasons why a noticeable noise at the moment of the impulse is a rather rare phenomenon, at least until school-age.

IMPLICATIONS OF FORM VARIANTS OF THE ATLAS

In our surgery, which is orientated towards conservative orthopedic and chiropractic medicine, the X-ray examination of both spinal poles is part of standard procedure in patients with corresponding complaints. As part of the clinical examination of our patients we frequently take X-rays of the spinal poles, i.e. the cervical spine and pelvic girdle, in order to obtain not only anatomical information but also an insight into the static situation.

The radiograph of the pelvic girdle is taken in a standing position, taking care to include the lumbar spine as far as L_1. This method makes it possible to obtain information about the lumbar column and the pelvis in one picture. We call this picture an LPH picture (lumbar area/pelvis/hip; see Gutmann and Biedermann 1990). Usually both junction regions of the vertebral column, at least in the case of adults, are thus simultaneously available for analysis and evaluation.

We had already noticed several years ago how often a hypoplasia of the arcus dorsalis atlantis was associated with disorders of the lumbosacral junction and asymmetries and that, in addition, these patients frequently had anatomically distinctive features of the hip joints, which were mostly flat on one side.

Quite early on it proved useful in our practice to look beyond the upper cervical region, in order to cope better with the clinical situation. In so doing, we repeatedly came across the simultaneous occurrence of minor varieties of the atlas, disorders of the lumbosacral junction and flat or dysplastic hip joints. In the examination, and particularly in the follow-up of patients where we found this combination of radiological findings, an abbreviation was found to be helpful. The acronym ALF (atlas–lumbar–femur) presented itself for this purpose.

Parallel to an evaluation of our own data, a literature search was carried out, which produced only relatively satisfactory results. In the 'classical' works (e.g. Wackenheim 1975, 1989) these form variations are scarcely mentioned; the emphasis is on the more serious deviations such as aplasia, fusions, etc. Hypoplasia itself is usually

not considered to be worth mentioning. Wackenheim (1983) writes characteristically of 'harmonious hypoplasia of the atlas'.

One of the few direct references was found in Köhler and Zimmer (1967): 'Therefore findings such as a narrow posterior arch of the atlas or comparable findings should be taken seriously and checked in detail for further radiological varieties and anomalies. Otherwise subtle clinical and neurological symptoms might not be identified.'

We examined the plates of 718 patients in our archive (Biedermann and Sacher 2002) to establish a base for a 'normally' developed atlas (Fig. 18.17). Based on these standard values, a group of 180 cases of hypoplastic atlas were examined further.

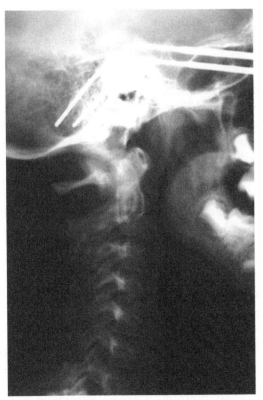

Figure 18.16 This 7-year-old boy categorically refused to take off his glasses. . . The radiologically relevant detail is the hypoplastic dorsal arc of C_1 which directs the attention to a static component of the headaches this boy was suffering from. As the lateral plate is taken in a sitting position, static imbalances show up here, and the scoliotic tilt between C_2 and the lower cervical spine is visible in the double projection of the articular surfaces.

FORM VARIATIONS OF THE ATLAS

Two forms of hypoplasia of the atlas (Köhler and Zimmer 1967, Wackenheim 1975) can be distinguished:

- hypoplasia of the anterior atlas arch, frequently accompanied by 'compensatory' hypertrophy of the posterior atlas arch
- hypoplasia of the atlas with a narrow posterior atlas arch, occasionally combined with hypertrophy of the arcus ventralis.

The posterior arch of the atlas can be hypoplastic on one or on both sides (Komatsu et al 1993). Other authors consider pronounced forms of hypoplasia of the posterior pedicle of the arch to be a gradual preliminary stage of aplasia of the atlas arch (Torklus and Gehle 1970) and refer to malformations over and above these, such as a combination with an os odontoideum. Bogduk and Twomey (1987) and also Riedel and Biedermann (1988) are of the opinion that such anomalies can interfere with the cervical balance and so be the cause of headaches. The term hypoplasia of the atlas with regard to cervical myelopathies (Inomata et al 1998, May et al 2001, Nishikawa et al 2001, Phan et al 1998, Yamashita et al 1997) refers rather to short posterior arches of the atlas that are

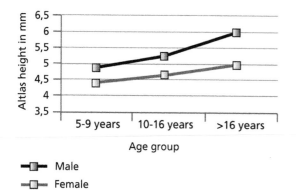

Figure 18.17   Average atlas height in different age groups.

possibly accompanied by hypoplastic anterior atlas arches, and the other way around, and so lead to a compression of the nerve structures.

The lumbosacral junction

There is a wide diversity of anatomical variations present in the lumbosacral region. Apart from pure asymmetries, i.e. functionally harmless presacral vertebra and tilted sacral bearing surface, there are numerous other variations with a bigger impact on the biomechanics of that region. The most frequent are defects of the arch of the presacral vertebrae (L_5 and S_1) as well as all types of lumbarization/sacralization. These may be associated with a malposition. But there are also cases where this defect of the articular surface has a symmetrical form. In such cases the articulation between the thickened transverse process and the ilium has to be taken into account. This leads to a marked biomechanical change in this area, especially if the defect is on one side only.

A symmetrical malformation does not lead to general static disorders but – depending on the form of this area – to a more or less clinically relevant instability of the lumbosacral junction.

Hip region

Similar to the lumbosacral junction region, two basic types are found when assessing the hip region: on the one hand changes that are relevant from a purely static point of view – i.e. differences in leg length – and on the other, morphological variations with and without effects on the static.

There are differences in the embedding of the femoral head in the pelvis and these basically depend on how deep the femoral head is located. If the femoral head is not located deep enough, this leads to increased disproportionate pressure between leg and pelvis and so to an incorrect stress or overstrain of the structures concerned. The first indication of this is usually an increase in the calcium salt in the area of the femoral head which is under strain. Sclerosis of the osseous cover of the socket is not in itself clinically relevant evidence, but during the examination, attention should be paid to the hip joint concerned and the adjoining muscles.

Usually a local hypermobility is found in hips with insufficient osseous support in the compensated phase, particularly when the internal rotation is tested. Quite often, this results in a lack of mobility when the symptoms of stress begin. So, in both cases, it is almost impossible to differentiate between purely functional and combined anatomical findings without a radiographic examination. In these cases it is advisable to examine in detail the relevant groups of muscles such as the adductors, the iliopsoas and the muscles attached to the trochanter.

PATHOGENETIC RELEVANCE OF FORM VARIATIONS OF THE ATLAS

For decades there have been controversial discussions about the question as to how much the form variation of the atlas itself is the cause of clinically relevant symptoms (see Gutmann 1983, Gutmann and Biedermann 1984). The assessment of the foramen retroarticulare atlantis (foramen arcuale) – a form variation in which the arteria vertebralis, which lies on the arcus dorsalis, is encased with bone – can serve as one example among many. Whereas in the 1970s and 1980s French authors in particular dealt with this topic, in the last few years some papers have come from China. These reported on an operative resection as a successful therapy for vertigo (Klausberger and Samec 1975, Li et al 1995, Limousin 1980, Piper et al 1979, Sun 1990), although in some papers only a small number of cases were used. These variants are visible at a very early age and help to classify postural problems found in these children more exactly.

Even if the clinical status does not seem to be clear, a foramen arcuale should at least raise the therapist's awareness that caution is essential, since serious complications after manipulation of the cervical spine are more likely in these patients (Cellerier and Georget 1984).

Slight form variations in the region of the atlanto-dental joint have a great effect on the tolerance of the head–neck aggregate, here particularly in the sagittal plane (Gutmann and Biedermann 1984). The anteflexion headache among schoolchildren, caused by inadequacy of the atlanto-dental connection, is one of the most frequent problems.

This knowledge of a connection between minor anatomical disorders at the level of C_1 and lumbosacral asymmetries resulted in a somewhat extended indication for lumbar/pelvis/hip X-rays of young people, for whom we otherwise keep these radiographs to a minimum in order to protect the gonads.

The same applies to more severe functional disorders, for example misalignments in the OC junction. As a rule, the palpatory findings point to painful tension in the short muscles close to a blockage rather than to a primary restriction of movement. This has normally been compensated by adjustments over several decades, to such an extent that no hints for it can be palpated.

Besides the counter-indications that can result from such findings, such a radiograph is valuable to the therapist by indicating a suitable form of treatment. It is only possible to make an adequate scientific evaluation of the findings and/or plan manipulation in the OC junction precisely if these defects can be excluded as much as possible or are included when planning the appropriate treatment.

If a routine X-ray reveals the presence of such a hypoplasia, more attention should be paid to possible static components of the child's complaints. In this way the influence of the tilted presacral bearing surface and/or a one-sided limited hip function on a primarily cervicogenic defect can be included in the diagnosis and the planning of the treatment. It has been known for decades that migranous headaches especially are influenced by static problems (Maex 1970).

THE ALF TRIAD

After the criteria had been defined for the presence of a hypoplasia of the atlas, the combination radiographs of 180 adult patients, which were available, were analyzed and evaluated (Tables 18.1, 18.2).

We cannot as yet offer an embryological model which might explain these interdependencies, but it seems probable that there is a strong family- and sex-specific component. We were able to record numerous cases where same-sex family members had comparable X-ray findings. Since systematic studies of this subject are out of the question for ethical reasons, this assumption cannot be checked statistically. Isolated literary references, however, confirm the large numbers of variations in the spinal form in families (Bogduk and Twomey 1987, Lang 1983).

The consequence for us in practice is that, in cases of known family occurrences of malposition and/or form variations of the atlas, we make a

Table 18.1 Distinctive features in the craniocervical junction ($N = 180$; M 73, F 107)

	M	F
Pronounced hypoplasia of the atlas	6	12
Borderline hypoplasia of the atlas	13	22
Other dysplasia (defects of the arch C_1)	1	1
Total $N = 55$	20	35

Table 18.2 Combination of distinctive features in patients with moderate hypoplasia of the atlas in a random sample of adults (N = 180; M 73, F 107)

	A	AL	AF	ALF
M (13)	1	2	1	9
F (22)	1	4	0	17
Total (35)	2	6	1	26

A, atlas; AL, atlas and lumbar; AF, atlas and hip joint (femur); ALF, triad of the three areas.

broad allowance for the indication of a radiograph of the lumbar/pelvis/hip region, whereas this X-ray is only taken in less than 20% of our cases before the patient has reached physical maturity.

A NEVER ENDING STORY

This chapter was one of the most difficult ones to finalize for the book, as new findings crop up almost every week. Time and again we changed, added or eliminated plates in order to keep the content as up-to-date (and concise) as possible.

Two aspects of the radiological examination of this area should be highlighted at the end:

- the interdependence between minor morphological findings, be it as the result of dysfunctional exertion or as an inherited trait, and the emerging functional patterns of the infant
- the dynamics of these morphological alterations which seem to be much more easily influenced by timely treatment than previously thought.

Both aspects need a lot more attention and the picture presented here can only claim to be a foretaste of a much more profound treatment of this complex topic. A well-read radiograph yields its secrets to the persistent inquirer. If some readers become interested in this not very easy task, they can be assured that their insight into the problems of their young patients will improve and thus the quality of their work – and their enjoyment, too.

References

Biedermann H, Sacher R 2002 Formvarianten des Atlas als Hinweis auf morphologische Abweichungen im Lenden/Becken/Hüftbereich. Manuelle Medizin 40:330–338

Bogduk N, Twomey L T 1987 Clinical anatomy of the lumbar spine. Churchill Livingstone, Melbourne

Cellerier P, Georget A M 1984 [Dissection of the vertebral arteries after manipulation of the cervical spine. Apropos of a case]. Journal of Radiology 65:191–196

Gutmann G (1953/1988) Die obere Halswirbelsäule im Krankheitsgeschehen. In: Biedermann H (ed) Von der Chiropraktik zur Manuellen Medizin. Haug, Heidelberg, p 81–114

Fried K 1963 Der Wirbelblock. Radiologia Diagnostica 4:165

Gutmann G 1975 Röntgendiagnostik der Wirbelsäule unter funktionellen Gesichtspunkten; Ergebnisse und Impulse für Klinik und Praxis. Manuelle Medizin 13:1–12

Gutmann G 1981 Funktionelle Pathologie und Klinik der Wirbelsäule. Vol 1. Funktionsanalytische Röntgendiagnostik der Halswirbelsäule und Kopfgelenke. G Fischer, Stuttgart

Gutmann G 1983 Die funktionsanalytische Röntgendiagnostik der Halswirbelsäule. Funktionelle Pathologie und Klinik der Wirbelsäule (Gutmann G, Biedermann H, eds), Vol. 1/2. Fischer, Stuttgart

Gutmann G 1987 Hirntumor Atlasverschiebung und Liquordynamik. Manuelle Medizin 25:60–63

Gutmann G, Biedermann H 1984 Die Halswirbelsäule, Part 2: Allgemeine funktionelle Pathologie und klinische Syndrome (Gutmann G, Biedermann H, eds). Fischer, Stuttgart

Gutmann G, Biedermann H 1990 Funktionelle Röntgenanalyse der Lenden-Becken-Hüftregion. Fischer, Stuttgart

Hartwig H 1964 Über Veränderungen an der Halswirbelsäule im Kindesalter unter besonderer Berücksichtigung des Sotterns. In: Müller D (ed) Neurologie der Wirbelsäule und des Rückenmarkes im Kindesalter. Fischer, Jena, p 343–357

Hollingworth W, Dixon A K, Todd C J et al 1998 Self reported health status and magnetic resonance imaging findings in patients with low back pain. European Spine Journal 7(5):369–375

Ingelmark B 1947 Über das craniovertebrale Grenzgebiet. Acta Anatomica (Suppl) 6:1

Inomata N, Hoshino R, Nishimura G 1998 Intractable apneic spells due to hypoplasia of the atlas in a patient with unclassifiable short-rib dysplasia. American Journal of Medical Genetics 76:276–278

Jacobi G, Riepert T, Kieslich M et al 2001 Über einen Todesfall während der Physiotherapie nach Vojta bei einem 3 Monate alten Säugling [Fatal outcome during physiotherapy (Vojta's method) in a 3-month old infant. Case report and comments on manual therapy in children]. Klinische Padiatrie 213(2):76–85

Jirout J 1990 Röntgenologische Bewegungsdiagnostik der Halswirbelsäule; funktionelle Pathologie und Klinik der Wirbelsäule (Gutmann G, Biedermann H, eds), Vol. 1/3. Fischer, Stuttgart

Kamieth H 1983 Röntgenbefunde von normalen Bewegungen in den Kopfgelenken. WS in Forschung und Praxis, Vol 101. Hippokrates, Stuttgart

Kapandji J A 1974 The Physiology of the Joints. Churchill Livingstone, London

Klausberger E M, Samec P 1975 Foramen retroarticulare atlantis und A. vertebralis-angiogramm. MMW Münchner Medizinische Wochenschrift 117:483–486

Koch L 1999 Differentialdiagnostische Probleme bei KiSS-Syndrom. In: Biedermann H (ed) Manualtherapie bei Kindern. Enke, Stuttgart, p 43–52

Köhler A, Zimmer E A 1967 Grenzen des Normalen und Anfänge des Pathologischen im Röntgenbild des Skeletts. Thieme, Stuttgart

Komatsu Y, Shibata T, Yasuda S et al 1993 Atlas hypoplasia as a cause of high cervical myelopathy. Case report. Journal of Neurosurgery 79:917–919

Lang J 1983 Funktionelle Anatomie der Halswirbelsäule und des benachbarten Nervensystems. In: Hohmann D et al (eds) Neuro-Orthopädie. Springer, Berlin, p 1–118

Lewit K 1985 Manipulative therapy in rehabilitation of the motor system. Butterworths, London

Lewit K 1994 The functional approach. Journal of Orthopedic Medicine 16:73–74

Lewit K, Sachse J, Janda V 1992 Manuelle Medizin. J A Barth, Leipzig/Heidelberg

Li S, Li W, Sun J 1995 Operative treatment for cervical vertigo caused by foramen arcuale. Zhonghua Wai Ke Za Zhi 33(3):137–139

Limousin C A 1980 Foramen arcuale and syndrome of Barre-Lieou. Its surgical treatment. International Orthopaedics 4(1):19–23

Maex L 1970 La Migraine et le Syndrome Cervicale comme Symptomes d'un Syndrome de la Statique. Belgische Tijdschrift Rheumatologie 5

May D, Jenny B, Faundez A 2001 Cervical cord compression due to a hypoplastic atlas. Case report. Journal of Neurosurgery 94:133–136

Murrie V L, Dixon A K, Hollingworth W et al 2003 Lumbar lordosis: Study of patients with and without low back pain. Clinical Anatomy 16:144–147

Nishikawa K, Ludwig S, Colon R et al 2001 Cervical myelopathy and congenital stenosis from hypoplasia of the atlas: report of three cases and literature review. Spine 26:80–86

Penning L, Wilmink J T, van Woerden HH et al 1986 CT myelographic findings in degenerative disorders of the cervical spine: clinical significance. AJR American Journal of Roentgenology 146:793–801

Phan N, Marras C, Midha R et al 1998 Cervical myelopathy caused by hypoplasia of the atlas: two case reports and review of the literature. Neurosurgery 43:629–633

Piper H F, Bastian G O, Warecka K 1979 Drehnystagmus und Hypoplasie des N. opticus in Kombination mit fehlendem septum pellucidum. Klinische Monatsblatter für Augenheilkunde 174:663–675

Riedel E, Biedermann F 1988 X-ray diagnosis of occipitocervical malformations. III. Atlas and axis malformations, segmentation disorders of the upper cervical spine. Radiologia Diagnostica 29:581–593

Sun J Y 1990 Foramen arcuale and vertigo. Zhonghua Wai Ke Za Zhi 636:592–594

Swischuk L 2002 Imaging of the Cervical Spine in Children. Springer, New York

Torklus D, Gehle D 1970 Die obere Halswirbelsäule: Thieme, Stuttgart

Valk J, van der Knaap M S, Grauw T et al 1991 The role of imaging modalities in the diagnosis of posthypoxic-ischaemic and haemorrhagic conditions of infants. Klinische Neuroradiologie 2:83–104, 127–137

van der Donk J, Schouten J S, Passchier J et al 1991 The associations of neck pain with radiological abnormalities of the cervical spine and personality traits in a general population. Journal of Rheumatology 18:1884–1889

Vojta V, Peters A 1992 Das Vojta-Prinzip. Springer, Berlin

von Lanz T, Wachsmuth W 1955 Praktische Anatomie 1/2: Der Hals. Springer, Berlin

Wackenheim A 1975 Roentgen Diagnosis of the Cranio-Vertebral Region. Springer, Berlin

Wackenheim A 1983 Roentgendiagnostik der Wirbel des Erwachsenen. Springer, Berlin

Wackenheim A 1989 Imaginerie du Rachis Cervical. Springer, Paris

Wood K B, Garvey T A, Gundry C et al 1995 Magnetic resonance imaging of the thoracic spine. Evaluation of asymptomatic individuals. Journal of Bone and Joint Surgery, American volume 77(11):1631–1638

Yamashita K, Aoki Y, Hiroshima K 1997 Myelopathy due to hypoplasia of the atlas. A case report. Clinical Orthopaedics 338:90–93

Chapter 19

The how–to of making radiographs of newborns and children

H. Biedermann

The radiograph of the spine, and especially that of the cervical spine, yields an amazing amount of information if analyzed thoroughly. The value of this information for diagnosis and treatment is often underestimated. The most plausible explanation may be that there are some thresholds to overcome before being able to enjoy the advantages of this tool. We have to convince the patient or the parents that it is useful to make the radiograph – in order to do that we have to give information about the risk of ionizing radiation and we have to put the doses used into proportion with the information gained.

We have to have the cooperation of the (young) patient for the plate, as the projection has to be thoroughly prepared and the error margin is not very large. We also have to be able to extract the information hidden in the plate. To do that one has to have looked at many radiographs of the spine and at even more of the cervical spine. In this chapter and Chapter 20 we shall try to give an overview of the complexity of this task.

If one of these obstacles is not mastered the entire endeavor fails. We have seen many plates that were technically so insufficient that there was no information to extract – and we have been presented with many plates which did indeed contain interesting and important information but the accompanying letter did not mention it.

In either case the result is discouraging for the one who tried and failed. The most likely reaction after having had this experience a few times is to say 'I don't need these plates anyway!' – and to abandon the arduous task. One can get away with this attitude for quite a while. But it limits the quality of one's work and the satisfaction of a job well done.

So we hope these chapters will convince those involved with manual therapy that it *is* worthwhile to make the effort and that at the end of this admittedly laborious path the reward will be worth the effort. These chapters will also serve as a refresher for those who know but have forgotten.

RADIATION PROTECTION

The best radiation protection is to take as few plates as possible. This principle is often forgotten, as it is easier to look at an isolated plate and check if it was taken *lege artis*. To come to a useful evaluation one has to first determine the structures which have to be depicted on the plate. Our plates of the cervical spine for example are 'unusual' in the sense that we do not cut off everything which is not cervical spine. Instead we insist on seeing the dental structures and the base of the skull. These structures help to evaluate the functional situation and the position of the head relative to the cervical spine (see Chapter 13).

On the caudal side we want to see as much as possible of the thoracic spine, as most of the hemivertebrae occur in the levels C_6/T_3. These are not visible on a 'normal' plate of the cervical spine as they are cut off in a misguided attempt to use as little radiation as possible. If this leads to a loss of important information, or to an additional plate being taken, this laudable effort to save radiation becomes counterproductive.

The same is true for the plates of the lumbar spine. In many cases, patients present one plate of the lumbar spine and one of the pelvis. Both plates could have been taken with one exposure, giving the examiner the additional benefit of seeing these functionally related structures in synopsis, which

makes the functional and static analysis much easier. So, again, the best way to use ionizing radiation sparingly is to take as few plates as possible and not to cut too much off the individual plate.

This holds true, too, for the (in)famous gonadic protection. The female model is completely useless: one or two kidney-shaped lead sheets are placed on the belly of a woman or girl. More often than not the structure in the radiation shadow of this sheet is a part of the small bowel, but not – as intended – the ovaries. In most cases these sheets block the view of the iliosacral joints and the presacral level, an important source of information for the assessment of the static situation.

With all this, a basic fact is forgotten: the biologically active radiation – i.e. the part of the spectrum which has the potential to cause damage to the cell and especially to the DNA – is the 'bremsstrahlung', which is triggered by the interaction of the primary X-rays with the tissue. This secondary radiation originates thus in the body and is therefore diffuse. It cannot be prevented from reaching the ovaries by shielding them from the primary radiation.

The only useful gonadic protection is the testicle cup, a lead 'bucket' wrapped around the testicles. This *does* protect the spermatopoietic tissue from ionizing radiation during a radiological maneuver. We tried to apply these when taking the plates of the lumbar/pelvis/hip region – and found out that to stand 'normally' with the testicle protection applied is impossible. This would mean that the picture we take is not reflecting the neutral stance we are seeking to depict but a more or less provisional position which depicts the pain-avoidance of the patient due to the discomfort of the appliance more than anything else. Therefore, we do not use it anymore.

Another similar problem is the use of lead gauntlets by the parents while stabilizing the head of their child for plates of the cervical spine. We saw that the loss of direct contact between the parent's hand and the child made it much more difficult to get satisfactory results. As we had to repeat

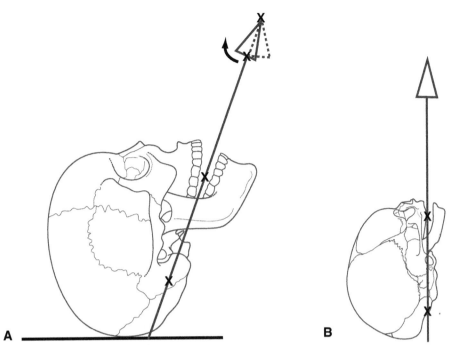

Figure 19.1 Schema for the a.p. projection of radiographs of the cervical spine. A: The situation in adults. To avoid overlapping between teeth and condyles one has to tilt the beamer ± 15°. B: In newborns the direction of the rays can be almost vertical. Between the two extremes one has to negotiate. A good guide is to stay a little caudally of the upper teeth and a little cranially of the protuberantia occipitalis externa, as shown for the adult's skull (A).

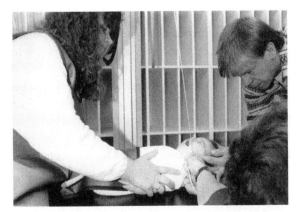

Figure 19.2 A concrete example of stabilization of an infant for radiography: the father holds the head, the mother stabilizies the trunk and the radiological assistant calibrates the tilt of the generator with the help of a string.

about 15% of the pictures, the additional exposure of the child's tissue more than outweighs the protection for the parent's hand. We dropped that procedure, too.

It goes without saying that we use lead sheets to cover the child's body while taking plates of the cervical spine and that the same holds true for any other regional plate taken (e.g. hands, knees, etc.).

WRITTEN CONSENT

How important is the documentation of the consent of the parents and how detailed should the information of the parents regarding the risks of manual therapy be?

Both questions depend crucially on the medico-legal context of one's work. Where I work (Germany, Belgium, Switzerland) I do not deem it necessary to let the parents sign a written form. All parents receive a folder explaining the procedure and the eventual reactions of the children. To our knowledge there are no serious side effects to manual therapy in children (MTC) if the guidelines laid down here are followed. Our archives comprise more than 25 000 children treated in our practice (as of July 2003) and another group at least as big as this one treated by colleagues who follow the same procedure.

Although it is not possible to categorically exclude any adverse effect of MTC on a child, with the material at our disposal it seems warranted to classify MTC as 'safe', certainly so as the energy used in the manipulation is well below any impulse which might cause soft tissue trauma, even in an anatomically unfavorable situation (Koch and Girnus 1998).

In all these years, three cases have come to our attention where children suffered seizure-like reactions after having been treated. In all three cases there was no mention of central nervous problems beforehand and the diagnostic procedures initiated after the parents' observation did not yield any usable indications.

So the jury is out on the question of *post hoc* or *propter hoc*, and the most we can assume is that MTC has as one consequence, an unspecific stimulation of the autonomic system and can as such trigger all sorts of reactions. The children are often tired or overexcited after treatment (see Chapter 11).

One might argue that a written consent form mentioning all problems known from manipulations of adults should be obtained beforehand to protect the therapist against eventual claims by the parents. Two points should be kept in mind when taking such a decision: how does such a form influence the relationship between therapist and parents, and does it really protect the therapist against these claims?

Any weighing up of these questions is a bit theoretical for us, as so far, we have not had any problems. So, there is a point in informing the parents as well and as honestly as possible, but based on our experience, the risks should not be exaggerated and it is certainly counterproductive for the eventual manipulation to apply schematically the incident reports from adults. The three most common risk factors in adults do not apply to children, at least not if the procedures outlined here are followed precisely:

- post-traumatic instability and/or angiological problems prior to therapy
- rotational manipulation and the application of excessive force
- frequently repeated manual therapy without a sufficiently large interval.

Almost all incident reports found in the literature show one or more of these risk factors. All of them are avoidable or non-existent in children. Lewit remarked already in the 1960s that one or two manipulations suffice to make the vertebrogenic problems disappear (Lewit and Janda 1964), so the most important risk factor should be avoidable in almost every case.

WHAT HAS TO BE SHOWN ON THE PLATE?

A very common answer to the difficulties of taking a plate of the cervical spine is to split the problem in two and shoot the condyles and upper cervical spine through the mouth and the rest of the cervical spine on a separate plate. Apart from the fact that this necessitates two doses of ionizing radiation and is thus not ideal because of radiation protection considerations, this method separates two adjoining and functionally closely linked regions, making the evaluation of the functional aspects of these plates unnecessarily cumbersome.

The radiation protection leads quite frequently to another deplorable situation: the cervical spine is barely visible on these plates, and a topographical orientation rendered difficult so that the base of the skull cannot be assessed.

Figure 19.3 Two attempts. A: The first time our little patient succeeded in closing his mouth just at the right (wrong) moment – even with his father's finger on his chin.
B: The second picture succeeded. The essentials are there from the condyles to C_2.

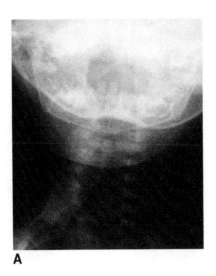
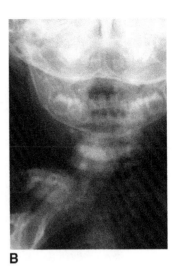

A   **B**

On the caudal side of the plate the important region of the cervicodorsal junction is often cut out. As most of the hemivertebrae leading to a fixed scoliosis of the neck are situated in this area (Wackenheim 1975), this is more than a trifling drawback, as this missing information prevents the correct diagnosis being found.

The condyles have to be seen as clearly as possible. This cannot always be achieved, as any shortening of the clivus leads to a superposition of the occipital mass and the joint C_0/C_1 – the lateral projection can be used to clarify such a situation. C_2 and C_3 are normally covered by the mandible, but in children its density is such that at least a cursory appraisal of these vertebrae is possible.

We would advise depicting the intraoral structures on the lateral plates. It is the norm that this area is cut out on the lateral plates, but the additional radiation load is minimal and the information obtained worth the small extra cost of a slightly bigger film.

Ideally we want a radiograph which shows the spontaneous position of the individual. Gutmann (1969) showed that for adults, this position is highly reproducible. In children – at least in those younger than 6–8 years – we cannot hope to convince them to assume such a posture. The best we can hope for is that they lie still. So the functional

aspect of these plates has to be taken with a grain of salt. As the functional aspect is in most cases much more clear-cut than in adults we are able to use these plates in most cases, anyway.
[fig 19.3]

THE POSITIONING OF THE CHILD

The unanimous judgment of our radiological assistants is that the age of 2–4 years is the worst time to take plates. Till the first birthday one can at least try to come to terms with the little patient and create a playful and relaxed atmosphere – as far as the constraints of the roentgen apparatus allow it. Around the first birthday (girls are, as always at that age, faster in that regard) the patient gets distinctively uncooperative.

We do ask two people well known to the child to accompany him the first time. In most cases these are the parents or one parent and one grandparent. It certainly helps to have two people, one grasping the head and the other holding the trunk. It also helps to explain the procedure carefully to these two helpers and motivate them beforehand. At least once a day we are confronted with one partner completely unable to handle the 'suffering' of the child – and you can be sure that

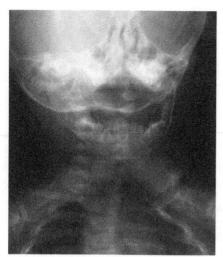

Figure 19.4 Rotation of the head. Such a picture is almost useless for functional analysis. Due to the rotation of the head the projection-faults eclipse the normal situation. Any statement about the relative positions of the suboccipital vertebrae is reduced to guesswork. The only useful information obtainable is on the morphological level, i.e. that no major malformations are present in the depicted area.

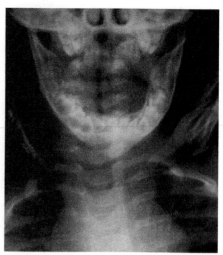

Figure 19.5 Beam direction too vertical. In this case the X-ray tube should have been tilted a little more to avoid overlapping of upper teeth and condyles. Due to the reduced bone density of infants as compared to adults, enough details are discernible anyway, so this radiograph is usable, albeit not ideal.

the infant has an immediate comprehension of this weakness, increasing resistance to the maximum to get where he wants to be, i.e. *not* on the radiological examination table.

As the a.p. projection is the most important plate at the cervical level we start there, and in quite a few cases we have to relinquish the lateral projection.

We use a wedge-shaped attenuation filter to compensate for the different density of the upper and lower cervical area. Digital equipment compensates for these steep gradients automatically.

SOURCES OF ERROR

Figures 19.5 and 19.6 show two a.p. plates which were taken too steeply and with too low an angle, respectively. The margin of error is not very big in the suboccipital area and especially so with children, as having to open the mouth is normally not to their liking.

Luckily the bone density of infants is inferior to that of adults and in many cases 'non-optimal' plates can still be used. We have to take into account that the resistance of the child is already provoked by the first attempt and the nerves of all others worn out to a certain extent. The threshold for requesting a new plate is therefore relatively high and we accept plates that would have to be refused in older children or adults. Figure 19.6 shows such a case: the projection is not ideal – to put it mildly – but everything essential can be examined at least well enough not to justify another exposure.

The most difficult age for any radiography is between the 1st and 4th birthdays. From the 8th–10th month on, babies start to be shy of strangers and a few months later their opinion of what is acceptable is quite developed – with girls a little earlier and more distinct than with boys. When the children reach preschool age they are much more open to persuasion. Quite a few pizzas or ice-creams have been successfully promised to achieve the cooperation of the little patients.

Besides this basic and most important obstacle to achieving a good plate, there are some minor

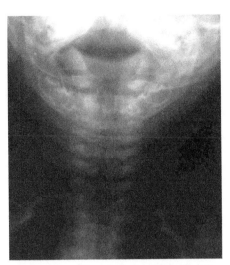

Figure 19.6 Beam tilt too much. This is the other extreme: here the tube was tilted too extensively, which leads to an overlapping between the mandibular bone and teeth and C_2.

and much more manageable details to keep in mind. One is the changing proportion of the skull base (see Chapter 4) in relationship to the cervical spine which necessitates different projection angles (see Fig. 19.1). Once the skull is aligned correctly we have to make sure that the mouth is opened sufficiently to allow an unhindered view of the condyles and C_1/C_2. In most cases the teeth and mandible cover the caudal part of C_2, but the functionally important aspect is the joint level C_1/C_2, which can normally be visualized without too much effort. Even when the mandible is projected onto a vertebra one should be able to see major pathologies, i.e. hemivertebrae, fusions and the like.

As already mentioned under the aspect of radiation protection, there is a widespread tendency to cut out as much as possible on these plates which sometimes leads to radiographs where the lowest vertebra of the cervical spine and the upper thoracic area are cut off even when it would have been perfectly possible to picture these vertebrae on the plate. As many congenital malformations are located in the cervicothoracic junction, this over-cautious approach can be one reason why such a diagnosis is overlooked. We would propose being very careful about cutting off areas which might yield useful information.

The eyes are one area one wants to shield from unnecessary exposure. Initially we tried to put a lead shield over the upper part of the skull and the eyes, but we quickly dropped this experiment as the children became so agitated by being blinded in this way that the double exposures which were thus necessary more than offset the apparent radiation-saving effect of this maneuver. We do try to use the diaphragms to reduce the radiation cone as much as possible but here, again, one has to take into account the movements of the children at the last moment and a little leeway has to be given to avoid shielding diagnostically relevant areas.

Once in a while, asymmetries of the structures of the skull base help in understanding the situation of the adjoining suboccipital level, one more reason not to shield this area on the plates.

PRACTICAL CONSIDERATIONS

Most radiological departments are located somewhere in the bowels of a hospital. Daylight is rare or non-existent on the premises and rooms displaying at least a basic client-friendliness are rare. The interior design is 'functional' and the colors used vary through the entire spectrum of gray to khaki. To my knowledge there is no regulation prohibiting the use of bright and friendly colors in radiological departments and a friendly picture on the wall does wonders to the mood of patients and personnel alike. Such a friendly layout is no miracle cure to achieve better compliance, but just one small detail helping to get there – and in any case, it does not make things worse.

Space, light and a friendly environment lay the groundwork for putting the children in a good mood. It is almost as important not to overburden the radiological assistants. Work with children is very demanding – in our consulting rooms it is considered almost as trying as telephone duty – and if possible one should try to rotate the tasks frequently during a working day. We try to assign another assistant every 3 hours in order to keep the spirits and friendliness level high.

Before and after taking the radiograph children should be given enough time to relax and adapt to all these strange things we want them to do. Often it helps to embellish the taking of the plates with a game or a challenge, like 'are you *really* able to lie still on the table even with the light on?'

As always the first and foremost step is to convince the parents that what we ask for is in the interest of the child and the quicker we get there, the better. It does not help to try to argue with children in such a situation. Yes, we explain what we want to do and what we have to ask the child to do in order to get there. But no, we shall not argue about the necessity of this with the child, as this inevitably leads to a quick escalation and never to a good radiograph.

It has to be clear for the accompanying adults that the doctor or radiological assistant responsible will explain and soothe, but at that point in time there is no place to discuss the principal necessity of such a picture. As soon as children sense a conflict between their care-givers and the person trying to take the plate they will exploit

Box 19.1 The ten commandments to achieve good radiographs

1. Take time.
2. Explain the why and how patiently.
3. A friendly and colorful room is not an option, but a must.
4. When taking the plates, be sure to be in command.
5. In case of doubt, it is better to cut off less rather than more.
6. When choosing the slope of the beam, it is better to incline a little too much.
7. Shoot the most informative plate first, i.e. in most cases the a.p. projection.
8. Take into account the age of the young patient when considering a repeat.
9. Be absolutely sure to have the parents on your side.
10. Take time.

this, and children are much more sensitive to these non-verbal clues than adults.

Following these rules is no guarantee for perfect plates – and even less so for a correct interpretation of them – but it goes a long way to avoiding frustrating experiences. And even then the road to an in-depth and complete evaluation of the plates is long . . .

References

Gutmann G 1969 Röntgendiagnostik der Occipito-Cervical-Gegend unter chirotherapeutischen Gesichtspunkten. Röntgenblätter 45–56

Koch L E, Girnus U 1998 Kraftmessung bei Anwendung der Impulstechnik in der Chirotherapie. Manuelle Medizin 36(1):21–26

Lewit K, Janda V 1964 Die Entwicklung von Gefügestörungen der Wirbelsäule im Kindesalter und die Grundlagen einer Prävention vertebragener Beschwerden. In: Müller D (ed) Neurologie der Wirbelsäule und des Rückenmarkes im Kindesalter. Fischer, Jena, p 371–389

Wackenheim A 1975 Roentgen diagnosis of the craniovertebral region. Springer, Berlin

Radiological examination of the spine in children and adolescents: pictorial essay

P. Waibel

CHAPTER CONTENTS

The most important imaging modalities to evaluate abnormal clinical symptoms or incorrect posture of the spine are conventional radiography, ultrasound, computed tomography and magnetic resonance imaging.

INDICATIONS

The following lists show the most important clinical signs for further imaging evaluation in relation to the anatomical level of the spine.

Cervical spine:

- torticollis
- trauma: persistent pain, neurological symptoms
- infections
- tumor.

Thoracic and lumbar spine:

- pain
- abnormal posture
- trauma: persistent pain, neurological symptoms
- infection/inflammation
- tumor.

TECHNIQUES

Conventional radiographic technique

The classic technique consists of static X-ray tubes with cassettes and analogous films. For the last 10 years the cassettes have been equipped with phosphor screens or function digitally.

With conventional technique it is possible to visualize the posture and the curvature of the spine. The technique allows depiction of the configuration of the vertebral bodies and arches as well as the bony structure of each element.

Ultrasound

The ultrasound picture is generated by transformation of transmitted and reflected ultrasound waves into a gray scale picture. The ultrasound waves are non-ionizing, which is especially important in children. Ultrasound waves are excellent for penetrating soft tissues. They are, however, fully absorbed by bony surfaces. High-frequency probes have a good spatial resolution but a reduced penetration depth. Ultrasound is examiner dependent. The incomplete depiction of the structure is a disadvantage.

Ultrasound is ideal for imaging the paravertebral soft tissues, the vessels and the spinal content in newborns.

Example: fibromatosis colli

Fibromatosis colli (Fig. 20.1) is a fibrous reaction probably to a birth trauma in the first weeks of life. It is a common cause of congenital torticollis and is present in approximately 0.4% of live births. Fibromatosis colli is hyperechogenic to normal muscles.

Other causes of extra-osseous structural torticollis that may be visualized by ultrasound include enlarged lymph nodes, benign congenital lesions (lymphangioma, hemangioma), and neoplasms (rare: rhabdomyososarcoma).

Computed tomography

Computed tomography uses a rotating X-ray tube. The opposite rotating detector measures the incoming radiation (which is partially absorbed by the patient) and reconstructs a two-dimensional picture which has the form of a slice of a few or several millimeters. With multi-slice helical technique, reconstructions in various planes are possible.

Computed tomography is most often used for depicting complex bony structures (e.g. preoperatively) or for the imaging of severe vertebral trauma.

Magnetic resonance imaging

This technique uses the influence of strong magnetic fields to the spins of unpaired atomic nuclei

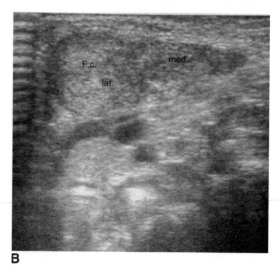

Figure 20.1 Fibromatosis colli, longitudinal aspect, right: transverse view with enlargement of only the clavicular part of the sternocleidomastoid muscle.

to image anatomical structures. The equipment consists of a coil with a static magnetic field (field strengths up to 1.5 T are used commercially), gradient coils, software installations and the terminals. Patients should not move during the sequences; so babies, infants and handicapped children must be sedated.

It is the method of choice for the demonstration of extensive structures, especially imaging of the spine and its contents, mainly soft tissues and neural elements. Ligaments and disks can be depicted in the case of a trauma.

The sequences and settings depend on the configuration (low/high field).

CONVENTIONAL RADIOLOGICAL TECHNIQUE: DETAILS

High speed screens should be used.

Wedge filters should be interposed to equalize the density between the different parts of the spine (especially the shoulder and the thoracolumbar transition. Immobilization and fixation devices are necessary for recumbent radiographs in small children and for handicapped patients.

For an erect view of the complete spine from C_1 to the level of the anterior superior iliac spine in older children a long cassette is mandatory (90×30 cm).

These cassettes are usually equipped with a fixed grid. Actually these projections are performed with digital radiography equipment in erect and recumbent positions. For imaging parts of the spine or a complete spine in preschool children, a wall Bucky is recommended.

The iliac crest and the ribs should be included on the initial study; in subsequent examinations they are radiographed on demand.

Radiation protection

The dose to the growing breast is markedly reduced when the patient faces the cassette in the posteroanterior projection. In anteroposterior projections the dose to the bone marrow of the spine is higher.

Table 20.1   Gonadal shielding

Examination	Male	Female
Cervical spine	Apron	Apron
Thoracic spine	Fixed shield	Fixed shield
Lumbosacral spine	Fixed shield	Shielding limited

Table 20.1 outlines the shielding required for the gonads.

What has to be visualized?

Cervical spine lateral:

- All seven vertebrae and cervicothoracic junction
- prevertebral tissue
- spinous processes, which should form a straight line
- margins of the lateral masses of C_1.

Thoracic and lumbar spine:

- visualization of the paraspinal lines
- posterior elements visible through the vertebral body.

DEVELOPMENTAL ANATOMY

All the vertebrae along with the occipital portion of the skull develop from primitive sclerotomes. For the upper cervical spine, the lower occipital and the upper cervical sclerotomes are important.

The atlas is formed from three ossification centers: the body (which is in fact the anterior arch) and the two neural arches.

The dens is actually the body of C_1 which separated in the development from the arch. The ossicle at the tip of the dens (os terminale) has derived from the fourth occipital sclerotome (known as the proatlas) (Fig. 20.2). The dens itself arises from two primordial centers in the frontal plane, which fuse with the os terminale to the mature dens.

During development the third to the seventh cervical vertebrae consist of six ossification centers. If one or more fail to develop, predictable

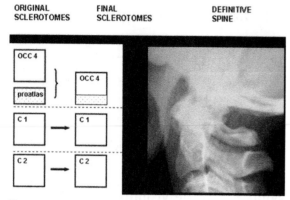

| ORIGINAL SCLEROTOMES | FINAL SCLEROTOMES | DEFINITIVE SPINE |

Figure 20.2 Developmental anatomy.

anomalous configurations result (see section on malformations).

Timing of ossification centers

Atlas: The anterior arch becomes visible in the first year of life. The posterior synchondrosis of the neural arches ossifies in the third year, the neuro-central synchondrosis in the seventh year.

Axis: Ossification center of the body in the fifth fetal month. Apical ossification of the dens occurs between the third and sixth year; fusion with the odontoid by the twelfth year. Fusion of the synchondrosis between the dens and the body occurs in the third to sixth year of life.

NORMAL VARIANTS

It is important not to confuse normal variants (Figs 20.3–20.9) with pathological entities. Normal variants are due to the complex origin of the spinal elements. They consist of variations in the shape and the size of the classically described anatomical forms.

MALFORMATIONS

Malformations are errors in development which lead to major abnormalities in the shape and the size of the vertebral elements (Figs 20.10–20.12). In most of the cases, an abnormal posture in the sagittal and/or frontal plane is encountered.

INFLAMMATION/INFECTION

Infections are diseases with causative agents. In cases without a known infectious agent, we can assume an inflammation. See Figures 20.13 and 24.14.

VERTEBRAL TUMORS

Primary vertebral tumors are rare. Ewing sarcoma, aneurysmal bone cyst, osteoblastoma (Fig. 20.15), osteoid-osteoma and osteochondroma are encountered.

Ewing sarcoma is generally sclerotic or mixed lytic-sclerotic. A neurological deficit is often present. Aneurysmal bone cyst is a radiolucent expanding lesion.

VERTEBRAL TRAUMA

The result of a trauma is not only a deconfiguration of the vertebral elements. Trauma also causes abnormal position of the vertebrae or pathological movement of the spine. For assessing the amount of the dislocation or abnormal movement, measurements are important. The most frequently encountered methods are shown (Fig. 20.17: posterior cervical line; Figs 20.18–20.21: predental distance).

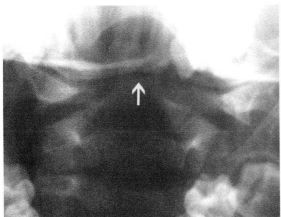

Figure 20.3   Tip of dens not yet ossified. Apical ossification of the dens between the third and sixth year; fusion with the odontoid by the twelfth year. The posterior arches of vertebra C_3 to C_7 fuse posteriorly by the second to third year. The synchondrosis between the body and the neural arches fuse between 3 and 6 years.

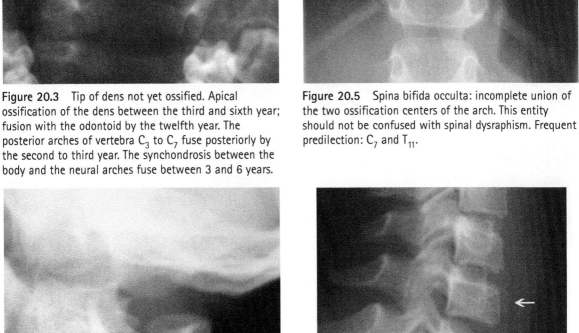

Figure 20.5   Spina bifida occulta: incomplete union of the two ossification centers of the arch. This entity should not be confused with spinal dysraphism. Frequent predilection: C_7 and T_{11}.

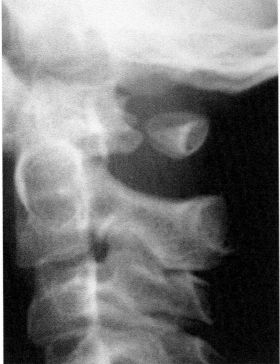

Figure 20.4   A posterior C_1 arch defect is the consequence of undermineralization of the cartilaginous anlage. The edges are smooth with well-corticated margins, so they are differentiated from fractures. Although defects can be large, these anomalies are stable.

Figure 20.6   Hypertrophy of the anterior tubercle of the transverse process may be noticed as a protuberance on palpation. It is the result of an uneven development of the ossification centers of the interarticular pars.

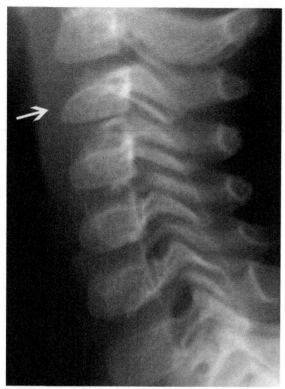

Figure 20.7 Anterior wedging is the hallmark of a fracture. However, in children it is seen more often as a normal finding. Physiological hypermobility leads to anterior growth impairment of the upper plate of C_3, producing a chronically wedged vertebra. Less frequently C_4 and C_5 are involved. In a traumatic situation, however, it becomes necessary to rule out a fracture. This can be done by CT. Note: in cases of severe hypotonia, several vertebrae may be deformed.

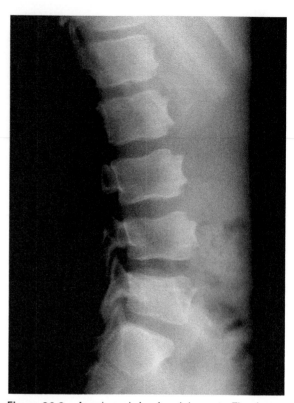

Figure 20.9 Apophyseal ring in adolescents. The rings are in a cartilaginous stage. Ossification begins in puberty and fuses definitively at 25 years. The development of the upper rims is advanced in comparison to the lower ones.

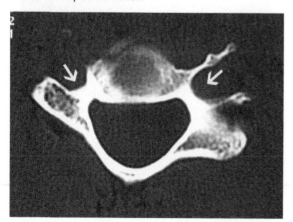

Figure 20.8 Asymmetrical growth of the chondrification centers of the interarticular pars leads to different length of the pedicles with some rotation of the arch in the transverse plane.

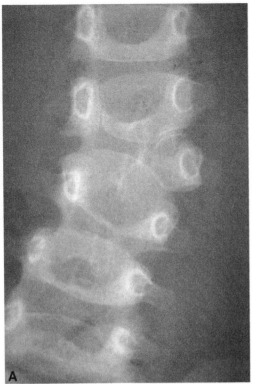
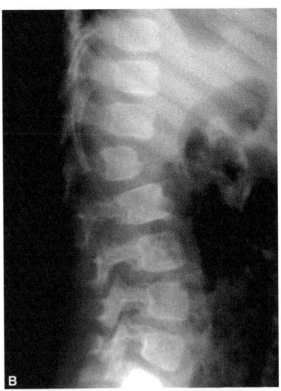

Figure 20.10 Asymmetrical undergrowth of one of the paired chondrification centers gives rise to hemivertebrae. Generally, the degree of the malformation depends upon the chondrification stage. A: Frontal hemivertebra. B: Sagittal hemivertebra. This entity may occur in combination with notochordal remnants.

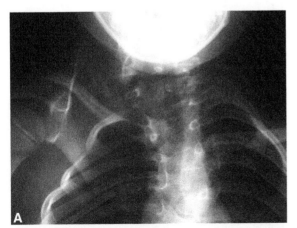
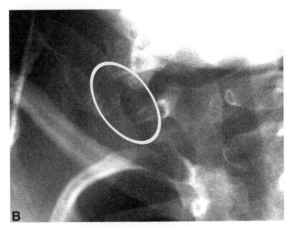

Figure 20.11 A and B: Klippel–Feil anomaly with Sprengel deformity. This is a congenital failure of descent of the scapula. In some patients, as in this case, the scapula is anchored to the spine by an anomalous omovertebral bone that articulates laterally with the medial border of the scapula and medially with one or more vertebral elements. This complex malformation is characterized by a very short neck and a high standing scapula on one side, resulting in a torticollis.

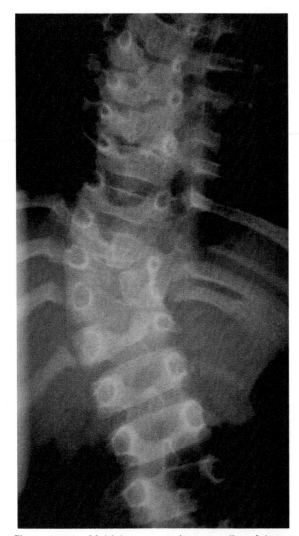

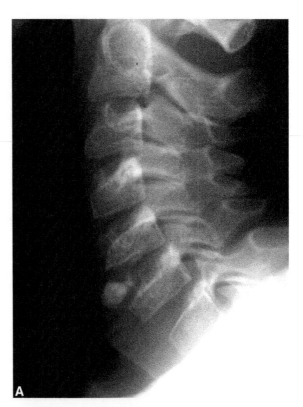

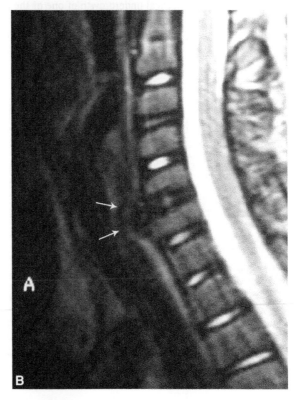

Figure 20.12 Multiple segmentation anomalies of the thoracolumbar spine. Segmentation anomalies occur with both horizontal and vertical fusions and separations of varying degree as a result of maldevelopment of the primitive sclerotomes of the spine. Vertebral malformations (single or complex) are an important part of the so-called VACTERL association (vertebral defects, anal anomalies, cardiac malformations, tracheoesophageal anomalies, renal malformations, limb defects).

Figure 20.13 A and B: The incidence of intervertebral disk calcification in children is low. Usually, except when present in the cervical region, they are not associated with local signs. Calcifications (arrows) are found in all components of the disks and may be single or in multiple sites. They disappear in most cases without sequelae. In MRI they are typically of low signal intensity in T1 and T2 sequences.

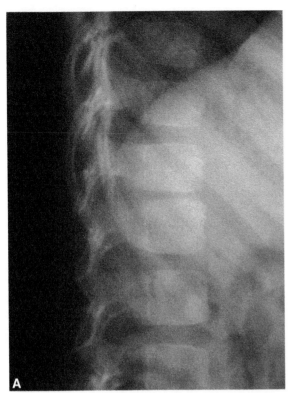

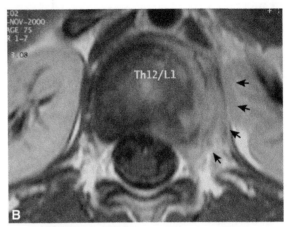

Figure 20.14   A and B: Narrowing of disk T$_{12}$/L$_1$, a result of inflammation and destruction. Diskitis is an inflammatory process of the intervertebral disk. It is considered by most to be a low-grade viral or bacterial infection and occurs most frequently in children from 6 months to 4 years of age with a second peak between 10 and 14 years. The infection probably comes through the valveless venous plexus. Symptoms may include fever, abdominal pain, back pain, limp and refusal to walk or to sit up. Despite the epidural effusion, there are only minor neurological signs.

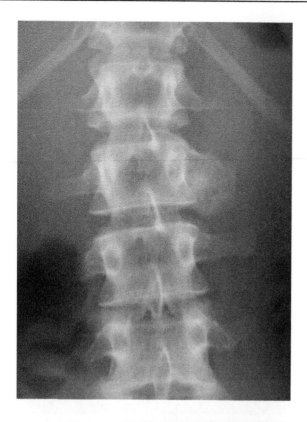

Figure 20.15 Osteoblastoma of the transverse process of L$_2$. It is like a giant osteoid-osteoma and has a predilection for the posterior elements, as in this case. Osteoid-osteoma causes back pain, worsening at night and with relief after aspirin. It may be associated with localized scoliosis. Osteochondroma may grow into the spinal canal. Hemangiomas are mostly incidental findings and cause a spongy osteoporosis of the vertebrae.

Figure 20.16 A: Long spine projection because of ill-defined thoracolumbar pain. B: Multiple collapsed thoracic and lumbar vertebrae. Diagnosis: lymphatic leukemia. Note: In cases of ill-defined pain localization it may be deceptive to perform overview radiographs of the spine. Involvement of the spine in Langerhans cell histiocytosis leads first to a cystic appearance. When collapse occurs a more sclerotic aspect predominates. Other metastatic lesions occur in leukemia, lymphoma, neuroblastoma and rhabdomyosarcoma.

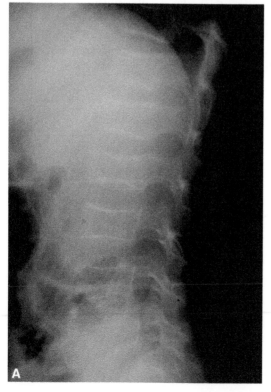

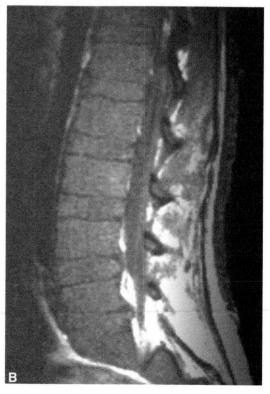

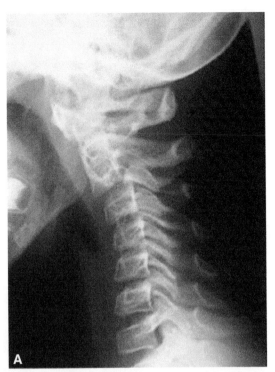 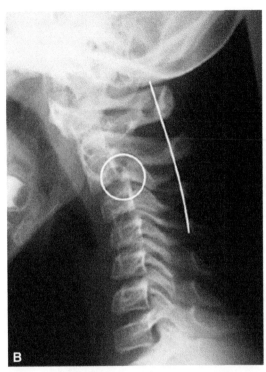

Figure 20.17   A and B: Posterior cervical line measurement. Anterior dislocation of C_2 on C_3 can occur with a hangman's fracture, but in infants and children it is far more common on a physiological basis. A line is drawn from the anterior cortices of the spinous tips of C_1 and C_3. If this line passes the anterior cortex of C_2 by more than 1.5 mm, a hangman's fracture should be suspected, otherwise the findings should be considered as within the physiological range.

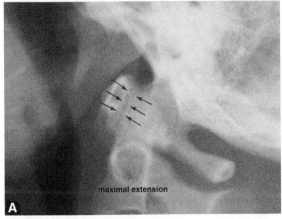 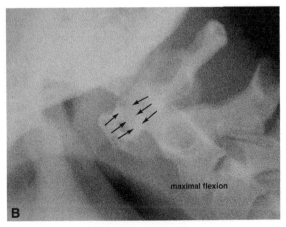

Figure 20.18   Predental distance measurement. A: Extension. B: Flexion. The maximum increase of C_1 to dens distance in flexion should not be more than 2 mm. Otherwise one should suggest an instability of the ligaments. These measurements are often done in children with Down syndrome or with mucopolysaccharidosis to exclude instability.

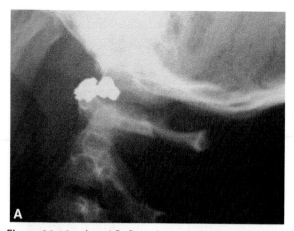

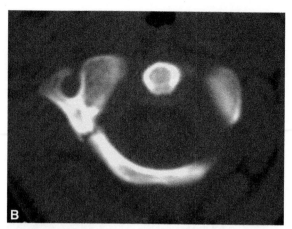

Figure 20.19   A and B: Posterior arch fracture. Note the sharp margins of the fracture. (Not to be confused with congenital defect of the arch, see Fig. 20.4.)

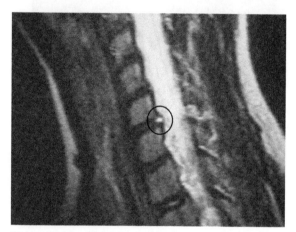

Figure 20.20   Disk injury without osseous involvement. High signal intensity of the posterior border of disk $C_{4/5}$. MR is superior to CT for depicting involvement of dural elements, tears and edema in the ligaments and muscles as well as avulsions of small osseous fragments.

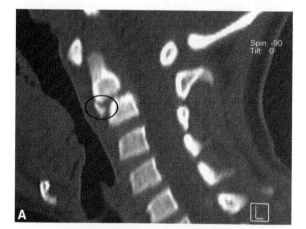

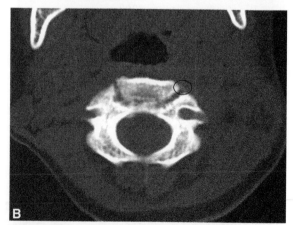

Figure 20.21   A: Sagittal reconstructed CT. B: Axial CT. Conventional radiograph was normal despite the epiphyseal fracture seen on sagittal reconstructed and on axial CT. The functional analysis revealed no instability, so it is a tight pseudarthrosis or non-union.

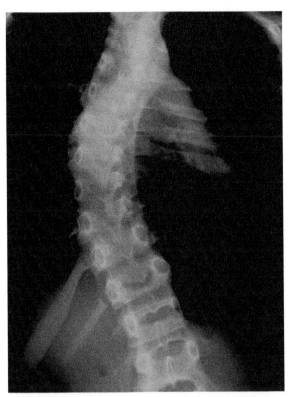

Figure 20.22 This is a typically right convex scoliosis. Torsion is evident in the structural scoliosis to the right, but not at the compensation curves. Scoliosis is defined as one or more curvatures of the spine. It is generally described in relation to the convexity of the angulation.

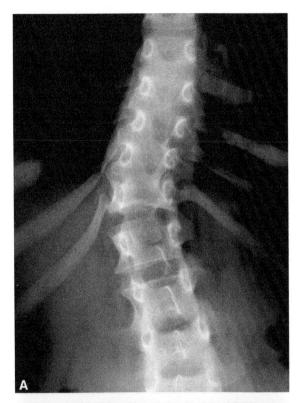

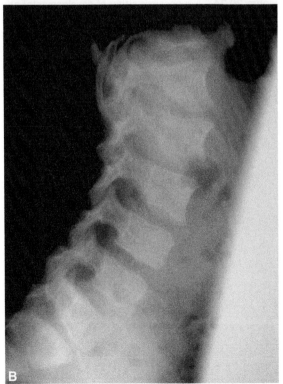

Figure 20.23 A and B: The anterior scalloping of some vertebral bodies suggests the diagnosis of neurofibromatosis. Depending on the etiology of the scoliosis, the shape of the vertebrae varies grossly. Neurofibromas lead to repetitive deconfiguration of primarily normal vertebral bodies and arches, depending on the size and the number of the lesions.

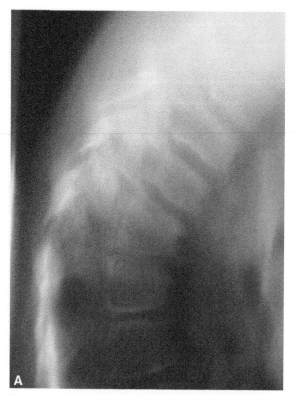

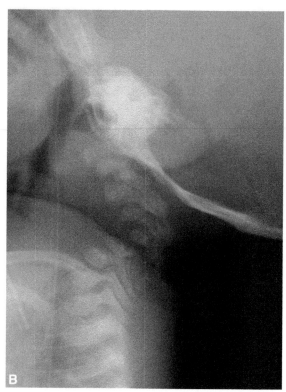

Figure 20.24 A kyphosis is either of developmental origin or the result of an acquired process. A: Hemivertebrae lead to a localized kyphosis. B: This is a complex malformation which will impair the medulla. The anterior wedging is part of malformation of the entire cervical spine. A regional skeletal dysplasia is likely. Some of them are distinct entities, such as the spectrum of the spondylo-epiphyseal or spondylo-metaphyseal dysplasias.

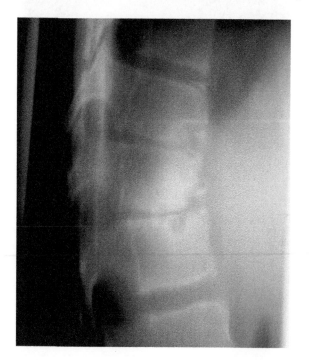

Figure 20.25 Scheuermann disease or juvenile osteochondrosis is the result of a degeneration and protrusion of the disk into the vertebral body. In contrast to diskitis the endplates of the vertebral bodies are not eroded but impressed. Typically the thoracolumbar transition is involved. The principal radiographic findings are progressive narrowing of one or more intervertebral spaces, deep irregularities of the edges and endplates as well as Schmorl nodes in the vertebral bodies, resulting in anterior wedging. Kyphosis is marked and is the lead symptom of the posture.

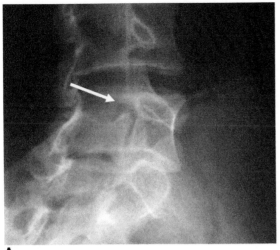

A

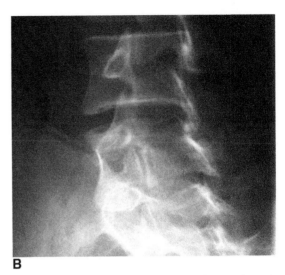

B

Figure 20.26 A and B: The radiographic hallmark of spondylosis is a lucency crossing the pars interarticularis at the neck of a 'Scottie dog' below the eyelike pedicles. This lucency looks like a collar. The oblique projections reveal in this case a unilateral spondylolysis. Once considered as a congenital defect, there is now some evidence of autosomal dominant transmission of the risk of developing this condition, probably on the basis of a dysplasia of the interarticular pars. The spondylolysis itself is considered to be a stress fracture. It appears in infancy to adolescence with an incidence of 5–6% after the age of 10 in white populations. The spondylolisthesis is most frequently the consequence of a spondylolysis.

SCOLIOSIS/KYPHOSIS

A scoliosis is a deviation of the curvature of the spine in the frontal plane, and kyphosis an abnormal amount of curvature in the sagittal plane.

Scoliosis and abnormal kyphosis are symptoms of an underlying disturbance of growth (Figs 20.22–20.26). There is a huge differential diagnosis.

Etiology:

- congenital scoliosis
- idiopathic

- neurofibromatosis
- post-irradiation
- neuromuscular
- compensatory (e.g. following trauma).

  Idiopathic:

- infantile <4 years
- juvenile 4–10 years
- adolescent >10 years; female : male = 4 : 1 to 8 : 1
- most cases: majority right convex.

Further reading

Burton E M, Brody A S 1999 Essentials of pediatric radiology. Thieme, New York/Stuttgart

Fesmire F M, Luten R C 1989 The pediatric spine: developmental anatomy and clinical aspects. Journal of Emergency Medicine 7:133–42

Godderidge C 1995 Pediatric imaging. Saunders, Philadelphia

Keats D R 1991 Practical pediatric imaging. Little, Brown and Company, Boston

Kuhns L R 1998 Imaging of spinal trauma in children. Hamilton: B C Decker

Roche C, Carthy H 2001 Spinal trauma in children. Pediatric Radiology 31:677–700

Silverman F N, Kuhn J P 1993 Caffey's pediatric X-ray diagnosis, 9th edn. Mosby, St Louis

Swischuk L E 2002 Imaging of the cervical spine in children. Springer, New York

Measuring it: different approaches to the documentation of posture and coordination

H. Biedermann, R. Rädel, A. Friedrichs

THE QUEST FOR THE GOLDEN RULER

At the beginning of the eighteenth century, several books dealt with the problems of children and their *education*, a word which had a much broader meaning at that time. These writers focused on the role of posture and gymnastics in the upbringing of children and gave copious advice on how to reach the ideal. In 1741 the French surgeon Nicolas Andry de Boisregard published a book about these topics which was translated into several other languages soon after. The English edition appeared in 1743 under the title: 'Orthopaedia: or, the art of correcting and preventing the deformities in children; by such means, as may easily be put in practice by parents themselves, and all such as are employed in educating children'. In the frontispiece of these books, a female figure – presumably an allegory of truth or science – holds a ruler with the inscription 'Hic est regula recti' – this is the right measure.

Andry de Boisregard was not the first to take a close look at the physical education of children. 'Paedotrophia' was a term coined in 1584 by Scaevola Samarthanus, and 'callipaedia' another one proposed in 1656 by Claudius Quillet (Wessinghage 1987). In the tradition of the Enlightenment, all these authors tried to look at their subject in a scientific way – and this included the attempt to quantify and measure whatever they were studying.

259

The yardstick remained the companion of all those trying to instill scientific thinking in the empirical science of medicine, and certainly those who made it their work to care for children. In the early twentieth century this led to extensive tables being compiled to provide a database for educators and doctors. Mostly these tables contained measurements of length and weight.

In the 1960s and 1970s a different approach gained ground. The ready availability of photographic documentation made it possible to combine radiographs and photographs to record the development of growing children. The most important single item for the prognosis of postural development and scoliosis was Cobb's angle, a measure of the degree of curvature of the spine used as a marker for the amount of postural problems to be expected (Deacon et al 1984, Greenspan et al 1978). Based on Lovett's 1907 publication, several generations of doctors had tried to develop treatment schedules to indicate where conservative treatment was sufficient and where an operation would eventually be inevitable. What became clear was that a single item like Cobb's angle would not be enough to evaluate the long-term perspective of the growing spine and the ensuing posture of the infant under observation.

It is not possible here to describe all the countless methods proposed to document and quantify the postural evolution of children in their adolescence. To get a feeling for the different approaches we shall present only a few representative examples:

- rulers
- photography
- Moiré tomography
- rasterstereography
- phase measuring triangulation
- four-quadrant weight scale
- cervicomotography
- ultrasonic skin distance measurement.

The most accessible means of documentation are standardized tables which document measurements of length and circumference in bilateral comparison. These items are completed by the measurement of the angles between joint partners, e.g. the tibio-femoral angle or Cobb's angle. The neutral-zero method of orthopedic documentation uses a similar approach. A standardized documentation of the normal movement range of the most important joints is compared to those of the patient. If measured at several instances, these data sheets give at least an indication of the direction of the evolution. The problem with this approach is that the generation of these measurements is interactive and it is easily imaginable that a gruff and indifferent examiner will document a wider range of joint movement than a more sympathetic doctor.

Widely used were spirit levels to judge symmetry and equilibrium. Figure 21.1 shows an Italian device to quantify the rib hump of scoliosis. The fundamental problem with all these tools was their direct contact with the patient and the fact that their application depended on the skill of the examiner, making the entire process error-prone.

The next step was the photographic documentation of the posture; the example shown here of a colleague in Milan (Fig. 21.2) indicates the amount of effort invested in these sheets (Neumann 1962). Whatever effort was taken, the best such a documentation was able to provide was a qualitative visual comparison of 'before' and 'after'.

A slight improvement on the simple photograph was Moiré tomography. Here the interference pattern of two light sources makes it possible to attribute bands of light and shadow to defined height profiles, thus giving at least an indication of the distances between different body regions. Moiré tomography made it easier to see the differences in bilateral symmetry, but an important drawback remained: this method did not yield sharp delimitations for the different height bands. A computer-aided processing of the resulting pictures was practically impossible. Several other approaches are currently commercially available. All intend to measure the surface of the back contact-free and in real time, thus obtaining a realistic picture of the person's momentary posture.

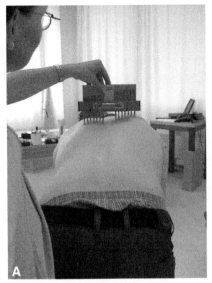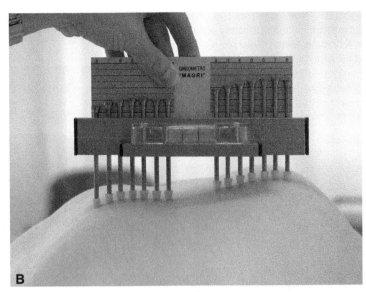

Figure 21.1   Gibbometro. This charming little device was used to document the amount of rib hump.

We are now in a position to be able to obtain data about the surface of the back with several methods. All these approaches have their drawbacks. Some are too slow to be used on freestanding patients, and some are too restricted in their application and allow only one position of the patient. But they all generate a three-dimensional point matrix which can be processed further. And that is where the real problem starts.

THE 'TYPICAL' POSTURE

A lot of work was invested in resolving the question of whether this short-term picture gave a reliable base to assess the individual's 'typical' posture – or at least the typical posture for a given situation.

It is – as usual – only in solving a given problem that one becomes aware of the intricate details of such an endeavor.

The easy part is the documentation of the situation 'as is' – but we will not get very far with this knowledge. We do know since systematic evaluation of radiographs of the vertebral spine are taken that there are different types which have quite diverging functional aspects and well-defined mor-

phological features, too. The best documentation of these types can be based on the form of the sacrum, as this determines the orientation of the lumbar spine and thus the form of the entire back.

In the 1990s we summarized the available evidence that these different types of sacrum were strongly associated with quite distinguishable types of clinical problems (Gutmann and Biedermann 1990). A pronounced curvature of the sacrum is a predisposition for a center of gravity in a more ventral position and a stronger muscular apparatus – the athletic type of the ancient world.

These observations date back decades (for a survey of this literature, see Gutmann and Biedermann 1990) but whenever one opens a book about vertebral pathology there is only 'the' standard type of vertebral spine presented. Small wonder that the majority of statistical evaluations looking for connections between a given pathology (e.g. discus degeneration) and clinical problems (e.g. low back pain) reach such contradictory results.

In dealing with the pathology of the hip joint, every orthopedic surgeon recognizes the importance of the femoral neck-shaft angle and its individual variations – but the enormous differences in the shape and structure of the components of

Figure 21.2 Standardized photodocumentation (courtesy of Dr Neumann, Milan). If we are really honest, all other methods are not that much better than this 40-year-old data sheet of an Italian specialist in manual therapy (Neumann 1962).

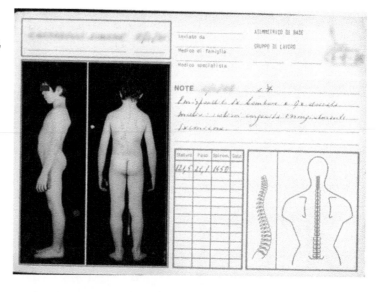

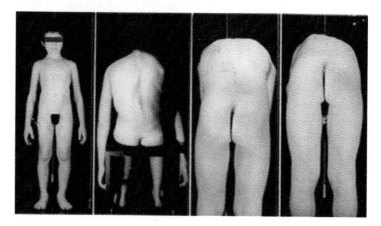

the vertebral spine are not recognized as having the same predictive relevance.

The evaluation of any documentation relating to the form of the back has to be seen as an extension of this scientific dispute. Without an agreement on the classification of the individual into the different postural types, no meaningful prediction about the pathogenetic potential of a given back form can be made.

We can even take this argument one step further. In accepting that there are different constitutional types we reach the perilous area of classification. Gould's polemic about cranial measurements is still vividly remembered (Gould 1981) and the political implications of these attempts as well. But it still holds true that there can be no meaningful interpretation of the human posture if the biotype of the spine under observation is not taken into account.

The research in this area is still incomplete, to say the least. So, yes, we do have some nice new tools to document the posture quantitatively, but not yet the necessary classification to work with these data in a meaningful way.

Take, for example, the measurements of motional stability obtained by four-quadrant scales (Lewit 1988, Vernon 1984) or the distance measurements of the ultrasonic devices (Friedrichs 2000).

Both approaches give an idea about the individual 'normal' position – which can be compared to an 'ideal' value. In the case of the four-quadrant weight scale, this would be a center of gravity in the midpoint of the scales. Most people deviate from this point. Does this indicate a pathology – or is it a normal variant with no diagnostic value?

In the ultrasonic distance measurements we see a similar distribution of the measurements. In most cases the measurements are not symmetrical and in many cases a clinical improvement of the patient coincides with a more asymmetrical peak of the curve than before.

The same is true for the postural symmetry of the back. We cannot assume that symmetry equals wellbeing and that asymmetry is a sure sign of pathology.

If we compare radiographs of the pelvic girdle and the lumbar spine with surface measurements we get a first clue: as soon as there is an anatomical basis for an asymmetry of the spinal orientation, this scoliotic posture is the most energy-efficient way of keeping upright. To obtain an 'ideal' (i.e. symmetrical) posture this individual would have to invest a lot more energy.

In another individual such a scoliotic posture might be an indication of an acute local irritation, be it vertebrogenic (blockage, disk protrusion, etc.) or abdominal, e.g. a kidney stone or appendicitis.

So the initial idea that we just have to enter the measurements of the form and/or function of the body into a computer to obtain a score for the wellbeing of the individual examined proves to be unrealistic. The best we can hope for is yet one more piece for our diagnostic puzzle.

In the case of the four-quadrant scale and the ultrasonic distance measurements the most important detail seems to be the stability of posture. The best indicator for an improvement was not necessarily a more symmetrical posture, but a more stable stance, indicated by a smaller deviation of the measurements from their midpoint. It seems appropriate to translate this basic finding from the weight scale research to the readings of the ultrasonic distance sensors. In the latter case, it

is possible to qualify the situation in different levels of the postural system, i.e. the different areas of the spinal engine (Gracovetsky 1988).

THREE-DIMENSIONAL MEASUREMENT OF THE BACK SURFACE

Based on the Moiré measurements, rasterstereometry (Frobin and Hierholzer 1981, Hierholzer and Drerup 1989) was an attempt to overcome the imprecise measurements inherent in Moiré topometry. The basic idea was to use a highly precise slide to create a pattern of light lines on the back of a patient and record this with a video camera. Through triangulation, a three-dimensional matrix was obtained and processed (Fig. 21.3).

As the workgroup of Drerup and Hierholzer is affiliated with an orthopedic clinic, quite a bit of research was done to find correlations between these measurements and the clinical problems of scoliosis or other problems of pathological posture (Hackenberg et al 2003). Other workgroups tried ultrasonic devices (Asamoah et al 2000) with basically the same methodological problems. Besides the psychological problem of acceptance by the scientific community the main obstacle was the

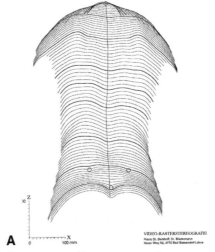

Figure 21.3   Rasterstereometric measurements.
A: The calculated data after filtering and smoothing.

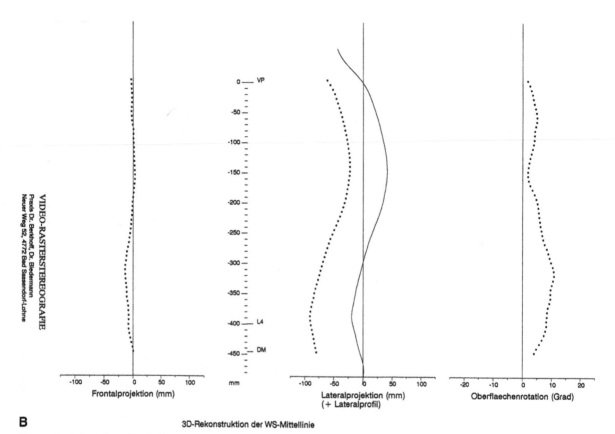

B   3D-Rekonstruktion der WS-Mittellinie

Figure 21.3 (continued)   B: The profiles derived from these data: midline of symmetry, sagittal shape of this midline (the dotted line indicates the probable situation of the midpoints of the vertebrae) and the rotations.

difficult reproducibility of the measurements on other machines and the fact that the installation was basically a one-trick-pony, i.e. usable for just this one measurement – and for that, rather expensive.

Attempts to use computers for the preparation and processing of the data did not yet lead to reliable results. A survey of the available literature confirms this (D'Osualdo et al 2002, Hackenberg et al 2000, Liu et al 2002, Pearson et al 1992, Samo et al 1997). While most papers are quite positive on first sight, the 'small print' gives a more sober appreciation: 'Anatomic alignment of the upper cervical vertebrae cannot be inferred from variation in surface measurement' (Johnson 1998).

Apart from optical methods, different kinds of instruments are available which record the shape of the spine by means of a sensor which has to be moved over the spinal midline. These measurements are even more problematic as they necessitate a longer measurement period and an interaction which tends to distort the data.

A new approach was the phase-triangulation device (Bohn et al 2000), which avoids many of the inflexibilities of rasterstereometry (Fig. 21.4). We were able to cooperate with a workgroup at the University of Nuremberg (Professor Häusler, haeusler@physik.uni-erlangen.de) who developed this application for various industrial and research purposes (www.3d-shape.com).

This instrument allows for high precision and great flexibility, but some principal problems persist, e.g. the penetration depth of the light into the skin and the movement of the patient during the recording.

The big advantage of this approach lies in its flexibility, allowing the recording of rather large

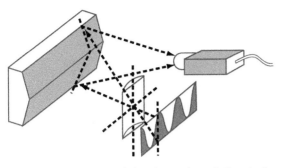

Figure 21.4   Principle of the phase triangulation device. The sensor is based on the principle of phase measuring triangulation. The binary mask is used to generate sinusoidal fringes by astigmatic projection. The accurate fringe pattern contributes largely to the accurate three-dimensional image.The mask is realized by a Ferro-Electric Crystal Modulator (FLC) to perform a phase shift. We acquire a sequence of eight different fringe patterns for one three-dimensional measurement.

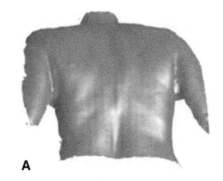

A

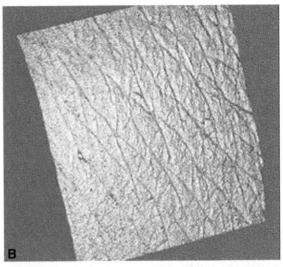

B

Figure 21.5   A and B: Two examples of three-dimensional measurements with fringe triangulation. Both pictures exist as a three-dimensional matrix and can be viewed from any angle with the appropriate software. The system makes it possible to obtain surface profiles at any position.

surfaces like the back and very small structures like the skin pores (Fig. 21.5). We were able to record facial features and the back using the same instrument (Fig. 21.6).

But here, too, the same problems persist to make progress slow and painstaking, to say the least. It turned out to be exceedingly difficult to find simple parameters linking the three-dimensional data to the clinical question at hand. We are able to record the shape of an individual back and we were able to show that this measurement was exact and reproducible to 1–2 mm, but beyond these measurements the real work starts. First attempts to compare surfaces taken several months apart showed that to compensate for the growth of the patient, it is not sufficient to just enlarge the initial dataset linearly. We have to take into account the different growth zones and maybe also different biotypes, too. What we know so far is how insufficient our current knowledge is (Nault et al 2002).

SONOGRAPHIC MEASUREMENT OF SHIFTS IN MOVEMENT PATTERNS

Using ultrasound to measure distances and changes thereof is new. The following paragraphs present 'work in progress' – and very thrilling work. The device presented here gives us a possibility to measure the behavior of parts of the body (in this case the spinal area) and to qualify it. This work builds basically on the experiences with the four-quadrant weight scale (Vernon 1984). These measurements showed that one of the best qualifiers for a clinical improvement is less swaying of the center of gravity, which may be interpreted as a more stable control of posture. We have known for many years, that lesions of the craniocervical junction influence balance and postural stability (Hülse 1998, Hülse et al 1998, Lewit 1988) and for many years, methods have been explored to

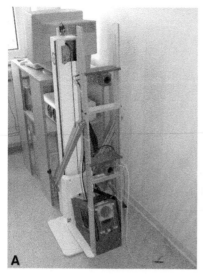
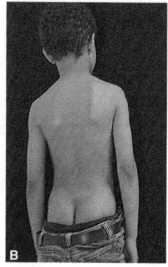
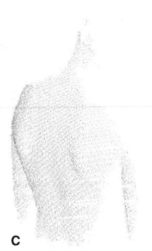

Figure 21.6 Setup of three-dimensional measurement (A). The equipment can handle two measurement areas; the upper one is calibrated for bigger surfaces like the back (B, C), the lower camera for faces.

document this (Norré 1976). Other methods were tried too; for example, poly-electromyograms (Stary et al 1964) yielded essentially the same results, that stability is a good measurement of the quality of the sensorimotor loop in postural control.

The advantage of this new approach is its portability and the fact that long-term recordings are possible without too much hindrance for the patient, as the recording gear can easily be put in a coat pocket.

Methodology

Skin generally has an elastic behavior, particularly across joints. With an alteration of the joint angle, the skin changes its length at certain positions near the joint (Derksen et al 1996, Friedrichs 2000, MacRae and Wright 1969, Snijders and van Riel 1987). The change in the tension of the skin is directly related to the angle alteration between the underlying structures (MacRae and Wright 1969, Snijders and van Riel 1987). This quality was described for the lumbar-region with a linear approximation (MacRae and Wright 1969).

The measurement device sonoSens is based on subcutaneous ultrasonic distance measurement (Friedrichs 2000). Two sensors per input-channel are placed on the skin, thus measuring the contraction and dilatation of the skin between them.

The instrument consists of a flat, lightweight unit with foil-keyboard, display and eight ultrasound transmitter-sensors (Fig. 21.7). The patient can easily carry it in a trouser pocket. For sensor fixation at the skin, special adhesive rings – comparable to those used for electrocardiography – are used. The velocity of the ultrasound in soft tissue is almost constant and within the range of 1500 m/s. The system measures the ultrasound underneath the skin. The time lags between different measurements make possible the calculation of the skin distance (Fig. 21.8). The device allows continuous monitoring of the posture for more than 48 hours with a sample rate of 1 to 10 samples/s.

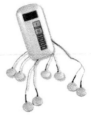

Figure 21.7 The sonoSens with four pairs of sensors.

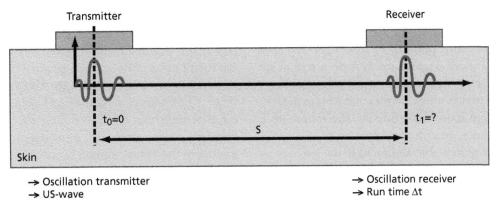

Transmitter

Receiver

Skin

$t_0=0$

$t_1=?$

S

→ Oscillation transmitter
→ US-wave

→ Oscillation receiver
→ Run time Δt

Figure 21.8 Principle of ultrasonic distance measurement. The travelling time of the ultrasound is measured between transmitter and receiver. Based on the known velocity of ultrasound through soft tissue the distance between both sensors is calculated. More information can be found at www.friendly-sensors.de.

A case example (Kelvin, 10 years)

History: The delivery was protracted; the mother reported a lot of crying during the first months. Later on, motor development was somewhat delayed which kept him from taking part in team sports. His social skills were also considered insufficient and problems were reported when he had to integrate into bigger groups. He had been on Ritalin medication for 2 years, after being diagnosed with ADHD. The reason why Kelvin was referred for manual therapy was pain in the right leg with no obvious cause.

On the first examination the boy made a somewhat tired impression. His muscular pattern seemed normal and his gait, too. The head was consistently tilted to the right and a slight cranial asymmetry was plainly visible. Standing on one leg was difficult for him, and with closed eyes it became impossible.

On examining the mobility of the spinal segments, an impairment of the left tilt and right rotation of the head of about one third was noted. The processus transversus atlantis was extremely painful on palpation.

These findings in the cervical level were accompanied by multiple blockages of the thoracic segments and the left sacroiliac (SI) joint. The os naviculare of the left foot was in a fixed position. The main finding was on the occipitocervical level. This blockage was removed.

Three measurements were made, before the treatment, 10 minutes later and 6 months later.

The sensors were placed bilaterally on three regions. They corresponded to the cervical, thoracic and lumbar spine, respectively. The measurements of the frontal plane (frontal movement index, FMI) were negative on the left side and positive on the right. In the sagittal plane (sagittal movement index, SMI) extension had negative and flexion positive values.

Table 21.1 shows the range of movement at the calibration.

Table 21.1 Range of movement at the calibration

Calibration values	Total	Cervical	Thoracic	Lumbar
Length at calibration	434 mm	52 mm	182 mm	200 mm
Flexion index frontal minimum	−9%	−6%	−14%	−8%
Flexion index frontal maximum	2%	17%	1%	6%
Flexion index sagittal minimum	−6%	−6%	−7%	−7%
Flexion index maximum	0%	4%	−1%	4%

Cervical FMI

The movement pattern of the cervical area (Fig. 21.9) shows a symmetrical pattern with wide margins before treatment. Immediately after treatment the peak is much sharper and a bit to the left, indicating a more stable stance. The follow-up 6 months later accentuated this even more: the posture is quite stable and more to the left.

The wide sway of the initial measurement was reduced immediately after the treatment and in the ensuing months the boy was able to optimize his gait even more.

Thoracic and lumbar FMI

The measurements of the thoracic area (Fig. 21.10) show a similar pattern: The initial curve is quite flat and a bit left-centered. After treatment the curve becomes much steeper (the movements thus more similar) and this development is accentuated in the last measurement, which shows an even steeper distribution of the measurements. The lumbar measurements confirm these findings (Fig. 21.11).

Sagittal SMI

Again the pre-treatment measurements show a flat distribution of the values. Positive values correspond to an increased length. The first graph (Fig. 21.12A) shows a symmetrical shape, indicating that stretching and shortening were approximately equally distributed. Immediately after the treatment the values shifted more to the positive side (Fig. 21.12B), indicating an increase of the stretching, while the distribution of the frequencies became more accentuated. The follow-up half a year later (Fig. 21.12C) shows an even sharper maximum in the middle range.

Lumbar SMI

Here, too, we see the same pattern on the two series for the lower spinal areas (Fig. 21.13). The main finding on all graphs is the sharper peak, an indication of the more stereotypical pattern of movements. It seems to be permissible to theorize that this decrease in sway can be used as a sign of a more efficient movement pattern, especially as it

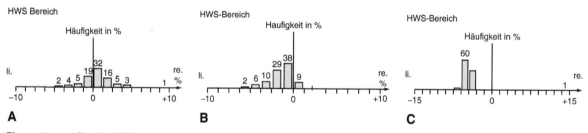

Figure 21.9 Cervical FMI. A: Before treatment. B: Immediately after treatment. C: Follow-up 6 months later.

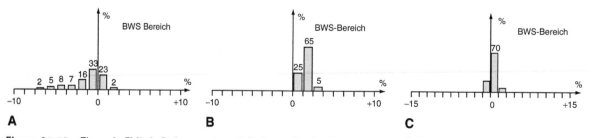

Figure 21.10 Thoracic FMI. A: Before treatment. B: Immediately after treatment. C: Follow-up 6 months later.

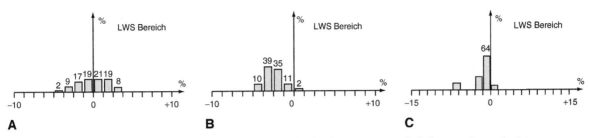

Figure 21.11   Lumbar FMI. A: Before treatment. B: Immediately after treatment. C: Follow-up 6 months later.

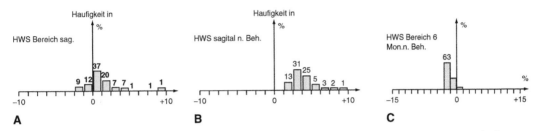

Figure 21.12   Sagittal SMI. A: Before treatment. B: Immediately after treatment. C: Follow-up 6 months later.

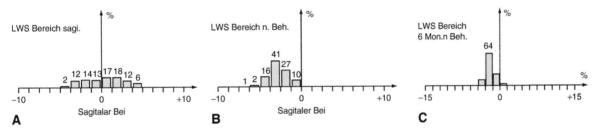

Figure 21.13   Lumbar SMI. A: Before treatment. B: Immediately after treatment. C: Follow-up 6 months later.

corresponds to a marked improvement of the subjective and objective situation of the patient.

The measurements shown here are fairly typical for children we treat for KIDD-related problems. Some observations can be made in almost all cases:

- The measurements are an objective documentation of the rapid changes which can be obtained by manual therapy of the OC junction.
- These changes influence not only the cervical coordination but the whole posture.
- The changes induced by one treatment can be documented months later and in most cases the situation is further improved, as indicated by an additional decrease in the measurement values.

This method has the potential to document objectively what we – until now – only surmised by clinical observation. To define useful patterns a lot more research will have to be done, but already now it seems clear that a decrease in sway (i.e. a sharper peak of the curve) corresponds well with better body control.

Last but not least we should report the outcome for Kelvin. He feels much better, has started to play soccer in a team – and is enjoying it. The suboccipital trigger points are no longer palpable and the Ritalin medication was reduced a lot.

A LONG WAY AHEAD

All these procedures are exciting and in trying to utilize them, a lot was learned. In order to use three-dimensional shapes for postural analysis we shall have to define the growth patterns of the vertebral spine, something not done yet. To make sense of the sonographic measurements of movement patterns we have to get a clearer idea about what to define as 'normal', etc. Only in trying to put our clinical observation on a solid, quantifiable and reproducible base did we learn *how* difficult such a quest will be.

For the time being, all these procedures are still highly experimental and the best one can say is that their use stimulates the analysis of the highly intricate mathematics necessary.

The main application for these computer-generated measurements will be in medical certificates or evidence used in court. For the day-to-day practice they will at best complement what an experienced practitioner grasps with his/her five senses and his/her intuition. Luckily orthopedic surgeons and chiropractors are over-represented in the group of admirers of mechanical toys, so there is hope of financing the costly development of the necessary hardware and software.

References

Andry de Boisregard N 1741 L'orthopédie ou l'art de prévenir et de corriger dans les enfants les difformités du corps. Vv Alix, Paris

Asamoah V, Mellerowicz H, Venus J et al 2000 Messung der Rückenoberfläche. Wert in der Diagnostik von Wirbelsäulenerkrankungen. Orthopäde 29(6):480–489

Bohn G, Cloutot L, Habermeier H et al 2000 Fast 3d-Camera for industrial and medical applications. University of Erlangen, Chair for Optics, Department of Optical Metrology, Erlangen, p 7

Deacon P, Flood B M, Dickson R A 1984 Idiopathic scoliosis in three dimensions. A radiographic and morphometric analysis. Journal of Bone and Joint Surgery British Volume 66(4):509–512

Derksen J C, van Riel M P, Snijders C J 1996 A new method for continuous recording of trunk postures while playing golf. Journal of Applied Biomechanics 12:116–129

D'Osualdo F, Schierano S, Soldano F M et al 2002 New tridimensional approach to the evaluation of the spine through surface measurement: the BACES system. Journal of Medical Engineering and Technology 26(3):95–105

Friedrichs A 2000 Neue Diagnoseverfahren für Biomechanik, Sport, Rehabilitation und Fahrzeugentwicklung. Friedrich Schiller University, Jena

Frobin W, Hierholzer E 1981 Rasterstereography: a photogrammetric method for measurement of body surfaces. Photographic Engineering and Remote Sensing 47:1717–1724

Gould S 1981 The mismeasure of man. Norton, New York

Gracovetsky S A 1988 The Spinal Engine. Springer, New York

Greenspan A, Pugh J W, Norman A et al 1978 Scoliotic index: a comparative evaluation of methods for the measurement of scoliosis. Bulletin/Hospital for Joint Diseases 39(2):117–125

Gutmann G, Biedermann H 1990 Funktionelle Röntgenanalyse der Lenden-Becken-Hüftregion. Fischer, Stuttgart

Hackenberg L, Hierholzer E, Potzl W et al 2003 Rasterstereographic back shape analysis in idiopathic scoliosis after anterior correction and fusion. Clinical Biomechechanics (Bristol, Avon) 18(1):1–8

Hackenberg L, Liljenqvist U, Hierholzer E et al 2000 Rasterstereometrische Oberflächenmessung bei Skoliose nach ventraler Derotationsosteosynthese. Zeitschrift für Orthopädie und ihre Grenzgebiete 138(4):353–359

Hierholzer E, Drerup B 1989 Assessment of three-dimensional scoliotic deformity by rastersterography. Biostereometrics. Proc SPIE 1030:9–15

Hülse M 1998 Klinik der Funktionsstörungen des Kopfgelenkbereiches. In: Hülse M, Neuhuber W L, Wolff H D (eds) Der kranio-zervikale Übergang. Springer, Berlin, p 43–98

Hülse M, Neuhuber W L, Wolff H D (eds) 1998 Der kranio-zervikale Übergang. Springer, Berlin

Johnson G M 1998 The correlation between surface measurement of head and neck posture and the anatomic position of the upper cervical vertebrae. Spine 23:921–927

Lewit K 1988 Disturbed balance due to lesions of the cranio-cervical junction. Journal of Orthopedic Medicine 58–61

Liu X C, Thometz J G, Lyon R M et al 2002 Effects of trunk position on back surface-contour measured by raster stereophotography. American Journal of Orthopedics 31:402–406

Lovett R E 1907 Lateral curvature of the spine and round shoulders. Blakiston

MacRae I F, Wright V 1969 Measurement of forecastle movement. Annals of Rheumatic Diseases 29:584–558

Nault M L, Allard P, Hinse S et al 2002 Relations between standing stability and body posture parameters in adolescent idiopathic scoliosis. Spine 27:1911–1917

Neumann C 1962 Differenze di lunghezza fra gli arti interiori e genesi delle scoliosi nell'età evolutiva. Ginnastica medica x:32–35

Norré M E 1976 Der Zervikalnystagmus und die Gelenkblockierungen. Manuelle Medizin 14:45–51

Pearson J D, Dangerfield P H, Atkinson J T et al 1992 Measurement of body surface topography using an automated imaging system. Acta Orthopaedica Belgica 58 (Suppl 1):73–79

Samo D G, Chen S P, Crampton A R et al 1997 Validity of three lumbar sagittal motion measurement methods: surface inclinometers compared with radiographs. Journal of Occupational and Environmental Medicine 39(3):209–216

Snijders C J, van Riel M P 1987 Continuous measurements of the spine movements in normal working situations over periods of 8 hours or more. Ergonomics 30:639–653

Starý O, Obrda K, Pfeifer I 1964 Polyelektromyographische Untersuchungen der propriozeptiven Analysestörungen bei beginnenden Bandscheibenschäden im Kindesalter. In: Müller D (ed) Neurologie der Wirbelsäule und des Rückenmarks im Kindesalter. Fischer, Jena, p 311–323

Vernon H 1984 The Four Quadrant Weight Scale: a technical and procedural review. Journal of Manipulative and Physiological Therapeutics 7:165–169

Wessinghage D 1987 Zur Herausgebe des Reprints. In: Wessinghage D (ed) Orthopädie oder die Kunst bei Kindern die Ungestaltheit des Leibes zu verhüten und zu verbessern (N Andry). Schattauer, Stuttgart

SECTION 5

Making sense of it all

SECTION CONTENTS

Chapter 22

Complexity theory and its implications for manual therapy

M. E. Hyland, H. Biedermann

INTRODUCTION

Manual therapy (MT) comes in two flavors. First, there is its use, increasingly accepted in many contexts, as treatment for the relief of everyday problems such as low-back pain; here MT coexists with other mechanical methods of treatment. The causal sequence often starts with a well-remembered accident ('I missed that step'; 'after one day of digging in the garden'), leading to a painful condition that forces the patient to seek help, followed by prompt relief after successful manipulation. This technical and well-delineated modus operandi of MT does not provoke too much resistance from conventional medicine and had we left MT there, harmony would reign supreme. This kind of MT may be called *trivial MT*.

The second course of action of MT is vastly different from the well-accepted 'technical' level. MT seems to be able to alter the course of an individual's development profoundly at some well-defined moments of ontogenetical development. Recent studies suggest that the first months after birth are as crucial as the intrauterine period for the long-term pattern of the individual's life. Out of a basket of basic developmental models a few are chosen and fixated, and these fixated patterns trigger life-long patterns of behavior with consequences decades later (Lopuhaa et al 2000, Roseboom et al 2000, Sival et al 1993).

Later in life this second, pivotal role of MT is much less frequently observed, but still occurs. In some cases of post-traumatic problems the role of MT in the individual's life can be dramatic, which is why we talk about *non-trivial MT* in these circumstances. The point of departure for this distinction were observations of the patients (and parents) themselves. When parents referring to the effect of MT talk about 'having another child' this reflects their observation of the profound alteration of the child's being in the full sense of the word.

In this chapter we want to discuss some theoretical considerations about how we can come to grips with this phenomenon, which is as bewildering for us professionals as it is for the parents and patients.

TWO LEVELS OF MANUAL THERAPY

Analysis and synthesis are two different ways of understanding the body, just as they are two different approaches to science. The study of anatomy is a good example of analysis. The aim of anatomy is to describe all the different constituent parts of the body. Biochemistry is another form of analysis, but this time at a more micro-level. Running through the analytical approach is the idea that by finding out about the 'parts' of a system it will be possible to work out how the whole functions. However, it has always been recognized by philosophers of science that analysis has its limitations. The reason is that sometimes properties 'emerge' from the constituent parts of a system in such a way that these emergent properties cannot be inferred from those parts in isolation. In order to understand these emergent properties, one needs a different kind of approach to study, that of synthesis. In the case of synthesis, an attempt is made to understand how the system operates as a whole.

Recent advances in complexity theory have been able to give greater substance to the philosophical assumptions underlying synthesis

(Cilliers 1998). Complexity theory has shown that certain sorts of complex system function in ways that are fundamentally different from simple systems (Bak 1996). What is important is the way the parts of the system are organized. Certain types of organization of the 'parts' of a system lead it to have properties that are not normally associated with either the parts in isolation, or the parts in simpler systems. One particular type of organization is that of a network. The brain is an example of a system that has a network structure. The brain consists of a series of neurons which are massively interconnected with other neurons by means of axons and dendrites. In fact, any system which consists of nodes massively interconnected by causal connections has the kind of organization that gives networks their special properties. What are these special properties? There are several types, but the ones relevant here are ones that give the functionality associated with intelligence (Ellis and Humphreys 1999).

People and animals are intelligent, largely we suppose, because of their brains. However, it is possible to simulate intelligence by using machines which, like the brain, have the capacity for parallel processing in a node-based structure. The study of artificial intelligence shows that parallel processing networks – rather than sequential systems – are the necessary structure needed to create 'intelligent' functions such as pattern recognition, problem solving and memory. The way memory is encoded is particularly important in the present context, because it is so fundamentally different from the way memory is encoded in unintelligent systems. This chapter is being written on a computer and the text is saved on part of the hard drive, with each letter occupying a physical space. Memory, in the computer, is spatially located, and that is a feature of all simple, sequential processing systems that have memory. However, in the case of network systems, memory is not spatially located. Instead memory is spread over many nodes as it takes the form of the activation between many nodes. Memory is in the whole system rather than in a part of the system.

So, losing a few cells in the part of the brain responsible for memory does not lead to loss of any specific memories associated with those cells. The brain, like all network systems, is comparatively insensitive to local error. Damage to the memory part of the brain leads to a gradual loss of memory of all kinds as the system gradually becomes degraded.

It is easy to accept that the brain is intelligent and a network system – people exhibit intelligence and the brain 'looks' like a network. However, network causal systems do not have to look like networks. All that is needed is that there should be massive causal connection between nodes, and this can be achieved in other ways, for example between ligands and receptors. Thus, the immune and endocrine systems can also be thought of as being network systems – and therefore exhibiting some of the intelligent functions associated with the brain. The intelligent body hypothesis (Hyland 2002) is the next logical step in the argument, and is based on the simple assumption that there are not several different networks (i.e. neurological, endocrine and immune) but one single network that has an overall integrative function within the body. The intelligent body hypothesis sees no dividing line between brain and the rest of the body. Just as mobile phones and landline phones connect seamlessly into a single phone system, the intelligent body hypothesis assumes that there is a seamless connection between the different systems of the body.

THE INTELLIGENT BODY

The intelligent body hypothesis suggests that the characteristic of intelligence normally associated with the brain is not specific to the brain, but is distributed throughout the whole body, forming an *extended network*. We talk about the *spinal memory* in dealing with the acquisition of sensorimotor skills. The extended network is an intelligent system that has the function of coordinating the different components of the body in an intelligent

manner. The extended network is an adaptive system. Just as the brain is capable of 'learning' and so enabling people to adapt better to their environments, so the extended network is adaptive (i.e. capable of learning) so that it can respond to external conditions. Normally this adaptive function leads to better self-regulatory control, but under specific circumstances, the reverse occurs and the system creates less effective self-regulation. These states of less effective self-regulation are the starting point for disease. According to this view, the error in the extended network can act as the distal point in the formation of disease.

Disease is a form of 'error' in the body. This error can take two forms. First, there is the system-specific, spatially located, disease entity error that is familiar to conventional Western medicine. Such error corresponds to 'broken parts' in a machine, and treatment involves correcting the disease entity. Whether it is a matter of killing bacteria by means of antibiotics, reducing inflammation by steroids, or substituting an artificial heart valve for a worn one, the principle underlying (classical?) medicine is to treat the part that has gone wrong. However, error in the body can also take another form, that of adaptive error in the extended network. Under these circumstances, there is no one part of the body that can be corrected (repaired), as information (and memory) is distributed throughout the extended network. The only way of correcting this second form of error is to engage with or communicate with the network.

The term 'robust therapy' may be used for therapies designed to correct disease entities (i.e. most therapies used in conventional medicine) and 'subtle therapies' for those therapies that involve therapeutic inputs into the extended network. Some of these inputs may involve lifestyle (e.g. psychological state, diet and exercise). Others may involve treatments found in MT. The aim of subtle therapies is to change the information that is stored in the extended network, and because networks respond to multiple inputs, it is likely that a combination of lifestyle change and other therapeutic techniques are most effective. Whereas robust therapies are supposed to function without regard for the interpersonal communication between therapist and patient, most subtle therapies – and MT with its direct therapeutic touch even more so – have to take into account the influence of this level of interaction.

THE 'PUSH' AND 'PULL' APPROACH TO THERAPY

How is it possible to change information stored in the extended network? From a theoretical perspective, there are two ways in which this can be done. The first way is to provide inputs that 'pull' the network back towards the desired direction. So, for example, if a person's health problem is the consequence of overwork, then a simple remedy is to rest, relax or meditate. Similarly, if a person's diet has created deficiencies, then some sort of supplement may be needed. The problem, however, is that many types of dysregulation in the network are deep-seated and, moreover, they exhibit a property which characterizes some network systems, they become 'stuck' in an unsatisfactory state. Simply pulling the network back in the right direction may not create sufficient energy to displace it from its dysregulated, stuck state. An alternative approach is to 'push' the network in the wrong direction, so that the network's naturally compensatory mechanism makes it spring back, back beyond its initial point so that the network ends up in a more regulated state. This push has to be carefully calibrated in order to exert enough energy to get the system out of its energetic trough, but not so irritating as to hinder the establishment of a new stability. Push therapies are familiar in psychology and immunology under the name of desensitization. In either case, a small 'dose' of an event that caused alarm within the body (an anxiety-provoking event in the case of psychology, and an immune-provoking event in the case of immunology) are presented under controlled situations so that the body can learn

that these events are no longer alarming. For example, if you are frightened of spiders, then desensitization might involve imagining a small spider far away while remaining calm, then imagining that spider a little closer while still remaining calm, and gradually a little closer still, and then in turn a real spider is brought gradually closer while you still remain calm. In fact, desensitization works better for anxiety reduction than it does for allergen desensitization, so clearly other inputs to the network are also important. However, what desensitization shows is that if the body is 'reminded' about traumatic events under carefully controlled situations, then the network may, if the conditions are right, adapt back towards a more regulated state.

One of the assumptions of subtle therapies, such as MT, is that trauma is in some sense remembered in the body, and that this traumatic memory is locked up in a stable state that creates disorder. Manual therapy can therefore be viewed as a way of reminding the body of that traumatic event, but in a kind of diluted form – in a way similar to desensitization. This recall of a trauma by MT allows the body, if the conditions are right, to compensate and stabilize the network in a new, more regulated state. One of the 'right' conditions is the right point in time to apply MT (see Chapter 17). The other essential condition is to give the body enough room to adapt and refrain from overloading the system. Dosage in robust therapies is often seen as something scalable (if one antibiotic did not suffice, let us use two). Non-trivial MT is very sensitive to over-dosage.

From a theoretical perspective, there are two important features about this process. The first is that eliciting the traumatic memory will lead to a temporary increase in symptoms, and so, consistent with clinical experience, patients can experience a deterioration before they improve. The second is that the context in which the therapy takes place is crucial to the end result. Although the manual therapist focuses on MT, the body is conscious of all possible inputs to the network – including psychological and nutritional inputs.

Providing a healing context is an essential part of the process, and this will include the right time in an intrinsically variable network to treat. Pull therapies are needed to help the push therapy to work, otherwise the push therapy simply creates an oscillation in deterioration and improvement. Pull therapies ensure that the network sticks in a healthy state after it has compensated for the push therapy.

These remarks based on complexity theory give us new insight into some puzzling observations when administering MT to small children. We obtain better insight into two faces of MT, one completely compatible with the 'robust' view on medicine, the other in line with a philosophy which tries to re-establish a new equilibrium.

The conclusion of this chapter is that MT should not be viewed as just a different technology compared with conventional pharmacological treatment (robust therapy), though in its trivial form (e.g. releasing a trapped nerve) it does work in this way.

Manual therapy, when acting as subtle therapy, works on the body in a fundamentally different way from that of conventional medicine. It works on the network rather than on a specific part or system in the body.

Manual therapy is not some mysterious, unscientific technique. It is a technique that is consistent with complexity theory and the assumption of the intelligent body hypothesis that the whole body operates, in part, as a complex system.

References

Bak P 1996 How nature works. The science of self-organised criticality. Copernicus/Springer, New York

Cilliers P 1998 Complexity and postmodernism: understanding complex systems. Routledge, London

Ellis R, Humphreys G 1999 Connectionist psychology; a text with readings. Psychology Press, Hove, UK

Hyland M 2002 The intelligent body and its discontents. Journal of Health Psychology 7:21–32

Lopuhaa C E, Roseboom T J, Osmond C et al 2000 Atopy, lung function, and obstructive airways disease after prenatal exposure to famine. Thorax 55(7):555–561

Roseboom T J, van der Meulen J H, Osmond C et al 2000 Coronary heart disease after prenatal exposure to the Dutch famine, 1944–45. Heart 84(6):595–598

Sival D A, Prechtl H F, Sonder G H, Touwen B C 1993 The effect of intra-uterine breech position on postnatal motor functions of the lower limbs. Early Human Development 32:161–176

Chapter 23

The big, the small, and the beautiful

O. Güntürkün

Ignoramus! Ignorabimus!

We do not know! We will not know! This was the final conclusion of Emil du Bois-Reymond at the end of his 1872 lecture on the 'Limits of Natural Science'. If the founder of modern physiology, a sworn natural scientist and atheist, sees no hope in our struggle to fully understand ourselves, our free will and our consciousness, we should pause for a moment to recapitulate on possible limits of knowledge. And we should look back at a discussion which started at the very dawn of modern science.

In 1776 the French mathematician and physicist Marquis Pierre-Simon de Laplace had proposed a radical idea, known as 'Laplace's Daemon': 'We may regard the present state of the universe as the effect of its past and the cause of its future. An intellect which at any given moment knew all of the forces that animate nature and the mutual positions of the beings that compose it, if this intellect were vast enough to submit the data to analysis, could condense into a single formula the movement of the greatest bodies of the universe and that of the lightest atom; for such an intellect nothing could be uncertain and the future just like the past would be present before its eyes.' In a continuation of this line of reasoning, Marvin Minsky (1985), one of the godfathers of artificial intelligence research, postulated pessimistically that in a world where action only occurs out of determinism or statistical noise, free will is a myth.

So, if we align with Laplace we should be able to extrapolate states of matter along scientific dimensions down to the core of our mind. However, if we go along with Bois-Reymond, we should face a border of explanation which we cannot surpass, regardless of our countless victories on the experimenter's bench.

Possibly an important problem elegantly swept away by Laplace is the problem inherent in extrapolations. Extrapolation is nothing more than the art of knowing the big from the small, or vice versa. It is easy as long as we can rely on simple linear relations. It becomes a mess with nonlinear interactions as exemplified by Edward Lorenz's butterfly which symbolizes the non-linear vision of chaos research. In 1972 the famous meteorologist Lorenz gave a talk entitled, 'Predictability: does the flap of a butterfly's wings in Brazil set off a tornado in Texas?' At the time, Lorenz did not in fact make any strong claims concerning the impossibility of reaching perfect prediction in theory. He did, however, suggest that not only do varying degrees of unpredictability reflect the varying degrees of human ignorance, they also reflect variations in the stability and complexity of the systems we wish to predict. For Lorenz and others, questions about inherent unpredictability were linked to questions about stability. Thus, he asked, 'is the behavior of the atmosphere stable with respect to perturbations of small amplitude?' If not, then we must seriously question the notion that perfect predictability is achievable even in theory. We shall return to this question later on. But for now let us first consider an example from neuroscience which is closer to the themes of this book than meteorology is.

The human prefrontal cortex is a vast territory with billions of neurons. It is heavily innervated by fibers from dopaminergic midbrain neurons. Only about 100 000 of these dopaminergic cells constitute this projection with each of them making more than 500 000 connections at cortical level. The prefrontal cortex and the dopaminergic neurons are reciprocally connected and most prefrontal cognitive operations depend on a precise and timely activation of the dopaminergic input. Therefore, the dopaminergic signal should be extremely fine-grained with respect to time and area to be able to modulate the prefrontal cortex with high precision. However, looking in more detail, it is easy to see that this cannot be the case. The projection from the cortical galaxy down to the minuscule dopaminergic cell group scales the activity pattern of a huge and fine-grained landscape down to a 'handful' of cells. Thus, the cortical signal cannot be about detailed contents but only about level of activity. Since each of the dopaminergic cells is hardwired to half a million of its own terminals in the cortex, its signal can also not convey a precise, detailed modulation but can only vary between 'less' and 'more'. But then, how is it possible that specificity emerges in this interaction? The solution might be simple. Every time highly interesting stimuli are processed by the prefrontal cells, cortical activity level increases. This increase is transmitted to the midbrain and the dopaminergic cells start firing. Their dopaminergic signal is broad and undifferentiated – but just in time. At the moment the dopaminergic signal arrives, several groups of internally reverberating neuronal circuits, the cellular assemblies, compete with each other for dominance in the prefrontal cortex. Dopamine further increases the activity level of highly active neurons while reducing the excitability of weakly active cells. In effect, it increases signal-to-noise ratio. This coincidence suddenly alters the game. The dominant cell group now plays 'winner-takes-it-all' and captures all relevant resources to hold them until internal processes or external stimuli trigger a new cortical activity carpet which then results in a new peak of activation. Taken together, in our example the scaling from a large system to a small one stripped away content descriptions and left only amplitude to work with.

Thus, the emergence of large-scale functions out of particle interactions is no playground for simple extrapolations. But its understanding is not beyond the reach of the human mind. This book on manual therapy testifies this in a beautiful way. In multitudinous ways the non-linear, unexpected but in the end understandable interactions of components that constitute our body become apparent. As long as we avoid simple-minded approaches, it is obviously possible to tease apart all the seemingly inextricably intertwined threads; one by one. What a beautiful and a quintessentially human quest!

Ignoramus! Scibimus!

References

Laplace M-S 1776 Mémoire sur l'inclinaison Moyenne des Orbites des Comètes sur la Figure de la Terre et sur les Fonctions, Mémoires de'l Academie royale des Sciences Paris, Savants étranges, 7: 503–524, oeuvres 8:279–324

Lorenz E N 1972 Predictability: does the flap of a butterfly's wings in Brazil set off a tornado in Texas? AAAS Meeting, New York

Minsky M 1985 The society of mind. Simon and Schuster, New York

Chapter 24

The KISS syndrome: symptoms and signs

A tool for the evaluation and assessment of the effects of manual therapy in small children

H. Biedermann

BEYOND THE SYMPTOMATIC APPROACH

One of the main intentions of this chapter (and the entire book) is to propose a long-term perspective for the functional disorders we find and treat in children and adolescents, the KISS syndrome. Having used this concept for more than 15 years we are still astonished how it renders otherwise incomprehensible effects of manual therapy in children (MTC) transparent, thus giving a better insight where (and where not) MTC may be usefully applied. Many problems which can at least be alleviated by MTC have a broad range of causal factors. Both to stay credible in one's therapeutic predictions, and to be effective in the choice of patients to be treated, it helps to use a diagnostic viewpoint that looks beyond the acute symptom for a broader pattern. The diagnostic procedure becomes more robust, too, as we do not have to rely on the current problems only but include the fourth dimension (time) in our reasoning.

Following this line of argument, a problem like colic is taken as the starting point of a diagnosis which starts with the moment of birth, or even earlier with the details of the pregnancy and – to make the range even broader – with details of the development of the siblings (see Chapter 26). We now know that children who have siblings with successfully treated KISS problems have a higher likelihood of developing similar problems themselves, even more so if the first one to be treated was of the same sex. This trend makes a genetic predisposition as one contributing factor very likely.

When treating adults by means of manual therapy we mostly start from a 'mechanical' complaint: 'my lower back hurts', 'I cannot move my arm freely', 'the headaches start from a feeling of tension in my neck' – that kind of complaint directs the attention of the therapist towards the musculoskeletal system as an important part of the patient's problems.

Not so in children. Some of the most impressive results are obtained in situations where the uninitiated do not see any connection with a biomechanical problem, let alone a disorder of the 'spinal engine' (Gracovetsky 1988).

This non-obvious connection between problem and (manual) therapy necessitates some conceptual changes. The two acronyms KISS and KIDD are not intended to offer yet another four-letter-word intimidation for parents and teachers alike. Maybe the most important advantage of MTC and the KISS concept is related to the fact that a treatment based on it is short, not onerous – and single. In most small children, one treatment suffices and in schoolchildren, two are the norm.

The first phase of applying manual therapy in a pediatric context was quite symptom-oriented and the European publications date back to the 1950s (e.g. Lewit and Janda 1964, Gutmann 1988). Gutmann, in particular, did a lot of research on the effects of manual therapy in schoolchildren and infants. In the 1960s Gutmann formulated a first framework to accommodate the observations in working with small children (Gutmann 1968). This work culminated in a monograph in 1984 which devoted two chapters to manual therapy in small children (Gutmann and Biedermann 1984). Some of the constituting details of KISS were already present there, especially the importance of the birth trauma in triggering the pathology. Due to the relatively small numbers of children treated (Gutmann saw 2–4 children per week) the broader pattern proved elusive, but these publications attracted the attention of some pediatricians and physiotherapists who sent more and more children. Unfortunately Gutmann fell ill and died in 1988 before the definite layout of this concept could be formulated.

Whereas there were some papers on MTC already in the 1950s and 1960s (Frymann 1966, 1976, 1988, Gutmann 1968, Lewit and Janda 1964, Upledger 1978), most papers dealing with manual therapy in infants were published more recently (Anrig and Plaugher 1998, Davies 2000).

The bulk of these publications follow the classic patterns of treatises about manual therapy in adults: the symptoms are topographically organized and the backbone of the paper consists of the different manipulation techniques for the different locations proposed by the author(s).

This approach misses the main point of diagnosing and eventually treating children and infants. In almost every case where manual therapy or a comparable procedure can be of help we found a typical developmental pattern. This

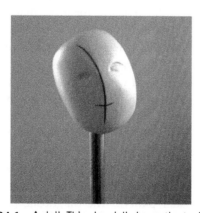

Figure 24.1 A doll. This clay doll shows the typical signs of cranial asymmetry found in KISS babies. In this case a left-convex case is shown. The statistics of these children show a left-convex posture of the trunk, retardation of hip development on the right, less spontaneous movements of the right arm and leg, inability to roll over to the right and to look to the right, as well as refusal to bend the head to the left. The morphological signs on the head are a less developed cheek on the right, a 'smaller' eye on the right, a c-shaped and left-convex facial midline (i.e. microsomia of the right half of the face) and a flattening of the left side of the occiput.

pattern is slightly different from one child to another, but a basic set of symptoms can be identified (Biedermann 1973, 1992, 1995).

THE FORMULATION OF A NEW CONCEPT

KISS = kinematic imbalances due to suboccipital stress.

The reason for this 'new' syndrome is that its definition gives us a taxonomic frame to accommodate the pathogenetic base (irritation of the suboccipital structures of the cervical spine) and the clinically dominant item, i.e. the fixed posture and the ensuing asymmetry.

We have to be careful not to over-emphasize the importance of the torticollis and/or C-scoliosis in the discussion of the KISS syndrome; it is like a self-

fulfilling prophecy to regard these signs as the most important. Most children are referred to manual therapy primarily because this kind of asymmetrical posture is apparent. To put these two specific conditions on top of the list is a circular argument: as we have noted they are the most prominent features, but not necessarily the most important causal agents. We saw that other less specific symptoms often precede the asymmetry and certainly the morphological changes of the skull.

Based on the rapidly increasing numbers of small children referred to us (we see 20–30 babies every day in a practice of 2–3 doctors) we proposed the KISS concept for the first time in 1990 (Biedermann 1990, 1991). The fixed posture was the last symptom in the clinical picture. Later on the initially homogeneous symptomatology was split into two groups, fixed lateralization (KISS I) and fixed retroflexion

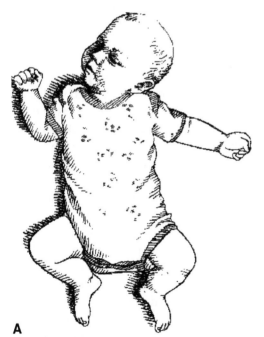

A

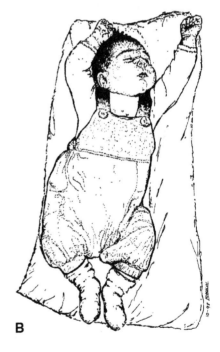

B

Figure 24.2 The KISS syndrome: clinical markers.

A: KISS I: fixed lateroflexion
- Torticollis
- Unilateral microsomia
- Asymmetry of the skull
- C-Scoliosis of neck and trunk
- Asymmetry of gluteal area
- Asymmetry of motion of the limbs
- Retardation of motor development of one side

B: KISS II: Fixed retroflexion
- Hyperextension (during sleep)
- (Asymmetrical) occipital flattening
- Shoulders pulled up
- Fixed supination of the arms
- Cannot lift trunk from ventral position
- Orofacial muscular hypotonia
- Breastfeeding difficult on one side

(KISS II). Figure 24.2 shows the main symptoms for these two groups schematically.

Since the first attempts to define this entity, the ever-increasing feedback helped to get a much clearer picture of the essentials of KISS. The initial emphasis on the mechanical aspect became much less important and the development over time came into the foreground. The first babies were brought to the consultation for treatment of their torticollis and this was reflected in the percentages we found in examining these children. Later on other symptoms gained more importance. Table 24.1 shows a comparison between data compiled in 1996 and a random sampling of 200 babies treated between January and March 2003.

Breastfeeding problems were not mentioned in our initial compilation as these complaints did not play a part at that time. It is also interesting to notice that the referral pattern changed: in the early days most children were brought on the advice of a physiotherapist and quite often in the face of objections from the pediatrician. This changed, and it is obvious that this influences the complaint patterns, too.

Table 24.1 Reported symptoms in children referred for manual therapy in 1996 compared with 2003

Spontaneous complaints reported by the parents	N = 263 (1996) (Biedermann 1999)	N = 200 (2003)
Torticollis	89.3%	53.2%
Reduced range of head movements	84.7%	78.3%
Cervical hypersensitivity	76.0%	64.7%
Cranial asymmetry	40.1%	67.6%
Opisthotonos	27.9%	44.8%
Restlessness	23.7%	39.2%
Forced sleeping posture	14.5%	45.7%
Unable to control head movements	9.5%	37.2%
Uses one arm much less than the other	7.6%	12.4%
Breastfeeding problems	–	18.4%

It is impossible to draw a clear line between symptoms caused by vertebrogenic functional disorders and neurological problems – the two overlap. The distinction between these two levels is even more difficult in young children as we know now how frequently trauma to the central nervous system happens and that these traumas leave no permanent lesions (Ratner 1991, Valk et al 1991) (see also Chapters 9 and 25).

In the cooperation with referring colleagues we see an almost identical pattern: in the beginning the children sent to us have a torticollis – later on all the other (and in our view much more relevant) symptoms precede this 'mechanical' indication, thus enlarging the scope of our treatment considerably. However, several details were not altered by these developments. During recent years we have examined a number of times the risk factors for KISS, and the associations that emerged were quite comparable. Prolonged labor, oblique presentation and multiple pregnancies came up consistently.

A fourth factor comes into play here: having treated one child, there is a high probability of seeing the next sibling, too, if he or she is of the same sex. As sexual dimorphism of the skeleton is well known, this finding does not cause too much surprise. We had to abandon our initial theory of the birth trauma as the only important risk factor and accommodate this additional – and quite important – contributing factor.

When the parents come to the consultation for the first assessment of their child they have to answer a questionnaire (Box 24.1).

The items in the questionnaire prompt quite a few parents to question us about their other children who they did not bring the first time, as they recognize the same pattern of symptoms in their case history, too. These children are mostly much older than the ones brought to be examined, i.e. are in primary school, and encounter the 'classic' problems we refer to in Chapters 10 and 25.

The impetus to think of manual therapy as *one* possible approach to these problems comes for the parents from learning about the pattern of symptoms presented in these KISS questionnaires, a welcome side effect of this evaluation procedure.

FUNCTION FIRST

One of the most important differences between the situation found in adults and that of the very young is the reversal of roles between function and form. In the newborn, morphology is soft, not yet defined in all details. We inherit pathways of development with our genetic makeup. The definite form of the adult body in its hardware and firmware (i.e. the automatic and autonomous level of control) is the result of this basic genetic layout and constant interaction with the environment. It is obvious that the external factors exert a greater influence in an 'unfinished' body. A premature baby who needs breathing assistance will develop cranial asymmetry after just a few days in a fixed position. An adult can tolerate the same position for a much longer time without any sign of an ensuing asymmetry.

This example may seem trivial, but it puts in a nutshell the difference between the two developmental periods. Function is in the lead, and morphology is to an important extent formed by it.

Almost everybody active in orthopedics and manual therapy starts their professional career examining and treating adults. What we see and learn there shapes our framework of expectations. It is very difficult to dissociate from that framework,

Box 24.1   Questionnaire for children

Birth:

- mother's age
- first/second/third . . . delivery
- duration of delivery (<1 h; 1–3 h; 3–6 h; >6 h)
    birthweight
    birth length
- oblique presentation
- twin
- forceps/vacuum
- cesarean (why?)

The first months:

- bad sleeper during first months – 6 to 12 months – later
- did/does the child often wake up at night?
- crying at night – how often?
- fixed sleeping pattern
- problems with breastfeeding on one side
- signs of colic
- orofacial hypotonus
- hypersensitivity of the neck region

Motor development: when did your child start to:

- crawl
- sit
- pull himself/herself up and stand
- walk

General health:

- bronchopulmonary infections
- headaches
- neurological disorders
- mouth is often open

Sensorimotor development slower than expected:

- posture and movement
- language
- concentration
- social integration

Asymmetry:

- visible immediately after birth?
- only later (when?)
- obstetrician/midwife saw it
- parents observed it first
- localization:
    arm
    trunk
    head
- baby looks only to one side
- moves only one arm/leg
- face is smaller on one side
- back of the head flat on one side
- has a bald spot on the back of the head

as we do need something to hold on to in order to understand whatever new facts we find.

One good example of this attitude towards children can be found in pharmacology: in order to find the correct dosage one is more often than not asked to multiply the dosage per gram by the body weight of the (small) patient. Studies about the effects of drugs in small children are rare and hard to come by.

An example closer to our topic is the heated discussion about the kinetics of the upper cervical spine, which arose after we published our findings about the movement patterns of the upper cervical spine (Biedermann 1991). It is a well-known fact that in adults, C_1 moves toward the concave side in bending of the head (Jirout 1990, Kamieth 1983), but we saw a different pattern in small children. In the vast majority of the small children we were able to examine (more than 20 000 until now), C_1 moves toward the convexity in side bending of the head. This is counter-intuitive at first sight, but even in adults this pattern can be found, albeit in only a few cases (Jirout 1990). Even with a condylar angle which is much less accentuated as in adults, the 'logical' movement pattern would be to recede to the concave side (see Chapter 18).

As this is not the case we have to ask what might be the reason for this pattern. For the time being, one can only offer an educated guess: during the first year the influence of gravity on the cervical spine is much less pronounced than after verticalization. The sensitivity of the newborn's spinal cord to mechanical irritation was brought to attention by some recent publications (Geddes et al 2001a, 2001b). In the light of these facts it is safe to say that the risk of injury to these structures is commonly underestimated. Taking into account this fragility, the paradoxical behavior of the cervical spine makes sense. Moving the atlas to the 'high' side of side-bending leaves more space for the intraluminal structures and minimizes their side-bending. We were able to verify in a large number of our radiographs that the condylar angle is much shallower during the first year (see Chapter 8), thus allowing this movement.

A WINDOW OF OPPORTUNITY

The acquisition of any skill requires a learning period and a predisposition to be acquired. The optimal point in time for a specific ability is embedded in the phylogenetically fixed development pattern. Language acquisition is the example we are frequently and painfully confronted with: whereas our children absorb another language without any effort, we grown-ups labor and toil and will never achieve the same level of effortless mastering our children grow into before puberty.

All our capacities, be they concerned with movement or perception, build on physiological and mental abilities learned beforehand. The earlier a basic skill's learning phase is situated in the 'normal' chain of events, the more its faulty acquisition will interfere with cognitive or motor developments later on (Miller and Clarren 2000).

Head control is situated very early on in this chain of events, which is one reason why the long-term consequences of its malfunctioning are so far-reaching. This is also the primary reason why we should check and treat even minor signs of asymmetry of the posture or form of the head: they may not look very impressive at that stage, but they can cause a derailment of the kinesiologic development and thus necessitate much more extensive treatment in later years.

Kinematic imbalances lead to behavioral and morphological asymmetries. 'Symmetric individuals appear to have quantifiable and evolutionary significant advantages over their asymmetric counterparts' (Møller and Swaddle 1997). We found signs of asymmetry and KISS in the newborn period of 72% of the schoolchildren we saw (and treated successfully) for headaches, postural and behavioral problems. The seeds of problems which surfaced at age 8 or 10 could be traced back to KISS symptoms before verticalization, i.e. during the first year (see Chapter 25). This is the main reason why it is necessary to have a vigilant attitude towards minor signs of functional asymmetry in this first stage of neuromotor development.

Even successfully treated babies continue to carry the imprint of their initial asymmetry with them. In times of exhaustion or after periods of rapid growth they will display the former asymmetrical posture again, at least temporarily. In most cases, these symptoms subside spontaneously and no treatment is necessary. Only if the asymmetry persists for more than a few days should one intervene therapeutically.

EVALUATING ASYMMETRY

It is very difficult to draw a strict line between 'normal' asymmetry and its pathological variant. For structures connected to sensory input, symmetry is more than an embellishment: most of the information has to be related to a three-dimensional analysis of its origin and here symmetry of the supporting structure simplifies processing. Strong asymmetry necessitates a higher level of 'input-correction' and is therefore an evolutionary disadvantage. According to Furlow et al (1997), 'fluctuating asymmetry could account for almost all heritable sources of variability in IQ'. This is but one hint of the importance of asymmetry as a marker or cause of other more fundamental problems. The impairment of sensorimotor development in KISS children seems to point to the same conclusions.

Complete symmetry is empty, dead (Landau 1989). A person or object needs a certain amount of symmetry to be considered beautiful, but the addition of a little bit of asymmetry can really make us like what we see (Swaddle and Cuthill 1995). Strong asymmetry on the other hand is seen as 'sick' (Parson 1990). Between these two extremes the ideal has to be found by intuition – or trial and error. A comprehensive treatment of symmetry and its evolutionary role can be found in Møller and Swaddle (1997).

One does not need to treat asymmetry in babies as such. However, the timely treatment to achieve a symmetrical posture and morphology goes a long way to preventing both current problems and later

complications. Having traced back a lot of schoolchildren's problems to initial asymmetries of posture (Biedermann 1996, Miller and Clarren 1959), one can attribute much more importance to them than their unremarkable symptomatology initially suggests. Asymmetry in posture and cranial configuration are a symptom, a sign calling our attention to the underlying condition that might be triggering it. By focusing on this prime mover we can successfully treat functional and morphological asymmetry as well.

When we began treating small children we did not draw a sharp line between different types of asymmetry; anything not symmetrical was considered to be of the same kind. It was only after having seen enough cases that we were able to distinguish between two types of asymmetry, one primarily located in the frontal plane – i.e. scoliotic posture – the other in the sagittal plane – i.e. hyperextension or ophistotonic posture. This led to the distinction between KISS I (fixed lateral posture) and KISS II (fixed retroflexion).

These two types of asymmetry can occur separately or together. The most common type combines a markedly scoliotic posture with a retroflexion component. Again this does not necessarily mean that this represents the majority of treatable cases, only the most easily perceptible and thus diagnosable clinical picture.

We see an interesting development in most of the contacts between us and pediatricians: the initial group of babies sent to us represent a fairly 'typical' collection of little patients with a 'classical' C-scoliosis (i.e. KISS I). After having seen the effects of treatment on these children, our colleagues are more aware of other signs connected to the KISS syndrome but less obviously cervicogenic at first sight.

These babies are then referred to us based on the less 'obvious' symptoms, but more specifically. It is less the screening for asymmetries than for the secondary symptomatology which becomes the dominant feature in the collaboration. These colleagues send babies with 'colic', cry-babies or children who have problems swallowing; they are *also* a bit asymmetrical, but this asymmetry is not such as to make the mother go to the pediatrician or make the latter think about referring the baby for manual therapy. It is not exaggerating to say that these babies – suffering from KISS II related problems – have a more relevant functional disorder than the KISS I cases.

We have to be alert to the range of problems originating from the malfunctioning of the cervical spine and the abnormal form of the cranium before we can recognize its therapeutic potential. The postural asymmetry and its morphological repercussions attract our attention to the cervical symptomatology, but the taxonomic frame is essential to be able to spot the problem. 'Words and taxonomies often exert a tyranny over thoughts. If you have neither a term nor a category for something, you may not be able to see it – no matter how largely or evidently it looms' (Steven Jay Gould 1997).

'MUSCULAR TORTICOLLIS' AND KISS I

Asymmetry in newborn babies is a well-known problem, and one which is often considered benign and disappearing spontaneously if left alone for long enough. It is certainly true that we have to be patient in the first days and weeks. After having passed through the birth channel, a realignment of the asymmetrical cranial bones and a resorption of soft-tissue edemas and/or hematomas takes time. An initially asymmetrical posture should be noted and observed, not more nor less.

If this asymmetry persists after 3–4 weeks, or additional symptoms appear, it is advisable to check if the range of movement of the head is impaired. This restricted movement is in most cases a sign for a protective immobilization of the upper cervical spine. For a long time this was linked to a malfunction of the sternocleidomastoid muscle, leading to the common diagnosis of 'muscular torticollis' (Binder et al 1987, Entel and Carolan 1997, Porter and Blount 1995, Robin 1996, Tom et al 1987, Vojta et al 1983). 'The etiology of

congenital muscular torticollis remains a mystery despite intensive investigation' is a commonly held view; like Davids et al (1993) most authors still put the blame on the trauma to the sternocleidomastoid muscle (Slate et al 1993, Suzuki et al 1984) – the most visible symptom was thought to be the cause.

At least in the early phases the shortened and thick sternocleidomastoid muscle is so prominent that it is a 'natural' culprit. Late cases of infantile torticollis often show a fibrosis of the sternocleidomastoid (Kraus et al 1986, Ljung et al 1989). The two facts were then easily combined: early hematoma results in later fibrosis.

Our experiences lead to different conclusions. There is no direct and linear connection between the initial hematoma and a late fibrosis. Children with an initial hematoma do not have a greater chance of developing a late fibrosis than newborns without a palpable tumor of the sternocleidomastoid. The connection between the two phenomena is much more intricate than such a linear concept suggests. The sternocleidomastoid is a co-victim of the underlying trauma to the articular structures of the cervical spine and as such, it is not a good starting point for therapy or analysis. It is far better used as an indicator of the improvement brought about by other therapeutic measures, as correct therapy of the suboccipital joints results in an alignment of the muscular tonus of the sternocleidomastoid.

There is a controversy about how to react to a fixed or asymmetrical posture in newborn babies. Some consider this a 'physiological scoliosis' and think it wears off without treatment (Bratt and Menelaus 1992, Kamieth 1988). More recent papers stress the importance of asymmetries in perception and posture for the development of more severe consequences later on (Keesen et al 1993). Asymmetry is frequently found in testing newborns (Groot 1993, Rönnqvist 1995) and its clinical significance has to be carefully examined (Buchmann and Bülow 1989). Seifert (1975) published data from unselected groups of newborn babies where she found that more than 10% of them showed signs of asymmetry in the functioning of the upper cervical spine.

In preparation for a study on MTC in newborns we examined a neonatal care unit and checked the 1–3-day-old babies for signs of impaired movement of the head or pressure hypersensitivity at the neck. More than half of those examined showed one or both signs and it quickly became clear that such an early intervention would not be useful. As more than three-quarters of these babies recover spontaneously, a standard examination and treatment at such an early point in time cannot be recommended. If there are other signs warranting examination and eventual treatment, such as breastfeeding problems or colic, the situation is different. In these cases we can examine and try to help.

Nobody advocates a treatment schedule where all these initially asymmetrical babies have to be treated routinely, but these babies should be re-examined later on and treated if the functional deficit has not subsided spontaneously after 4–6 weeks. We would propose taking a large margin, especially as MTC is a low-risk procedure, quite uncomplicated and does not have to be repeated more than once or twice. Anything improving the symmetry of sensory input early on can only exert a positive influence on the further development of the child.

Keessen et al (1993) show that the accuracy of the proprioception of the upper limb is reduced in cases with idiopathic scoliosis and spinal asymmetry. As we know that the proprioception of the arms depends heavily on a functioning suboccipital region (Hassenstein 1987), functional deficits in this region should be corrected as soon as possible.

As is often seen in the history of medical knowledge, our frame of reference changed over time: already in 1727 Nicolas Andry de Boisregard, who coined the word 'orthopedics', had mentioned the treatment of torticollis as one important field of this new discipline (Andry de Boisregard 1741). In going back to the roots we understand that good posture in children was at the forefront of orthopedic diagnostics and treatment: Ortho-Pedics – 'rightening the young' was so important for Andry that he used this concept as the definition of the medical procedures he published in his book. This fundamental underpinning of the new discipline was lost in later centuries and Andry's eminently functional approach had to make way for the mechanistic paradigms which have dominated orthopedics in the last decades.

Figure 24.3 Two KISS babies with their cranial asymmetries. Both pictures were taken by the parents and are reproduced here with their friendly permission. They show in both cases a right-convex KISS situation with the accompanying cranial scoliosis, microsomy of the left side of the face, flattening of the right occipital region and a seemingly asymmetrical positioning of the ears. All these morphological asymmetries need many months to subside. The important sign at the check-up 3 weeks after the initial treatment is the free movement of the cervical spine.

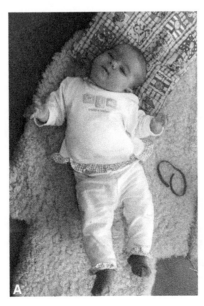 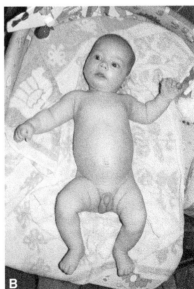

PLAGIOCEPHALY AND KISS II

Unilateral flattening of the head is an almost inevitable symptom in children with KISS II. The amount of asymmetry can be quite remarkable and it is understandable that parents are worried about this. In recent years we have seen more and more clinics advising parents to use helmets or bands to correct this (Aliberti et al 2002, Clarren et al 1981, Draaisma 1997, Teichgraeber et al 2002), while other authors stress that this treatment of non-synostotic plagiocephaly does not offer a marked improvement over simple handling advice (Bridges et al 2002).

In order to come to a proper assessment of an asymmetrical skull, a synostotic plagiocephaly has to be excluded, as this is a clear indication for surgical treatment. But the synostotic form is very rare – Mulliken et al (1999) found only 1 in 115 cases of plagiocephaly – so it is safe to assume that the sign of plagiocephaly should first and foremost be a motivation to look for other symptoms indicating a functional vertebrogenic disorder, i.e. in most cases KISS II.

One reason why many orthopedic specialists have such problems with this approach may be found in the ingrained preference of our colleagues for redressement as a basic therapy (Fig. 24.4).

Influencing the morphology through treatment of the functional disorders takes time, the more so if the intended change affects osseous structures. The cranial asymmetries are a good example of that. While we see changes in unilateral facial microsomia in weeks, the same change on the occipital side takes months. The facial asymmetry is primarily located in the soft tissue and seems to be controlled by asymmetrical activity of the ganglion stellatum. Here the changes in autonomic regulation influence the soft tissue turgor and act relatively quickly. On the other hand, the osseous structures of the occipital bones have to adapt their morphology to the changes in the muscular structures attached to them and this process is closely linked to the growth of the skull, which leads to a time frame of months, or even years, for the normalization of the skull's form.

It demands a lot of confidence on the part of the parents just to wait. The idea that doing too much might endanger the final result is difficult to grasp, even more so when such an invasive therapy is proposed by authoritative proponents.

We have to make a clear distinction between asymmetry as a symptom of an underlying functional deficit and a residual asymmetry where the functional base was successfully treated. We shall come back to the problem of relapsing asymmetries (see Chapter 25). Especially after having seen the

Figure 24.4 A: Treatment of a baby with scoliotic posture in the 1950s (Mau and Gabe 1962). The basic idea of redressement is clearly visible. B: The physiotherapy accompanying this bedding followed the same lines. Analyzing the pictures of the physiotherapy with hindsight one sees that some of the procedures advocate manual therapy of the suboccipital structures – these parts of the therapy may have been the most effective.

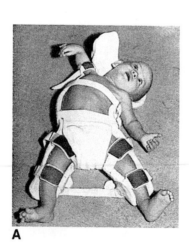

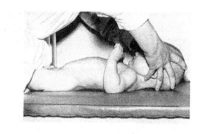

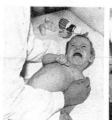

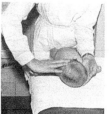

A   B

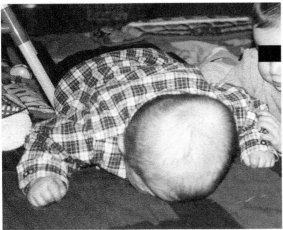

Figure 24.5 A typical case of KISS II with flattened occipital area. These asymmetries are easy to observe but difficult to document on photos.

sometimes dramatic improvements of their children, the parents tend to be very anxious when they encounter even a modest relapse. Good counseling is very helpful in preventing this kind of overreaction.

COLIC

One example of symptoms not readily attributed to functional disorders of the vertebral spine is colic (Fig 24.6). Through the observations of the parents we had the idea to check systematically if and how much we were able to relieve the sufferings of 'cry-babies' (i.e. colic). Initially quite a few of these small children were referred to us for treatment of postural asymmetries only and the accompanying colic was not mentioned by the parents during our interviews.

But in the questionnaire we ask the parents to send back to us 6 weeks after their visit they mentioned that the babies were much calmer and slept better.

Later on we found in a simple retrospective evaluation that up to 55% of those who said that incessant crying was one of the main reasons their child was presented in our consultation, registered an improvement of more than two-thirds in the week after treatment (Table 24.2) (Biedermann 2000).

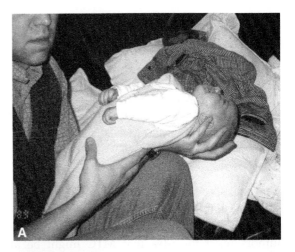

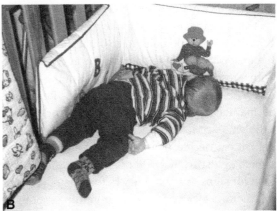

Figure 24.6 Two examples of babies with colic. Most infants with colic belong to the group of KISS II children. Overextension (A) and the sleeping position (B) are fairly typical.

In recent years there have been more publications about the role of physiotherapy or MTC in the treatment of colic (Klougart et al 1989, Olafsdottir et al 2001, Wilberg et al 1999). The least we can state is that this approach is worth trying, as one treatment suffices to see if any effect can be obtained.

The pathomechanism linking a disorder of the upper cervical spine and colic seems to be the faulty regulation of the abdominal muscles. Most babies where colic symptoms were successfully treated by MTC showed a KISS II symptomatology, i.e. forced retroflexion of the head and trunk, orofacial hypotonia and problems in connection with swallowing and excessive vomiting. Several

Table 24.2   Results of treatment (interviews with parents) (Biedermann 1999)

Sympton	(Very) good result after:				Improved	No change	Total
	1 day	1 week	2 weeks	3 weeks			
Torticollis	78	28	33	19	40	25	223
Ophisthotonos	10	6	5	7	12	5	45
Restless/crying	26	5	6	2	6	7	52
Fixed sleeping posture	16	3	3	6	4	1	33

studies of specialized pediatric clinics hint at least that muscular imbalance plays a part in the etiology (von Hofacker et al 1999), even if these authors reject the idea that MTC might be an effective tool in the treatment.

The basic trigger which makes pediatricians send the babies to a specialist in manual therapy is the hypersensitivity of the neck region in combination with a restricted range of movement of the head.

Those who have already observed the success of manual therapy in cases of colic or feeding problems are looking actively for these signs to help them decide if it is advisable to refer these babies to a specialist. Others find it easier to first look for signs of asymmetry before they take manual therapy as a treatment option into account. In both cases, it helps to have the pattern of typical KISS complaints present, even if not all symptoms can be found in an individual case.

Restlessness and excessive crying are symptoms which make quantitative measurements difficult. Even the inter-personal 'standards' may be difficult to evaluate. Wessel et al (1954) postulated an average of over 3 h/day for more than 5 days as a definition, similar to Brazelton (1962). Zeskind and Barr (1997) remarked that cry-babies have a phonatorily different crying pattern (see Geertsma and Hyams 1989, Hülse 1998). Betke (1997) and Spock (1944) drew attention to the different course of the baby's crying during the first 3 months with a maximum during the sixth week. Most crying happens in the afternoon or evening, regardless of whether the children are breastfed or not, or are the first-born or came later (St James-Roberts and Halil 1991).

These contradictory observations put pediatricians in an unenviable situation. They do not have much to offer to those parents who come with colicky children. Small wonder, then, that the most often used line is 'wait and see', and it is not surprising that one of the frequently used arguments of pediatricians is the well-known 'over-anxious mother'. The corollary of this line of reasoning is the disturbed mother–child relationship, another popular catch-all for functional problems without an attributable morphology.

As in the case of colic, this approach is not very satisfactory, to say the least. It puts the blame on the mothers and weakens (or destroys) the confidence between parents and doctor.

Some authors consider this excessive crying as something 'physiological' as it subsides in most cases after the third month without specific intervention (Betke 1975), a similar argument as is used for the scoliotic posture of the newborn in general (e.g. Gladel 1977). Even if one concedes that the crying stops one day, Lucassen's argument holds: 'I am too impressed by the parental feelings of helplessness and hopelessness, by their sentiment of anger and fright, their idea that something is seriously wrong with their child to be able to leave them alone with this essentially self-limiting problem' (Lucassen 1999).

Brazelton (1962) and Wessel (1954) are the main points of reference in the classic approach to colic. Quite a few diverse factors are accused of being at the root of the problem. Lucassen (1999) sees a cow-milk allergy as the root cause while von Hofacker et al (1999) dispute this. The American Academy of Pediatrics (1989) discouraged the use of hydrolyzed baby's milk for years and Brazelton had already written in 1962 that it was best 'to keep nutritional advice as vague as possible'.

The best approach to this problem is to take the complaints of the parents seriously. If a mother says she thinks her child is unhappy, restless and cries too much – believe her. There are a few cases where an overly concerned parent is the main problem, but even in these cases, it helps more to take these complaints seriously than to ridicule the worried mother.

It may sometimes just be enough to support the insecure mother with one's empathy and willingness to listen to her. If it helps to prevent turning her fear into a self-fulfilling prophecy – so much the better!

When we listen carefully to the reports of the parents we encounter a lot of symptoms reminding us of KISS. Often the children hate to be put to bed, and their mothers have to carry them in their arms till they fall asleep. Only then can they try to put them down carefully, always hoping they do not wake up suddenly.

Once they are asleep these children are restless, moving around in their bed. They often assume a stereotypical posture, mostly with a forced retroflexion of the neck and a tilt to one side. They wake up several times, crying, and have to be taken out of the bed and into the arms of the parent to calm down.

The symptoms compiled by a pediatric clinic in Munich specializing in the treatment of these cry-babies support this (von Hofacker et al 1999):

- hypotonia of the trunk
- (unilateral) muscular hypertonia of one extremity
- shoulder retraction
- postural asymmetries
- impaired postural control
- non-ideal quality of the spontaneous movements
- tendency to premature and non-optimal verticalization.

The least one can say is that these symptoms make a functional disorder of the sensorimotor apparatus a prime suspect. And once we get that far it seems obvious to think about checking the upper cervical spine.

By far the most important argument to examine and treat these cry-babies lies in the fact that we found episodes of crying at an early age in many cases where the children came years later for problems of cervico-cephalgia or sensorimotor disorders. In an almost identical manner the parents of these children report excessive crying, colic and fixed posture during the first year.

In a small sample of 100 babies who were referred to us with the initial diagnosis of 'excessive crying', we came up with the following results (Biedermann 2000):

- boys were – as with KISS in general – over-represented (58 : 42)
- 63 parents reported improvement after our treatment
- this improvement was arbitrarily quantified by them as 81% (median 80%)
- the time-lapse between treatment and improvement was 4 days (median 3 days)
- the average period of excessive crying before treatment was 4 weeks
- the average duration per day was 3–5 hours.

This list of results suffers from all the weaknesses of a retrospective compilation, but it shows a tendency that is reported from others active in the field, too, and should be adequate as a base for a rigorous prospective study. Those pediatricians who are already aware of the possibilities of MTC now routinely check their cry-babies for symptoms of KISS, especially KISS II.

DIFFERENTIAL DIAGNOSIS

Asymmetry – at least temporarily – is very often present during the child's development. If it was the only diagnostic criteria to filter out functional problems of the vertebral spine we would be in a difficult situation. Luckily we have an assortment of clues to rely on for a reasonably precise diagnosis. Nevertheless it is only after having evaluated the eventual result of a manipulation that the relevance of functional disorders of the suboccipital region for a given problem can be assessed. The threshold for intervention is relatively low as there are no known risks as long as the proper procedure is followed.

One of the most important diagnostic problems is the detection of spinal tumors. The severity of these cases and the need for timely intervention attributes much more importance to their detection than the rarity of their occurrence might suggest (5/100 000, of these 10–20% in children; Obel and Jurik 1991). Some of the signs are quite specific, e.g. a protrusion of the optic disk or impairment of the pyramidal tract. Others are far less specific and can easily be confused with functional problems. Even specialists note that a wrong initial diagnosis is the rule and not the exception (Matson and Tachdjinan 1963).

Quite often the first symptoms that attract attention are secondary problems due to functional disorders, i.e. a torticollis (Bussieres et al 1994, Shafrir and Kaufman 1992, Visudhiphan et al 1982). These symptoms are identical to those caused by primary vertebrogenic factors and may even improve at first. Gutmann published such a case of a young boy he treated – initially successfully – for headaches and neck pain (Gutmann 1987). After a complete remission the problems reappeared, seemingly after a minor trauma, as happens quite frequently. When the boy came back a third time – again after some minor knock on the head – Gutmann insisted, nevertheless, on an MRI, which resulted in the diagnosis of a tumor.

One caveat is a crescendo of symptoms: most functional disorders show a flat curve of development and are often traceable back to an initial trauma. If the pain pattern or the amount of dysfunction shows a rapid increase, further diagnostic measures are necessary. As much as conventional X-ray plates of the cervical spine are essential for the evaluation of functional disorders of the spine, they do not furnish the necessary information to diagnose intramedullary tumors. MRI scans are by far the best method. As soon as we discover details

in the case history or in the clinical examination which point towards an origin of the problems beyond the functional level, a neuro-pediatrician should be consulted.

In a recent publication we summarized the items necessitating further diagnostics as follows (Biedermann and Koch 1996):

- inadequate trauma
- late onset of symptoms
- multiple treatments before first presentation
- crescendo of complaints
- 'wrong' palpatory findings.

This last item is by far the most important and in those cases where I had to diagnose a tumor it was this 'wrong' feeling which alerted me. This impression is difficult to describe; one has to examine many necks to calibrate one's hands finely enough in order to filter out these cases. In two of them the main area of pain sensitivity was unusually low, in another case the sensitivity was so extreme that even after trying to palpate gently the hyperesthesia persisted. These three children were referred to a neuropediatrician and the preoperative diagnosis was mainly based on MRI.

In 1997/8 we asked for MRI scans in 12 cases (of a total of 2316 children examined). In two cases a tumor was found (1 hemangioma, 1 astrocytoma). It has to be added that most of the children we see have already been examined by a pediatrician and the normal waiting period for an appointment is 2–4 weeks. This filters out all those cases where the rapid deterioration necessitates immediate action.

In our aim to find the few cases with a serious background we cannot rely on an initial trauma as an exclusion criterion against tumor. In several of these cases where we had to diagnose a tumor in the end, an 'appropriate' trauma was reported.

A second important group are cases with an inflammatory component. This is quite rare during the first year but gets much more relevant from the second year on. A typical problem of the childhood years is Grisel's syndrome. This condition was first described in 1830 (Mathern and Batzdorf 1989) and is much more frequent in children than in adults (Martinez-Lage et al 2001, Okada et al 2002, Robinson and De Boer 1981, Watson-Jones 1932).

The diagnosis of Grisel's syndrome is often done in the context of an AARF (atlanto-axial rotary fixation) (Kawabe et al 1989, Roche et al 2001, Waegeneers et al 1997) which produces signs of a fixed torticollis. Here the case history is most valuable, as these children have a comparatively short duration of complaints, no significant signs of KISS-related problems previously and often a history of tonsillitis or otorhinological treatments (Samuel et al 1995).

Other diagnoses are even rarer at that phase of the development. One fact often overestimated at that age is the role of strabismus. Before verticalization, this does not cause any relevant torticollis. Afterwards it is sometimes difficult to distinguish between cause and effect, as proprioceptive problems of the neck can worsen a heterotropy at least as much as vice versa. Strabismus is in any case not an absolute contraindication for MTC.

These 'hard' differential diagnoses have to be kept in mind permanently. But at the same time it has to be emphasized that they are exceedingly rare. We see more than 2000 babies every year and about one or two of these cases surface.

Besides these cases of tumor or inflammation (Grisel's syndrome) there are 'soft' contraindications for MTC. This group comprises osseous malformations (see Chapter 18), neuromuscular syndromes and the large group of cerebral and spinal palsy.

In the next chapter, some of these are discussed in more detail.

Box 24.2 lists the absolute and relative contraindications for MTC in babies.

THE 'SPONTANEOUS SUBSIDING OF THE SYMPTOMS' – A QUESTION OF THE VIEWPOINT

The disappearance of any clinical problem around the first birthday is one of the strongest arguments

---

Box 24.2   Absolute and relative contraindications for MTC in babies

Absolute contraindications:

- tumor
- inflammation (e.g. Grisel's syndrome)
- extreme hypermobility
- extreme osseous malformation
- trauma and instability

Relative contraindications:

- syndromes associated with hypermobility (e.g. Down syndrome)
- cervical fusion syndrome (Klippel–Feil)
- current infection, especially naso-bronchial
- any treatment of the neck during the previous 1–2 weeks

---

of the school of thought which still treats many KISS-associated symptoms as 'physiological', be it the fixed posture, the initial colic signs or the delayed motor development. The second and third years of a child can be quite normal even after such a difficult first year. Those problems encountered later on – coordination weakness, headaches or hyperactivity – are rarely seen in connection with the earlier signs of autonomic dysregulation, asymmetry and problematic motor development.

One of the main motivations for proposing KISS as a classification tool is just this long-term view of apparently disjointed phenomena. We do treat babies to help the parents with their sorrows about colic or sleeping problems, but the deeper motivation is the knowledge of those long-term problems apparently connected with KISS.

Today we cannot be sure that it is enough to make the initial KISS symptoms disappear to avoid these later difficulties, and it is unlikely that we will be able to verify this conjecture in a rigid scientific manner. We would have to diagnose KISS in newborns and just wait – an unrealistic proposal. We toyed with the idea of using the (few) children whose parents did not want a treatment. But these cases are far too few to serve as a valid group and it would not be a random sample but a very skewed group.

So one day we shall probably be able to use epidemiological tools to render weight to this argument. In the meantime it seems safest to treat those children who find their way to a specialist in MTC and keep an eye open for subsequent problems. At least the parents of these children are already alerted to the potential of vertebrogenic disorders (and their simple remedies), a fact which speeds up the eventual diagnosis of such problems.

The cessation of an apparent symptomatology around the first birthday is one of the reasons we propose a differentiation between KISS (till at most the second birthday) and KIDD (from preschool age till the end of adolescence (see Chapter 25). KISS happens during an ontological stage where the functional problems and the ensuing pathology can be described with reasonable precision (Box 24.3). The main symptom – fixed and asymmetrical posture – is clear enough and the effects of MTC can be seen in days or weeks.

In KIDD (KISS-induced dysgnosia and dyspraxia) the situation is more complicated. Not only are the patients older – between 4 and 15 years approximately – but the external influences which complicate the clinical and nosological picture are multilayered and much less easy to decode than in KISS. The next chapter deals with what we know – and with the many exciting 'loose ends' we hold in our hands.

Box 24.3 Typical sequence of KISS–related symptoms

> 1–2 months: dysphoria, breastfeeding problems, colic
> 3–4 months: asymmetry develops, e.g. unilateral retardation of hip development
> 5–9 months: signs of asymmetry and retarded sensorimotor development
>   During all this time sleeping problems play an important role, be it difficulties in putting the child to sleep or frequent awakening during the night

References

Aliberti F, Pittore L, Ruggiero C et al 2002 The treatment of the positional plagiocephaly with a new thermoplastic orthotic device. Childs Nervous System 18(6–7):337–339

American Academy of Paediatrics 1989 Committee on Nutrition: hypoallergenic formulas. Pediatrics 83:1069–1086

Andry de Boisregard 1741 N L'orthopédie ou l'art de prévenir et de corriger dans les enfants les difformités du corps. Vv Alix, Paris

Anrig C A, Plaugher G 1998 Pediatric chiropractic. Williams & Wilkins, Baltimore

Betke K 1997 Rezidivierendes Bauchweh bei Kindern und die sogenannte Säuglingskolik. Pädiatrie Praxis 53:473–480

Biedermann H 1990 Das Atlas-Blockierungssynsrom des Neugeborenen und Kleinkindes: Diagnostik und Therapie. KG-Intern 11–15

Biedermann H 1991 Kopfgelenk-induzierte Symmetriestörungen bei Kleinkindern. Kinderarzt 22:1475–1482

Biedermann H 1992 Kinematic imbalances due to suboccipital strain. Journal of Manual Medicine 6:151–156

Biedermann H 1993 Das Kiss-Syndrom der Neugeborenen und Kleinkinder. Manuelle Medizin 31:97–107

Biedermann H 1995 Manual therapy in newborn and infants. Journal of Orthopaedic Medicine 17:2–9

Biedermann H 1996 KISS-Kinder. Enke, Stuttgart

Biedermann H 1999 KISS-Kinder: eine katamnestische Untersuchung. In: Biedermann H (ed) Manualtherapie bei Kindern. Enke, Stuttgart, p 27–42

Biedermann H 2000 Schreikinder: Welche Rolle spielen vertebragene Faktoren? Manuelle Therapie 4:27–31

Biedermann H, Koch L 1996 Zur Differentialdiagnose des KISS-Syndroms. Manuelle Medizin 34:73–81

Binder H, Gaiser J F, Koch B 1987 Congenital muscular torticollis: results of conservative management with long-term follow-up in 85 cases. Archives of Physical Medicine and Rehabilitation 68:222–225

Bratt H D, Menelaus M B 1992 Benign paroxysmal torticollis of infancy. Journal of Bone and Joint Surgery 74-B:449–451

Brazelton B T 1962 Crying in infancy. Pediatrics 29:579–588

Bridges S J, Chambers T L, Pople I K 2002 Plagiocephaly and head binding. Archives of Disease in Childhood 86(3):144–145

Buchmann J, Bülow B 1989 Asymmetrische frühkindliche Kopfgelenksbeweglichkeit. Springer, Berlin

Bussieres A, Cassidy D, Dzus A 1994 Spinal cord astrocytoma presenting as torticollis and scoliosis. Journal of Manipulative and Physiological Therapeutics 17:113–118

Clarren S K, Smith D W, Hansen J W 1981 Helmet treatment for plagiocephaly and congential muscular torticollis. Journal of Pediatrics 1:92–95

Davids J R, Wenger D R, Mubrak S J 1993 Congenital muscular torticollis: sequela of intrauterine or perinatal compartment syndrome. Journal of Pediatric Orthopedics 13:141–147

Davies N 2000 Chiropractic pediatrics. Churchill Livingstone, Edinburgh

Draaisma J M T 1997 Redressie Helm Therapie bij Plagiocephalie. In: Voorkeurshouding bij Zuigelingen. VCNN, Lustrum, NL

Entel R J, Carolan F J 1997 Congenital muscular torticollis: magnetic resonance imaging and ultrasound diagnosis. Journal of Neuroimaging 7(2):128–130

Frymann V 1966 Relation of disturbances of craniosacral mechanisms to symptomatology of the newborn. Journal of the American Osteopathic Association 65:1059

Frymann V 1976 The trauma of birth. Osteopathic Annals 4:8–14

Frymann V 1988 Learning difficulties of children viewed in the light of osteopathic concept. In: Retzlaff E W, Mitchell F L Jr (eds) The cranium and its sutures. Springer, Berlin, p 27–47

Furlow F B, Armijo-Prewitt T, Gangestad S W et al 1997 Fluctuating asymmetry and psychometric intelligence. Proceedings of the Royal Society of London. Series B Biological Sciences 264(1383):823–829 [cited in Blickhorn S 1997 Symmetry as destiny – taking a balanced view on IQ. Nature 387:849–850]

Geddes J F, Hackshaw A K, Vowles G H et al 2001a Neuropathology of inflicted head injury in children. I. Patterns of brain damage. Brain 124(Pt 7):1290–1298

Geddes J F, Vowles G H, Hackshaw A K et al 2001b Neuropathology of inflicted head injury in children. II. Microscopic brain injury in infants. Brain 124(Pt 7):1299–1306

Geertsma M A, Hyams J S 1989 Colic – a pain syndrome of infancy? Pediatric Clinics of North America 36(4):905–919

Gladel W 1977 Überlegungen zur Spontanheilung der sogenannten Säuglingsskoliose. Zeitschrift für Orthopädie 115:633

Gould S J 1997 Evolutionary psychology: an exchange. New York Review of Books 9 October

Gracovetsky S A 1988 The spinal engine. Springer, Vienna

Groot L 1993 Posture and motility in preterm infants. In: Fac Bewegingswetenschappen. Frije University, Amsterdam

Gutmann G 1968 Das cervical-diencephal-statische Syndrom des Kleinkindes. Manuelle Medizin 6:112–119

Gutmann G 1987 Hirntumor Atlasverschiebung und Liquordynamik. Manuelle Medizin 25:60–63

Gutmann G 1988 Die obere Halswirbelsäule im Krankheitsgeschehen. In: Biedermann H (ed) Von der Chiropraktik zur Manuellen Medizin. Haug, Heidelberg, p 81–114

Gutmann G, Biedermann H (eds) 1984 Die Halswirbelsäule. Part 2: Allgemeine funktionelle Pathologie und klinische Syndrome. Fischer, Stuttgart

Hassenstein B 1987 Verhaltensbiologie des Kindes. Piper, Munich

Hülse M 1998 Klinik der Funktionsstörungen des Kopfgelenkbereiches. In: Hülse M, Neuhuber W L, Wolff H D (eds) Der kranio-zervikale Übergang. Springer, Berlin, p 43–98

Jirout J 1990 Röntgenologische Bewegungsdiagnostik der Halswirbelsäule. In: Gutmann G, Biedermann H (eds) Funktionelle Pathologie und Klinik der Wirbelsäule, Vol 1/3. Fischer, Stuttgart

Kamieth H 1983 Röntgenbefunde von normalen Bewegungen in den Kopfgelenken. WS in Forschung und Praxis, Vol 101. Hippokrates, Stuttgart

Kamieth H 1988 Die chiropraktische Kopfgelenksdiagnostik unter funktionellen Gesichtspunkten nach Palmer-Sandberg-Gutmann aus schulmedizinisch-radiologischer Sicht. Zeitschrift für Orthopädie 126:108–116

Kawabe N, Hirotani H, Tanaka O 1989 Pathomechanism of atlantoaxial rotatory fixation in children. Journal of Pediatric Orthopedics 9(5):569–574

Keesen W, Crow A, Hearn M 1993 Proprioceptive accuracy in idiopathic scoliosis. Spine 17:149–155

Klougart N, Nilsson N, Jacobsen J 1989 Infantile colic treated by chiropractors: A prospective study of 316 cases. Journal of Manipulative and Physiological Therapeutics 12:281–288

Kraus R, Han B K, Babcock D S et al 1986 Sonography of neck masses in children. American Journal of Roentgenology 146:609–613

Landau T 1989 About faces. Doubleday, New York

Lewit K, Janda V 1964 Die Entwicklung von Gefügestörungen der Wirbelsäule im Kindesalter und die Grundlagen einer Prävention vertebragener Beschwerden. In: Müller D (ed) Neurologie der Wirbelsäule und des Rückenmarkes im Kindesalter. Fischer, Jena, p 371–389

Ljung J G B M, Guerry T, Schoenrock L D 1989 Congenital torticollis: evaluation by fine-needle aspiration biopsy. Laryngoscope 99:651–654

Lucassen P 1999 Infantile colic in primary care. Faculteit Geneeskunde, Vrije University, Amsterdam

Martinez-Lage J F, Martinez Perez M, Fernandez Cornejo V et al 2001 Atlanto-axial rotatory subluxation in children: early management. Acta Neurochirurgica (Wien) 143(12):1223–1228

Mathern G W, Batzdorf U 1989 Grisel's syndrome. Cervical spine clinical, pathologic, and neurologic manifestations. Clinical Orthopaedics 244:131–146

Matson D D, Tachdjinan M O 1963 Intraspinal tumors in infants and children. Postgraduate Medicine 34:279–285

Mau H, Gabe I 1962 Die sogenannte Säuglingsskoliose und ihre krankengymnastische Behandlung. G. Thieme, Stuttgart

Miller R I, Clarren S K 2000 Long-term developmental outcomes in patients with deformational plagiocephaly. Pediatrics 105(2):E26

Møller A P, Swaddle J P 1997 Asymmetry, developmental stability and evolution. Oxford University Press, Oxford

Mulliken J B, Vander Woude D L, Hansen M et al 1999 Analysis of posterior plagiocephaly: deformational versus synostotic. Plastic and Reconstructive Surgery 103:371–380

Obel A, Jurik A G 1991 Alternating scoliosis as a symptom of spinal tumor. Fortschritte der Röntgenologie 155:91–92

Okada Y, Fukasawa N, Tomomasa T et al 2002 Atlanto-axial subluxation (Grisel's syndrome) associated with mumps. Pediatric International 44(2):192–194

Olafsdottir E, Forshei S, Fluge G et al 2001 Randomised controlled trial of infantile colic treated with chiropractic spinal manipulation. Archives of Disease in Childhood 84:138–141

Parson P A 1990 Fluctuation asymmetry: an epigenetic measure of stress. Biological Review 65:131–145

Porter S B, Blount B W 1995 Pseudotumor of infancy and congenital muscular torticollis. American Family Physician 52(6):1731–1736

Ratner A J 1991 Zur perinatalen Schädigung des zentralen Nervensystems. Kinderarzt 22:205–215

Robin N H 1996 Congenital muscular torticollis. Pediatric Reviews 17(10):374–375

Robinson P H, De Boer A 1981 La maladie de Grisel: a rare occurrence of 'spontaneous' atlanto-axial subluxation after pharyngoplasty. British Journal of Plastic Surgery 34(3):319–321

Roche C J, O'Malley M, Dorgan J C et al 2001 A pictorial review of atlanto-axial rotatory fixation: key points for the radiologist. Clinical Radiology 56(12):947–958

Rönnqvist L 1995 A critical examination of the Moro response in newborn infants – symmetry, state relation, underlying mechanisms. Neuropsychologia 33:713–726

Samuel D, Thomas D M, Tierney P A et al 1995 Atlanto-axial subluxation (Grisel's syndrome) following otolaryngological diseases and procedures. Journal of Laryngology and Otology 109(10):1005–1009

Seifert I 1975 Kopfgelenksblockierung bei Neugeborenen. Rehabilitacia. Prague (Suppl) 10:53–57

Shafrir Y, Kaufman B A 1992 Quadriplegia after chiropractic manipulation in an infant with congenital torticollis caused by a spinal cord astrocytoma. Journal of Pediatrics 120:266–269

Slate R K, Posnick J C, Armstrong D C et al 1993 Cervical spine subluxation associated with congenital muscular torticollis and craniofacial asymmetry. Plastic and Reconstructive Surgery 1187–1195

Spock B 1944 Etiological factors in the hypertrophic stenosis and infantile colic. Psychosomatic Medicine 6:162

St James-Roberts I, Halil T 1991 Infant crying patterns in the first year: normal community and clinical findings. Journal of Child Psychology and Psychiatry 32(6):951–968

Suzuki S, Yamamuro T, Fujita A 1984 The aetiological relationship between congenital torticollis and obstetrical paralysis. International Orthopaedics (Germany) 8:75–81

Swaddle J P, Cuthill I C 1995 Asymmetry and human facial attractiveness: symmetry may not always be beautiful. Proceedings of the Royal Society of London, Series B, 261:111–116

Teichgraeber J F, Ault J K, Baumgartner J et al 2002 Deformational posterior plagiocephaly: diagnosis and treatment. Cleft Palate–Craniofacial Journal 39(6):582–586

Tom L W, Rossiter J L Sutton L N et al 1987 The sternocleidomastoid tumor of infancy. International Journal of Pediatric Otorhinolaryngology 13:245–255

Upledger J E 1978 The relationship of craniosacral examination findings in grade school children with developmental problems. Journal of the American Osteopathic Association 77(10):760–776

Valk J, van der Knaap M S, de Grauw T et al 1991 The role of imaging modalities in the diagnosis of posthypoxic-ischaemic and haemorrhagic conditions of infants. Clinical Neuroradiology 127:83–140

Visudhiphan P, Chiemachanya S, Somburanasin R et al 1982 Torticollis as the presenting sign in cervical spine infection and tumor. Clinical Pediatrics 21:71–76

Vojta V, Aufschnaiter D V, Wassermeyer D 1983 Der geburtstraumatische Torticollis myogenes und seine krankengymnastische Behandlung nach Vojta. Krankengymnastik 35:191–197

von Hofacker N, Papousek M, Jacubeit T et al 1999 Rätsel der Säuglingskoliken. Monatsschrift für Kinderheilkunde 147:244–253

Waegeneers S, Voet V, De Boeck H et al 1997 Atlantoaxial rotatory fixation. A case report and proposal of a new classification system. Acta Orthopaedica Belgica 63(1):35–39

Watson-Jones R 1932 Spontaneous hyperaemic dislocation of the atlas. Proceedings of the Royal Society of Medicine 25:586–590

Wessel M A, Cobb J C, Jackson E B et al 1954 Paroxysmal fussing in infancy, sometimes called 'colic'. Pediatrica 14:421–434

Wilberg J, Nordsteen J, Nilsson N 1999 The short-term effect of spinal manipulation on the treatment of infantile colic. Journal of Manipulative and Physiological Therapeutics 22:517–522

Zeskind P S, Barr R G 1997 Acoustic characteristics of naturally occurring cries of infants with 'colic'. Child Development 68(3):394–403

Chapter 25

KIDD: KISS-induced dysgnosia and dyspraxia

How functional vertebrogenic disorders influence the sensorimotor development of children

H. Biedermann

FROM KISS TO KIDD

Since we first used the term KISS internally in our office some 15 years ago, it quickly turned into a handy shortcut to describe a vertebrogenic problem. Later on, when the acronym was used in communications with other colleagues, too, they sent children for treatment with the remark: another 'KISS kid'. This label – originally intended only for smaller children – underwent an almost inflationary usage and had to serve as a catch-all for any functional disorder of spinal origin.

But too much usage renders such a concept useless. In the 1990s we differentiated between KISS I and II on the basis of the main symptoms these two types display, i.e. fixed lateroflexion for KISS I and fixed retroflexion for KISS II. This differentiation loses its meaning after verticalization, as the influence of the upright stance modifies the basic conditions to such an extent that the fixed posture is almost completely abandoned. 'After the first birthday the children (seem to) recover spontaneously' (von Adrian-Werbung 1977, Gladel 1977) – which is the main reason why many pediatricians have difficulties considering a fixed posture during the first year as warranting therapy. Like colic, this is thought of as 'self-limiting' and a 'wait and see' attitude is recommended.

The more subtle diagnostic tools of recent years and the epidemiological tools used in the search for long-term effects have shown that the underlying assumption does not hold true any more. Some publications link early plagiocephaly to later school problems (Miller and Clarren 2000) and others show similar findings for asymmetrical use of the extremities during the first year (Handen et al 1997, Hatwell 1987).

And those looking closely enough realized that the infants did not lose their asymmetry altogether. Parents reported that they observed a head tilt or a difference in shoulder height intermittently, mostly when the children were tired or some other stress occurred. But the 'simple' phenomenology of KISS mostly disappeared and what was left showed some connection to the initial asymmetry, but the range of symptoms was much wider and even less precise than at the infant stage.

With the knowledge gained about the first year, and the normalization we were able to initiate by removing functional disorders, new light was shed on the disabilities of older children. To put this diverse information into a viable concept we first have to step back a bit and look at the conceptual level of the problem.

THE *GESTALT* PROBLEM

Diagnostic procedures use basically two paradigms:

- On one side is the 'scientific' approach which tries to find one parameter to validate the diagnosis. This being an often impossible quest, one settles for the minimal combination attainable. This adaptation of Occam's razor to the medical reality has its charm: if we are able to give such a standard solution to our diagnostic problems, all our work as members of the healing profession can be put to a test, quantified and compared with others.

- On the other side are those who use an approach usually characterized as 'holistic', i.e. trying to grasp the complexity of the patient's situation and ailments as a whole. The advantage of this approach lies in its openness, which usually offers alternative choices for understanding and eventual treatment.

Both approaches are valid and have to be used appropriately. There are situations where the scientific approach leads to a quick and efficient treatment – think of a bacteriological infection – and there are occasions where the second approach offers a better base. A prime example of this is the diffuse problems many parents of schoolchildren are confronted with. Books like *Tom Sawyer* give an idea of the amount of energy in boys of school age and their problems dissipating it a hundred years ago, and times are not kinder to these boys today.

So what we are dealing with is a complex situation, an interdependence of external influences and the several phases of development children undergo before reaching puberty (not that it gets any better, then). Kühnen describes some cases in her chapter (see Chapter 10) and reading these pages gives a first clue about what to look for.

To find an appropriate name for such a complex disorder was not easy. First and foremost it had to reflect the interdependence of cervical function disorder, perception problems and the ensuing motor phenomena which are in most cases what parents and teachers recognize first.

We decided to call this disorder KISS-induced dysgnosia and dyspraxia (KIDD) to highlight the importance of the upper cervical spine for a smooth functioning of perception (gnosis/gnosia) and motor control (praxis/praxia). Needless to say that these two cannot be separated – there is no perception of any kind without at least a minimum of motor control and vice versa. But for all practical purposes the perception precedes the efferent impulses. The fascinating discovery was that there was a common denominator for many apparently diverse problems, once they were looked at with this concept in mind.

There is no 'hard' test in screening children for an eventual involvement of the cervical spine. The item list offered here is but a very global framework and – as often – almost too all-encompassing to be usable without some qualifying remarks. It is important to keep in mind that there are some 'first-rate' symptoms (primarily postural or motional asymmetry) and some items in the individual case history (KISS-related problems during the first year of life) that are in the foreground, but even these have to be complemented by other supporting findings to make a firm diagnosis of KIDD. At the end of the day, it is the success of the ensuing manual therapy which delivers the conclusive evidence. Lewit (1988) called this the *test manipulation*.

SYMPTOMATOLOGY OF KIDD

The second to fourth years in the life of a child are rather uneventful seen from the viewpoint of functional disorders. The development of children at that age is so rapid and yet so variable that a clear-cut pathology is rarely seen. This does not mean that such problems are completely absent, but they do not manifest themselves in a relevant way. Children are mostly at home or in the protected atmosphere of a kindergarten and any non-standard behavior is attributed to external influences.

In our statistics this age group forms a dip as compared to the first year or the period after the fourth birthday. Deliberately over-simplifying the situation, we can compile the following scheme:

- First year of life: the classic KISS symptoms of fixed lateroflexion or fixed retroflexion with the accompanying symptoms of dysphoria, swallowing problems and asymmetrical motor development.
- Second to fourth years: the 'silent' period, i.e. not many obvious problems reported.
- Fourth to sixth years: complaints about 'clumsiness' or slow motor development; first remarks about 'difficulties with other children'. Sleep disorders. Very rarely headaches.
- First school years: the lack of fine motor skills comes to attention; drawing and writing are difficult for the child and often refused. Global motor skills are also lacking; these children attract (negative) attention because they cannot sit still, and their poor coordination at sports makes them the butt of jokes – or they try to cover up by playing the 'clown' themselves. Headaches are mentioned more frequently.
- Pre-adolescence: difficulties regarding social interaction are in the foreground. The pupils are described as being unable/unwilling to fulfil the requirements of school. Headache is almost always mentioned.

When these children are examined for the first time, we find a whole range of symptoms (see also Chapter 10):

- imbalance of the muscular coordination with asymmetrical tonus of the postural muscles
- shortened hamstrings
- kyphotic posture with hyperlordosis of the cervical spine and hypotonus of the dorsal muscles of the thoracic area, often accompanied by orofacial hypotonia
- scoliotic posture in sitting and/or standing position
- shoulders at different height
- sacroiliac (SI) joint mobility asymmetrical often with asymmetry of leg rotation
- balance tests insufficient and mostly asymmetrical
- insufficient coordination of vestibular input, e.g. standing with raised arms and closed eyes difficult
- acoustic orientation laborious; locating the source of an 'interesting' noise difficult
- combination of arm and leg movements difficult, e.g. jumping-jack test
- fidgeting and restlessness, sometimes tics
- using eye control to compensate for lack of proprioception, refusing to lie down supine, clinging with one hand to the examination table

- decompensation when the close range is invaded by the examiner; wild resistance against palpation.

It is important to distinguish between the basic personality of a child and these superimposed functional disturbances. Depending on the character frame of an individual, one child may react aggressively and become uninhibited and hyperactive while another child reacts to the same disturbances by withdrawing. There is no score, no single test, but a *Gestalt* – and we can train our clinical view to recognize this.

The four most reliable items to look for in order to validate the assumption of a KIDD component are:

- a case history with the relevant KISS symptoms during the first year
- asymmetry of posture and movement during examination
- a sufficient number of symptoms from the list above
- the palpation of restricted movement and hypersensitivity to palpation in the suboccipital area.

If these four items can be found, it is almost always worth treating the functional impairment of the upper cervical spine (item four on the list) and then seeing if and how much the other symptoms react to this. The older the children are the more time should be allowed after the manipulation before any other treatments are resumed. In many cases the family comes back for the check-up 2–3 months later and the parents report that 'nothing changed'. When we examine the children we often find that the initial asymmetry of the posture or the balance problems are not detectable any more. Once we point that out to the parents, they reply by saying 'well, he can bicycle now' or 'in the last month she finally got her swimming medal' – thus acknowledging improvements in coordination not mentioned initially. Coming back 2–3 years later for a routine check-up, the same parents quite often say that 'since the first meeting the entire development went into fast track', or something similar.

It is thus important to document the initial situation as precisely as possible in order to detect these gradual improvements which the parents often do not see because they are confronted with their children every day. Sometimes it is the remark by a visiting aunt who sees her niece only rarely that opens the eyes of the parents to the progress made since our intervention.

KIDD IS AN AGGRAVATING FACTOR BUT RARELY THE STRUCTURAL SOURCE OF A PROBLEM

Usually we tell parents that we do not treat dyslexia or ADHD or headache. We try to influence the prevailing conditions and in eliminating some of the irritation in a complex system we create the more stable background against which children are able to re-equilibrate their homeostasis.

The same is true for migraine: if our treatment is successful, the frequency and strength of the attacks is significantly reduced but the migraine rarely disappears completely. For all practical purposes, this suffices and the children and their families are content.

Once we see KIDD as an additional stress factor and not as the prime mover it becomes clearer that there is no such thing as a 'KIDD test'. It is good news and bad news at the same time: if we find signs of asymmetry and functional impairment we can be sure that there is a KIDD component to the problem at hand – but we cannot be sure how much of it will change once we have treated these functional impairments.

There are many approaches which link the group of conspicuous symptoms to sensorimotor disorders. The Blythes (www.inpp.org.uk) propose the model of 'persistent primitive reflexes' as the reason for quite similar symptoms, Harold Levinson (www.levinsonmedical.com) has a similar concept. A lot of exercise-based treatments show improvements when the children are tested afterwards, and this extends to the effect of learning to play an instrument or singing as a means to connect the motor sphere and the perceptive level.

Many educational systems took advantage of the intimate connection between motor capabilities. Montessori, Orff, Steiner and other eminent figures in this field proposed combinations of music, exercise and handiwork to help children overcome their school problems.

So there are many roads which lead to Rome, and the one advantage of our proposition is that it acts fast and it does not interfere with other attempts which may be used to complement it.

We often recommend these additional therapies, adapting to the possibilities and needs of the individual children. One child may need a re-education of the orofacial muscles by specialized physiotherapeutic protocols (e.g. Padovan or Castillo-Morales). Others can use a combination of sport and remedial medicine, e.g. hippotherapy or speech therapy. All these methods can be used to attain the goal of normal function and development more easily, and in many cases we ask the specialists who take care of the children to decide when another session of manual therapy may be necessary.

The reason why we propose starting with the examination and eventual treatment of the spinal system is that these problems can be dealt with fairly easily by an experienced specialist, and this initial removal of vertebrogenic disorders facilitates (and in many cases makes possible) the ensuing therapies. These therapies have training as their main component and need to be repeated often in order to lead to a lasting improvement. Manual therapy based on the KIDD concept, on the other hand, has the big advantage of being discreet. In most cases a yearly follow-up of our young patients is enough.

In addition to Kühnen's chapter (see Chapter 10) we want to elaborate on one of the main symptoms which makes parents bring their children for our treatment: headache.

HEADACHE AS A LEAD SYMPTOM

In small children it is the torticollis which alerts doctors and physiotherapists to the idea that manual therapy might be an option. These children have in almost every case other problems, too, which were not reported on the first occasion as the family surmised that 'there is anyway nothing to be done about it' – quite comparable to the restlessness of the newborn baby which was not mentioned in the beginning.

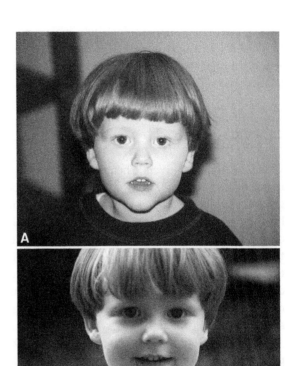

Figure 25.1 A and B: This boy's facial expression changed after he was treated at the upper cervical spine to relieve his headaches. When the mother sent me these pictures she wrote in the accompanying letter: 'His face became alive'. This new dimension of non-verbal communication will help him to develop his social skills. The orofacial hypotonia is still evident even after the treatment, albeit clearly attenuated.

So headache functions as a catalyst to facilitate the contact between the young patient and the specialist in manual therapy. Adults often project on the young ones their own experiences with headaches. How questionable this might be cannot be discussed here; but we know that lumbago-like complaints by children and juveniles are assimilated completely differently from the way adults deal with them. Children say, for example, 'it's tickling' and mean: this palpation hurts (see Harbeck and Peterson (1992) for comparison); they say 'I have headaches' and mean 'my neck feels sore'.

So, instead of a clear-cut definition we are now faced with a vague description: complaints by schoolchildren, whereby the main complaint is located inside their head.

Commonly proposed pathogenetic concepts

When dealing with juvenile headaches generally – in the same way as with adults – a mainly vasogenic/migraine model is favored: 'Vasomotor headache and migraine are frequent among children, the former considerably more frequent than the latter . . . usually it affects bright, often ambitious, at the same time sensitive and unbalanced children, not rarely with different manifestations of a "neuropathic" resp. neuro-vegetative diathesis' (Schulte et al 1992).

Lance et al (1965) found, when evaluating 2000 patients at a clinic dealing with headaches, 5% 'diseases of the cervical spinal column and the sinuses, systemic and psychiatric disorders' – i.e. the remainder after migraine (53%) and tension headaches (41%) had been deducted. Similar statistics can be found elsewhere (e.g. Chu and Shinnar 1992, DiMario 1992, Sillanpaa et al 1992). In none of these works is any thought given to a cervicogenic factor, while Rabending and Quandt (1982) at least accept 'radiation from myogelotic or cervical postural stress or spondylitic developments' as the second most important factor after vasomotor dystonias.

Using these statistics as a base, every manual therapist or physiotherapist would have to withdraw timidly from treating headaches. But nevertheless these are – independent of the 'exact' diagnosis, which was handed out elsewhere – next to dizziness, one of the most successful areas of manual therapy. It is always a question of the point of view . . .

The child whose parents are classical migraine patients and who is complaining about headaches has a high chance of inheriting vaso-frailty. One should not lament fatalistically this fate and retreat to drug therapy, but should search for other – and more accessible – co-factors and try to eliminate them.

Without neglecting the other causes or even downplaying them, it seems realistic to claim that vertebral factors are by far the leading cause. Maybe a dentist would say the same about dental factors, the nutritionist would point out the influences of food, the allergenic specialist his specialty; all true and all are right. In the individual case the simplest approach to the problem will be chosen.

Together with Gutmann we reported on the different kinds of vertebrogenic headaches (Gutmann and Biedermann 1984). In our view, they represent the largest contingent of headaches, but even initial success of the manual therapy should not block the view on intracranial problems behind them (Gutmann 1987).

The term 'school-headache' coined by Gutmann (1968) was especially created for those headaches occurring among adolescents – the anteflexion-headache. The triggering mechanism is the forward bending during reading or writing in order to bring the viewing axis into an angle of 90° to the document. Today this request of the eyes to look straight onto something is widely ignored; most schools procure flat tables. The good old school-desk with its inclined writing surface would do more good for the posture and muscular balance of the pupils than 'anatomically adapted' chairs. If this is not taken into consideration the supportive structures of the neck are overloaded and react with pain. The younger the children, the less they will complain of pain and the most visible sign that something is wrong may be a slumped posture, fidgeting or reduced attention span.

The anatomical correlate of this is the nodding movement at the suboccipital level, stretching the interspinal ligaments and the linea nuchae. These structures cannot take much when it comes to bending and shearing, and certainly not over longer periods of time.

If the anteflexion of the head does not happen harmoniously, kinking stresses occur, which can rarely be tolerated.

When does such a situation arise?

One cause can be found in variations of the dens (see Chapter 18). This uneven anterior surface prevents the slipping of the frontal bow of the atlas during anteflexion. This is not as rare as it appears at first sight; those children already conspicuous during the postnatal period, and who were not treated at their cervical spine, seem to be predestined for it.

Block vertebrae in the area of the upper cervical spine lead to a disturbed harmony in movement (see Chapter 18). Through radiological changes among older patients, it can be observed how the surrounding segments of movement react with structural loosening on the additional burden of work, be it the osteochondrosis of the intervertebral disk or arthrosis of the vertebral joints. Most of the time these secondary symptoms are not yet visible among children.

The constitutional hypermobility leads especially with adolescents to a situation where maintaining a posture with the head bent forward exceeds the abilities of the passive support structures of the neck. In these children we often find an interspinal pain when palpitating between the processi spinosi. The unfavorable ratio between the weight of the head and mass of muscles as well as age-related increased mobility make children and juveniles (girls even more than boys) vulnerable to it.

Trauma – e.g. accidents with frontal crashing – can cause this scenario, too. Even well-intended physiotherapy (isometric exercises or similar) makes the complaints chronic when applied too early. Children are especially vulnerable to this overload.

One should not have any illusions about protective possibilities when fastening seatbelts for children (or infants); the smaller the child the higher the risk of a massive injury of the cervical spine. A blockage of the occipitocervical joint after a trauma is obligatory and often triggers symptoms only after a long incubation period. This is also the reason why other authors are much more reluctant in judging the importance of traumas in the genesis of cervical complaints (Kamieth 1990).

Lumbosacral asymmetries can be caused either by true differences in leg length or by asymmetries in the transitional zone between lumbar spine and sacrum. In children, there is in most cases a functional component, too, e.g. SI joint blockage. Not *every* migraine is caused by statical asymmetries, but every case like this ought to be checked, especially if signs of a hypoplastic arcus dorsalis C_1 can be found (see Chapter 18).

Restricted movement of the thorax, e.g. a scoliosis there, can lead to additional stress on the cervical spine, forcing it to do more than it should.

One problem in schoolchildren is that the symptoms of vertebrogenic origin are so multifaceted.

Flehmig sums up these children as follows (Flehmig and Stern 1986):

- poor impression of themselves
- quickly frustrated and attempt to avoid new situations
- frequently late, forget easily
- easily distracted, unable to concentrate on one topic.

When comparing these descriptions with the criteria which Schulte et al (1992), for example, use as a baseline for children likely to develop vasomotor headaches, it is obvious how much these groups overlap each other; with this evidence we would see KIDD as the most probable background irritation.

ADVICE FOR THE CASE HISTORY

Frequently the children's ability to provide information is underestimated; especially when relatives start talking and attempt 'to cut a long story short', a lot will be missed. It is preferable to obtain a written report from the parents first and then to inquire from the children themselves what their complaints are. The parents can then be consulted again for details of the early infancy.

Especially important are details of the delivery, early kinetic development, eventual traumas and naturally the family history. Often the first suspicious moments are already showing up.

Caution is required if the complaints have a crescendo character; if these are increasing continuously during the observation period, they indicate an intra-cerebral event. Also complaints that are occurring constantly and do not alter much when changing positions, or according to the time of day or stress, should be treated with caution.

These days the typical ante-flexing-headache is not limited to school any more; one can speak as well of a 'Gameboy' headache, to name just one example. Space for outdoor playing is often lacking; activities at home are frequently linked with fine-motor and bending forward, which brings with it the same stress for the cervical spine, and the classical picture of the 'pure school-headache' blurs (Fig. 25.2).

Often statical complaints can be interpreted better and hence the differentiation between true differences in length of legs (occurs only when standing or walking on horizontal ground, not for example when hiking) and lumbar-sacral asymmetries (complaints also when sitting).

The accompanying symptomatic is multifaceted and does not yield much: besides neck and back pain, dizziness or problems in coordination may also be reported ('he is constantly falling down'). In principle all kinds of headaches ought to be investigated for a cervicogenic component; even if they are not dominant for the individual case, the complaints are at least lessened and/or other therapies made easier if they are treated with manual therapy.

Other pathogenetic factors should not be neglected. Manual therapy is generally the least time-consuming treatment and therefore ought to come first. But, depending on the examination, other sites have to be taken into account, too:

Figure 25.2 (A and B) Subtle signs of postural disorders as in these two examples should alert the pediatrician to consider the musculoskeletal system when examining an adolescent, even if the symptoms reported by the family are on another level.

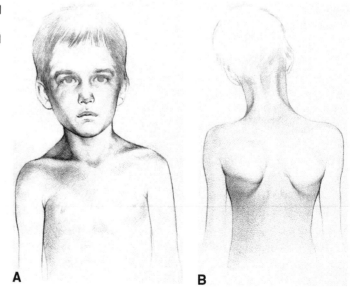

A **B**

- palpating a tension of muscles used for chewing and of the inner lower jaw, it is obvious to consult a dentist or orthodontist
- when encountering hypotonic muscles, one thinks of specific targeted physiotherapy
- if we find hypersensitive and/or hypotonic abdominal muscles, dietetic measures should be considered.

Prime candidates for treatment are – even more than with adults – the two poles of the spine. The suboccipital area and the SI joints interact functionally and we advise focusing on the cervical spine, first. If a correlate can be found there – e.g. restriction of mobility – the treatment should start here. After this initial manipulation, one should wait for around 3 weeks. The younger the patient, the more important it is to keep this rest period. It is astonishing how many of the other symptoms will have disappeared spontaneously.

KIDD AS *ONE* COMPONENT IN A COMPLEX SITUATION

The observations regarding headache should have shown how this 'established' indication for manual therapy opened the possibilities to reach children whose other disorders seemed more important for them, but nobody had considered manual therapy an option for their treatment.

In a pilot study at a school for children with learning problems we were able to show that practically all children with KISS items in the case history gained from manual therapy (Biedermann 2001). During the discussions with the teachers which preceded the treatment of the children, the argument of those professionals was that most of the children came from dysfunctional families, or had documented neurological deficits – so how did we think we could help them? We pointed out that we were indeed unable to improve the alcoholism of the father or the fact that the divorced parents were constantly quarreling, but that we did intend to improve on the sensorimotor equilibrium of the children. The follow-up showed that the school results of these children did actually improve.

The logical consequence is to immerse manual therapy for children into a wider concept (as already mentioned above) and to keep in mind how simple such an attempt is.

The KIDD concept does not claim to replace other approaches (see e.g. for ADS, Chapter 12) but it completes our therapeutic and diagnostic arsenal, thus giving all involved one more option to bring into play. And more often than not the improvement we can furnish motivates child and family to muster the energy for a more energetic push ahead.

References

Biedermann H 2001 Manual therapy in children. In: Vernon H (ed) The craniocervical syndrome. Butterworths, London, p 207–230

Chu M L, Shinnar S 1992 Headaches in children younger than 7 years of age. Archives of Neurology 49:79–82

DiMario F J 1992 Childhood headaches: a school nurse perspective. Clinical Pediatrics 31:279–282

Flehmig I, Stern L 1986 Kindesentwicklung und Lernverhalten. Child Development and Learning Behaviour. Fischer, Stuttgart

Gladel W 1977 Überlegungen zur Spontanheilung der sogenannten Säuglingsskoliose. Zeitschrift für Orthopädie 115:633

Gutmann G 1987 Hirntumor Atlasverschiebung und Liquordynamik. Manuelle Medizin 25:60–63

Gutmann G 1968 Schulkopfschmerz und Kopfhaltung. Ein Beitrag zur Pathogenese des Anteflexions-Kopfschmerzes und zur Mechanik der Kopfgelenke. Zeitschrift für Orthopädie und ihre Grenzgebiete 105:497–515

Gutmann G, Biedermann H 1984 Die Halswirbelsäule Part 2: Allgemeine funktionelle Pathologie und klinische Syndrome. Fischer, Stuttgart

Handen B L, Janosky J, McAuliffe S 1997 Long-term follow-up of children with mental retardation/borderline intellectual functioning and ADHD. Journal of Abnormal Child Psychology 25(4):287–295

Harbeck C, Peterson L 1992 Elephants dancing in my head; a developmental approach to children's concepts of specific pains. Child Development 63:138–149

Hatwell Y 1987 Motor and cognitive functions of the hand in infancy and childhood. International Journal of Behavioral Development 10:509–526

Kamieth H 1990 Das Schleudertrauma der Halswirbelsäule. WS in Forschung und Praxis, Vol 111. Hippokrates, Stuttgart

Lance J W, Curran D A, Anthony M 1965 Investigations into the mechanism and treatment of chronic headache. Medical Journal of Australia 2:909–914

Lewit K 1988 Disturbed balance due to lesions of the cranio-cervical junction. Journal of Orthopedic Medicine 58–61

Miller R I, Clarren S K 2000 Long-term developmental outcomes in patients with deformational plagiocephaly. Pediatrics 105(2):E26

Rabending G, Quandt J 1982 Kopfschmerz und Migräne. In: Quandt J, Sommer H (eds) Neurologie Grundlagen und Klinik. Fischer, Stuttgart

Schulte F J, Spranger J, Feer E 1992 Lehrbuch der Kinderheilkunde. Fischer, Stuttgart

Sillanpaa M, Piekkala P, Kero P 1992 Prevalence of headache at preschool age in an unselected child population. Cephalalgia 11:239–242

von Adrian-Werbung H 1977 Beobachtungen an 108 Kindern mit Säuglingsskoliosen. Zeitschrift für Orthopädie 115:633–634

Chapter 26

The family dimension
How birth trauma and family history complement each other in facilitating functional vertebrogenic disorders in children

H. Biedermann

Twelve years ago the etiology of KISS seemed to be clear: the entire problem was related to birth trauma and the 'usual suspects' were all there: prolonged labor, breech position, extraction aids and twin pregnancies (Biedermann 1991). Time and again we saw the same results when analyzing our data (Biedermann 1996, 1999). But meanwhile another puzzling detail came to our attention: more and more often we saw the siblings of the children we had treated – and they, too, had quite similar problems. In the beginning we attributed this to the fact that the parents involved had seen the effects of MTC and were therefore more prepared to think of vertebrogenic problems when dealing with whatever came their way.

This notion certainly plays a part in the set-up, but contrary to that we noticed another little detail: we saw far more children of the same sex than those of the opposite sex. Had it only been an enhanced awareness on the part of the parents, this should not have played such a prominent role. In an ad-hoc compilation done between September and December 2002, we saw that siblings of the same sex comprised 84% while a cross-over (i.e. a sister coming after a brother had been or vice versa) occurred in only 16% of the cases.

And it went even further than that. Almost stereotypically we are confronted with the question 'do you treat adults, too?' – and when we say yes we get the panoply of problems of the parents. But here, again, a trend was perceptible: in the wake of the baby boy came the father, and after the little girl was taken care of, the mother arrived with her migraine (Fig. 26.1). This trend was less pronounced than in the siblings, but the ratio was by no means 50:50, more like one-third to two-thirds.

What we are talking about here are trends, impressions. It seems unlikely that there will ever be a database to test this hypothesis. But for all practical purposes this does not matter too much. It is simply worthwhile to think about such a family trait when discussing functional disorders with the parents.

As we ask for two adults to accompany the infants we treat, we often see both parents. In quite a few cases, one of the parents cannot come and in these cases it is the grandparents who accompany the young patients. If the 'right' grandparent is present we ask about the early days of the father or mother, and it is striking how

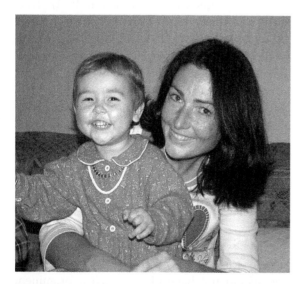

Figure 26.1 A fairly typical example of the 'family dimension': after the little girl was successfully treated for her KISS-related problems, the mother came to have her neck strain and headache examined. Both have a similar facial asymmetry and the cross-bite of the daughter should disappear in the following months.

often one gets told that 'he had the same problems', 'she was difficult with breast-feeding, too' or something in that vein. There are entire families where it is known that they do not crawl before starting to walk or where certain movement patterns reappear generation after generation.

In a family where there is a history of scoliosis we would screen the children *very* carefully for an asymmetrical posture; if we know that one member of the family suffered from KISS-related problems we do the same.

Since we encourage this 'screening' by the parents and those in contact with the children – i.e. kindergarten teachers, coaches or physiotherapists – we see more children where the vertebral connection is not that obvious for the uninitiated.

Anybody whose sight is diminished tends to recognize people not only by their faces but by their gait and other movement patterns. These people tell you that they sometimes have difficulties distinguishing between members of the same family as 'they walk alike'.

Radiographs tell the same story: block vertebrae are clustered in families and tend to stick to one sex (von Lanz and Wachsmuth 1955, Wackenheim 1975).

In the light of these insights we had to revise the assertion made in the beginning: a birth trauma *and* a genetic predisposition cooperate to produce KISS, and both aspects of this etiology combined give our diagnostic efforts a more solid base.

THE FAMILY WAY

Having said that, we turn to another dimension of the influence of family on the individual's health. Wolf and Bruhn (1997) dedicated an entire monograph to the influences that the family and social environment have on the general health situation of an individual. Wilkinson applied epidemiological and statistical methods to do research on the level of entire societies (Wilkinson 1996). These studies showed in convincing detail how much of the health and wellbeing of an individual and even more so of a child depends on the stability, warmth and support of the immediate and wider environment.

Every day one encounters families where even an outsider can feel the tension and 'bad vibes' raging inside this little group. How much of the jerkiness of the young adolescent, and how much of the migraine of the schoolchild is due to these factors, which are way beyond our influence?

The very big and the very small – society and family – play important parts in determining the wellbeing of a child, and our contribution to that wellbeing depends crucially on these external factors.

Some of these influences can at least be modified. A single child needs the contact in kindergarten or in an informal day-care group much more than another one with several siblings; in town – and even more so in high-rise apartment buildings – the space for open play is much more restricted than in a rural setting. We have to encourage the mothers to give their children a chance to play, even if this contains the risk of a few bruises once in a while.

From primary school age on we encourage sports and preferably sports together with the parents. It is much more reassuring for a 6- or 8-year-old to be sporty (in following judo or athletic courses) than to need constant treatment (in having to go to physiotherapy regularly). If the latter is unavoidable it helps to try to 're-package' it as athletics or training, as well.

There are families – and certainly mothers – where one look tells that they are already over-stressed by their accumulation of responsibilities. In these cases we have to take care not to further these stresses. In many other cases, it is advisable to design routines which integrate the parents into the therapy. This can be done by suggesting they do sport together with their child, or by asking them to join their child in out-door activities.

Certainly with hyperactive children, it helps to have the parents draw up a weekly plan and look at how many meals were taken together, how many hours of TV were noted and how many hours of 'quality time' their child had with one or both of them. The results are sometimes astonishing for all concerned.

KISS IN THE GENE POOL

Having got so far, one question arises: if there is a predisposition for KISS and if this predisposition is genetic – i.e. not induced by external factors such as living conditions – how come this short-coming was not weeded out by evolutionary pressure? Or, to ask the other way round: what is the positive side of this trait?

At first we thought that problems related to KISS were only apparent in our society of relative abundance. Deliberate search in other cultures demonstrated, however, that the torticollis neonatorum is by no means confined to industrialized societies. From the tikis of Polynesia, who display the same symptoms (Fig. 26.2), to the baby massage in India described by Leboyer (1976), examples abound to show that KISS is much older than the twentieth century.

Andry describes in detail the problems of the torticollis neonatorum and the amount of space dedicated to this problem alone indicates that it was important more than 250 years ago (Andry de Boisregard 1941).

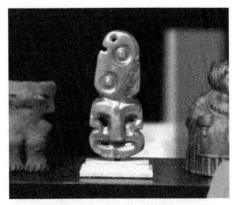

Figure 26.2 A Polynesian tiki. This photo from an art fair shows a Polynesian amulet which allegedly displays a totemistic figure of a newborn baby with a tilted position of the head in order to protect against evil spirits.

Our data and the research of others indicates that about a third of all newborn babies have reduced mobility of the head and cervical spine immediately after birth (Buchmann and Bülow 1983, Güntürkün 2003, Seifert 1975). Six weeks later this figure has reduced to about 10%. After simple remedies are used, such as changing the orientation of the bed relative to the window or favoring the other side for feeding the child, half of these infants return to a symmetrical posture and roughly 5% of all infants need some form of professional help. This is a sizable proportion.

It should be noted that there is a distinction to be made between a postural preference and a fixed position. The former being a normal aspect of all infants, it is the latter which hinders neuromotor development and needs our attention.

If a left-handed person writes about the bilateral organization of the brain and its consequences, one can be sure that he will find some positive things to say – besides all the well-known facts of increased mental disorders and all the accidents we left-handers seem to be so much more prone to than right-handers (Goldberg 2001).

A similar situation is true for the 'KISSed'. If one finds ample evidence in one's CV that fits the KISS pattern, it seems natural to look for the positive side of it all. In the preparation of this book Ramirez (see Chapter 5) and I found out that we were fellow-sufferers in this regard: clumsy youths with a fear of heights, lots of problems with sports and other 'mechanical' activities – but nevertheless a reasonably successful journey through life.

The KISS predisposition does not entail long-term difficulties per se, which is one reason why its effects on sensorimotor development took so long to decipher. As the above-mentioned members of the author team of this book proudly assert, there is life beyond KISS even without specific treatment. But, looking back at my own unhappy times in the gym or on the dance-floor (not to mention the terrible challenge of staircases, ladders or balustrades), I would go to great lengths to alleviate the fate of my young

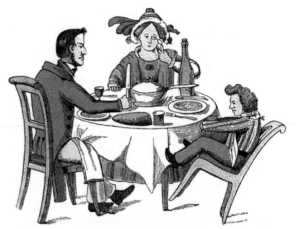

Figure 26.3　Fidgety Philip; the Struwwelpeter (Hoffmann 1846) contained an entire collection of stories about 'difficult' children. It was published a hundred and fifty years ago by a medical doctor working in a lunatic asylum. He hadn't yet heard of ADD . . .

fellow-sufferers – as I did with my son, who has inherited the same 'talents' and was delivered with the help of a vacuum extractor. The insight of somebody who knows these problems from first-hand experience is helpful in getting a feeling for the intricate problems of children with KISS.

Most of what follows here is speculative. Even though it is based on the many thousand young ones we saw during the last decades we do not have the rigorous protocol to be able to offer more than presumptions.

The genetic makeup predisposing for KISS seems to contain an inability to develop automatisms and a difficulty in relegating acquired micropatterns to the subconscious level. The negative side of this phenomenon is that these patterns are close to conscious control and have to be activated at will, i.e. not automatically. This enables the bearers of these traits on the other hand to re-examine these automatisms and improve them.

Secondly, there is something one could call the 'Wilma Rudolph effect' – the famous sprinter who overcame a crippling polio infection to become a top athlete. Some KISS kids bite through their obstacles, and, having got to the other side of that challenge, they have a better control of this part of their sensorimotor apparatus.

This phenomenon is quite common in actors or musicians, too (and politicians, for good measure). Like Demosthenes – who fought his stammering by exercising his speech with a pebble in his mouth – those with a challenge grow on it while they fight it – if they succeed.

But this positive line of events rests on a few assumptions. The families and the school environment have to be supportive to help the affected children tackle the difficulties of their predisposition.

As with dyslexic children, it would help a lot if we were able to use the label 'attention deficit disorder' (ADD) in a non-negative way. It is true that these children are very often difficult to handle, but it is equally true that they often display talents which we should not overlook. If we take into account how different the percentage of children diagnosed with ADD is in populations with very similar genetic makeup it seems at least farfetched to attribute ADD solely to a genetic factor. This one-dimensional explanation also runs counter to the fact that ADD is diagnosed with a steeply increasing frequency, without any change in the underlying gene pool. Even gross underdiagnosing would hardly suffice to explain an over 100-fold increase in the use of Ritalin during the last decade in the USA alone.

If the proponents of a genetic factor in ADD were correct, the question immediately arises why this allegedly very negative item in our heritage was not weeded out by evolution a long time ago. Careful studies showed time and again that even lethal genetic factors bestow competitive advantages on their bearers: the gene for sickle-cell anemia protects in a heterozygous carrier against malaria, and the gene for cystic fibrosis increases resistance against typhoid fever. If we were to accept that there is such a thing as 'genetic programming' for ADD, we have to do our best to understand the eventual advantages such a gene might carry as 'collateral advantage' lest we prevent the adaptation of children treated with psy-

chopharmaceuticals to their inherited genetic makeup.

Let us get back to the problem of the left-handed. Boys are over-represented in the KISS collective, and it is more likely for a KISS kid to be left-handed, so it seems an interesting point of departure to find out if there are other problems with the same profile. There we arrive at the 'terrain minée' of ADD. It is true that ADD – if ever we accept it as a valid diagnosis at all – is found predominantly in boys and that left-handed boys seem to be even more predisposed (Golderg 2001). Many publications about ADD and similar conditions (MCD, POS, etc.) stress the fact that the children affected have problems with proprioception and movement control (DeGrandpre 1999, Faraone 1995, Shaywitz et al 1995). And, like KISS, ADD 'runs in families', i.e. a predisposing factor is very probable (Faraone et al 1995, Schweitzer and Sulzer Azaroff 1995).

Schoolchildren with an initial diagnosis of ADD represent the bulk of our patients of that age group. And in a sizable proportion, the disappearance of the functional vertebrogenic problem helps sufficiently for them to reach a higher level of self-organization. It seems fruitless to discuss if the initial diagnosis was wrong or if manual therapy can indeed help to alleviate the symptoms of ADD in general. As far as our patients are concerned the most precise indicator that an attempt with manual therapy should be made is the early history. If signs of functional disorders are to be found, a closer examination should follow and – even if the other indications are quite inconclusive – a test manipulation (Lewit) should be tried.

In all these years we could not find *the* item to predict the outcome of our therapy. There were children who fitted the picture perfectly, a fixed position during the first year of life, colic and sleeping problems, and last but not least the 'right' segmental findings with irritable trigger points, and movement restrictions in the occipitocervical region. Everything seemed to indicate that the treatment would be a success and change the situation profoundly – but, alas, nothing remarkable happened. At the follow-up examination the segmental restrictions proved to be absent, but the behavior of our young patient had not changed a bit. Here the functional hindrance on the vertebral level was clearly present, but irrelevant.

On the other hand, we had children who were treated more or less haphazardly – for example because another family member had to come. Some of them showed amazing reactions to manual therapy. After many similar experiences we tend to treat as soon as we find at least some signs of early asymmetry, a reduced mobility of the cervical spine and local trigger points.

Contrary to pharmacotherapy in ADD, which normally does not influence long-term performance, schoolchildren who react positively to manual therapy show improvement in their reports, and more often than not, these improvements last. So, although we cannot offer a wonder cure for ADD, we do have a sizeable group of children usually labeled as ADD whose response to manual therapy gives them a chance to get onto a new track in their development. This chance is even greater if the child in question shows symptoms of KISS or has a sibling who was treated for it.

GROWTH AND DEVELOPMENT

Studying the early months of human development focuses the attention on the very special situation of the individual. As long as we live we develop, but much more so in this first phase. Simply taking into account the rapidly increasing body mass – an admittedly rough yardstick – one has to determine how this process is organized. On one hand there is the notion of growth, i.e. augmentation of cell mass and cell number tightly regulated by genetic control with minimal external input. Maturation is a similar concept, indicating a slightly different path. On the other hand 'development is not just more than growth – it is more than maturation, requiring constant negotiation with the environment' (Konner 2002).

As soon as we accept the paradigm of development, the pathways of the input come under close scrutiny. From the first cell division after fertilization the specific environment of the developing organism plays an important part in this process. The simplistic notion of a rigid genetic program unfolding almost automatically was elegantly refuted by J.-P. Changeux (1984) who remarked on the impossibility of determining the structure of 10^{11} cells of the central nervous system with 10^{15} connections by means of the 30 000 genes present in the human genome. A lot of this complexity is left to chance and even identical twins develop different neuronal structures a long time before being born. Slight influences in this initial phase are amplified by the extreme sensitivity of the developing sensorimotor apparatus, and a minute alteration of the input may result in a dramatically different path of development – or may be adjusted by the internal stabilizing factors.

Once the primal influence of the environment for the development of the newborn is established the question of how this environmental factor exerts this influence becomes paramount. During the intrauterine period, chemical stimuli – transmitted via the placenta – are in the foreground. Every mother can tell stories of how the child reacted to food during the pregnancy. Many other stimuli are transmitted via endocrine messengers, e.g. the mother's adrenaline or other stress factors.

But even in the uterus, external sensory stimuli are capable of reaching the fetus, as extensive literature documents.

The sensory stimuli gain a much bigger influence after birth. Basic reactions to noise and light are easy to accept for the amazed observer, but it is even more startling to realize that newborn babies are able to react in a coordinated way to the complex stimulus of a smiling face, even imitating the facial movements presented to them a few hours after birth (Kugiumutzakis 1988). Eye contact with the care-giver is an essential ingredient for this communication and the quality of sustained eye contact helps, for example, to transmit the soothing gestures of a mother (Trevarthen 1979).

The 'hardwired' mechanisms which allow a newborn baby to recognize a face as something important and which supply at least a basic meaning to facial movements form the base on which the newborn starts its learning process.

Besides the skin sensitivity and the primary sentiment of being protected by close contact, it is the acoustic and optic input channel which determines the amount and quality of the external input of the rapidly differentiating neural system of the infant.

Here the quality of the cervical system comes into play, as a proprioceptive organ and as an effector of head movements directing eyes and ears towards a point of interest. It is easy to imagine that difficulties in locating and fixating such a source of interest impede the social and motor learning and we have already mentioned how a tense muscular tonus in the newborn baby can hinder bonding by giving the mother the impression that the child rejects her – something we heard time and again, especially as a relieved remark after the improvement a manipulation was able to bring.

As we know now how the feedback of the mother's encouragement facilitates the acquisition of all complex capabilities (Cleary et al 1997, Goldstein et al 2003, Tessier et al 1998, Teuchert-Noodt and Dawirs 2001) we realize how even a minor interference in this primal relation can have wide-ranging consequences. If we are only able to improve this bond a tiny bit by taking away the muscular tension of the newborn – not to mention nerve-racking conditions like colic – we can ease the first steps into life of our young patients considerably.

References

Andry de Boisregard N 1741 L'orthopédie ou l'art de prévenir et de corriger dans les enfants les difformités du corps. Vv Alix, Paris

Biedermann H 1991 Kopfgelenk-induzierte Symmetriestörungen bei Kleinkindern. Kinderarzt 22:1475–1482

Biedermann H 1996 KISS-Kinder. Enke, Stuttgart

Biedermann H 1999 KISS-Kinder: eine katamnestische Untersuchung. In: Biedermann H (ed) Manualtherapie bei Kindern. Enke, Stuttgart, p 27–42

Buchmann J, Bülow B 1983 Funktionelle Kopfgelenksstörungen bei Neugeborenen im Zusammenhang mit Lagereaktionsverhalten und Tonusasymmetrie. Manuelle Medizin 21:59–62

Changeux J P 1984 L'homme neuronal. Fayard, Paris

Cleary G M, Spinner S S, Gibson E et al. 1997 Skin-to-skin parental contact with fragile preterm infants. Journal of the American Osteopathic Association 97(8):457–460

DeGrandpre R 1999 Ritalin nation. W W Norton, New York

Faraone S V, Biederman J, Chen W J et al 1995 Genetic heterogeneity in attention-deficit hyperactivity disorder (ADHD): gender, psychiatric comorbidity, and maternal ADHD. Journal of Abnormal Psychology 104(2):334–345

Goldberg E 2001 The executive brain. Oxford University Press, Oxford

Goldstein M, King A, West M J 2003 Social interaction shapes babbling: Testing parallels between birdsong and speech. Proceedings of the National Academy of Sciences USA, 2003, online

Güntürkün O 2003 Human behaviour: Adult persistence of head-turning asymmetry. Nature 421(6924):711

Hoffmann H 1846 Der Struwwelpeter. Literarische Anstalt, Frankfurt/Main

Konner M 2002 Weaving life's pattern. Nature 418:279

Kugiumutzakis G 1988 Neonatal imitation in the intersubjective companion space. In: Braten S (ed) Intersubjective communication and emotion in early ontogeny. Cambridge University Press, Cambridge, p 63–88

Leboyer F 1976 Shantala, un Art traditionel: le massage des enfants. Seuil, Paris

Schweitzer J B, Sulzer Azaroff B 1995 Self-control in boys with attention deficit hyperactivity disorder: effects of added stimulation and time. Journal of Child Psychology and Psychiatry 36:671–686

Seifert I 1975 Kopfgelenksblockierung bei Neugeborenen. Rehabilitacia, Prague (Suppl) 10:53–57

Shaywitz B A, Fletcher J M, Shaywitz S E 1995 Defining and classifying learning disabilities and attention-deficit/hyperactivity disorder. Journal of Child Neurology 10 (Suppl):50–57

Shaywitz B A, Fletcher J M, Shaywitz S E 1997 Attention-deficit/hyperactivity disorder. Advances in Pediatrics 44:331–367

Tessier R, Cristo M, Velez S et al 1998 Kangaroo mother care and the bonding hypothesis. Pediatrics 102(2):e17

Teuchert-Noodt G, Dawirs R 2001 Malfunctional reorganization in the developing limbo-frontal system in animals: Implications for human Psychoses? Zeitschrift für Neuropsychologie 12:8–14

Trevarthen C 1979 Communication and cooperation in early infancy: a description of primary intersubjectivity. In:

Bullowa M (ed) Before speech. Cambridge University Press, Cambridge, p 321–372

von Lanz T, Wachsmuth W 1955 Praktische Anatomie 1/2: Der Hals. Springer, Berlin

Wackenheim A 1975 Roentgen diagnosis of the cranio-vertebral region. Springer, Berlin

Wilkinson R G 1996 Unhealthy societies: the afflictions of inequality: Routledge, London

Wolf S, Bruhn J G 1997 The power of clan: the influence of human relationships on heart disease. Transaction, New Brunswick

Epilogue

H. Biedermann

Science is the art of not fooling yourself
R. Feynman

Working in several European countries, I am acutely aware how much the cultural and political context one works in influences what can be achieved. Manual therapy has different flavors in different countries, being a domain of neurologists in the Czech Republic and of rheumatologists in Denmark. In Belgium and the Netherlands most of the work is done by specialized physiotherapists, and in the USA, chiropractors and osteopaths are in the foreground.

As diverse as the professionals who treat children (and adults) are the techniques used. For the moment the trend in manual therapy is towards 'gentle' procedures, admittedly a little more time-consuming, but often achieving the same results. The remarks of Lynn Pryor (1988) about the different cultures of looking at healing and disease are as true for our specialty.

It is true, too, that the social environment plays an enormously important role. Wilkinson (1996) argued convincingly that 'social, rather than material factors are now the limiting component in the quality of life in developed countries'. The Dutch cardiologist Dunning gives a nice example of the ideal beauty: 'the tall, thin and brown of today as contrast to the pale, pudgy and plump of Rubens and Rembrandt' (Dunning 1990). We have to keep these 'big' frames of reference in mind in order to put what we can do for our patients in realistic proportions to the cultural context, limiting and enabling our work.

These are the constraints of medical work or rather healing in general. For manual therapy with its functional approach, another difficulty arises.

THE TWO FLAVORS OF MANUAL THERAPY

The special character of manual therapy can be seen from two points of view, giving it two very different flavors. From inside out it is a wonderfully all-encompassing variant of the healing professions, enabling those proficient in it to solve problems from fields as far away from each other as otorhinology (vertigo, tinnitus) (Hülse 1998), internal medicine (pseudo-angina pectoris, vegetative dystonia) (Kunert 1963) or – to approach the main topics of this book – pediatrics.

Seen from the outside, this very ability turns manual therapy into an unwelcome guest (to use the least unfriendly definition) of one's own field of work. 'How dare those people claim to solve problems which have been hounding us for many years', these specialists exclaim, branding those intruders as confidence tricksters unable and/or unwilling to use a rigorous and 'scientific' approach.

In Europe, where chiropractors are not as prominently in the picture and therefore attract much less criticism, this discussion is waged well inside the medical profession. Especially in Germany, those doctors busy with manual therapy are firmly inside 'mainstream medicine' and not considered so much part of an alternative circuit as in the UK, for example.

Two factors contribute to this situation – viewed as a challenge or a nuisance (again depending on the viewpoint):

- Manual therapy, if seen as more than a minor treatment technique, deals with functional pathology and stands as such in a certain contradiction to the mostly patho-morphological viewpoint of more traditional medicine. Moreover, drug treatment is central in internal medi-

cine, whereas it is at best a subordinate therapeutic modality in manual therapy in children (MTC). Insight into the dialectics of functional stimulation and the resulting morphology opens up new approaches to problems seemingly unrelated to vertebrogenic disorders.

- Manual therapy is a specialty whose practitioners are to be found in private practices – and that is where most of the research pertaining to this field comes from. This causes a visceral mistrust in those members of the healing professions who are accustomed to consider universities as the source of knowledge.

Universities are by definition institutions which have to convey generally accepted wisdom on to the next generation. This leaves just enough space for gradual changes, incremental improvements on an idea commonly accepted as valid. To embrace a new point of view these institutions need a hard push, which in turn requires a lot of energy and persistence from those who want to bring about such a change.

Far from pretending to offer a radically new view we tried to show that manual therapy in children can look back on a long history. What is comparatively new (and one of the main points of discussion) is the much broader perspective which is applied nowadays, conceding a much deeper and more far-reaching influence to apparently 'minor' functional problems.

It is in this light that the subtle interpretation of functional findings in X-rays acquires a new role as indicators directing the clinician's attention towards vertebrogenic pathology, and that pathologies of (for example) persistent primitive reflexes (Goddard Blythe and Hyland 1998) are reinterpreted as caused by functional disorders of the cervical spine. When we propose a functional level to many pathologies it is not to replace whatever concept might prevail in a given context, but to complement it with another one in order to open additional therapeutic avenues. As this goes beyond the 'commonly accepted practice' such a new concept has to prove its value.

REQUIREMENTS FOR A NEW CONCEPT

In order to be accepted, such a new mode of explanation has – first and foremost – to facilitate the treatment of the patients in question (more) successfully than others. Without this first step nobody will even bother to think about dropping an entrenched point of view. Secondly the success in daily practice has to be used to construct a working model of what happens and why.

Inertia is a very laudable quality of the scientific consensus. A new concept, be it therapeutic or diagnostic, has to fulfill some minimum conditions in order to merit broader acceptance (Ruse 1999). The more general a new proposal is, the better it has to fulfill them to overcome the force of habit.

These basic requirements can be subsumed under three main headings:

- internal coherence and external consistency
- unificatory power and elegance (simplicity)
- predictive accuracy and fertility.

Coherence: Ideas and concepts have a tendency to wear out. In the beginning, one is confronted with a clear-cut structure, black or white and with no loopholes. Almost any classification sooner or later suffers from the fact that new knowledge necessitates fudging its principles to accommodate the implications of the new knowledge. The more we get used to a concept the easier we accept these exceptions. But when starting out with a new way to explain everything, we would not accept this.

Consistency: If we are asked to accept a new explanation for a well-known problem, the least we can ask for is that the (new) explanation offers a consistent mode of interpretation of the facts, including – for good measure – those facts which we had to classify as 'untypical' or 'non-relevant' in order to make the commonly established theory fit the practical situation.

This leads to the next item, the unificatory power one asks of a new concept. If someone proposes a new view on problems we handle with a well-established concept, this new approach has to offer enough good arguments to abandon our habitual view. One of the most convincing points in such a discussion is the capability of a new theory to integrate facts which were until then beyond the scope of a given theoretical frame. This inclusion should flow naturally from the basic framework of such a new theory in order to be convincing – what one would call elegance.

Any new medical theory should offer us a tool leading to a better therapy. To achieve this, a newly proposed concept has to offer tools to predict developments on the basis of a given clinical situation and to spawn new diagnostic and therapeutic insights. This fertility of a new concept is in my view the most attractive component.

Only if we feel that a new way of classification gives us a more lucid description of the enormously complex clinical reality we are confronted with every day, do we make the effort to leave well-known models behind and embark on the acquisition of something new.

We hope to have demonstrated that this can be applied to our model. It helps to explain 'old' problems from a new viewpoint (like colic or 'muscular' torticollis) and the therapy derived from this concept is successful and efficient. We are now at a point in time where the publication of this book seemed the right thing to do.

If not overdone, the model of KISS and KIDD should help to ask new and interesting questions. This in turn should help us to further improve our understanding of the interdependence of (mal-) function and the morphological differentiation in adolescence.

'The mark of a healthy research field is that there is never a good time to write a book about it' (Bengtson 2003) – very true for manual therapy in children, too. In the 3 years it took to write and compile this book, quite a few details were added to our model and I am sure that in the time passing between the submission of this text and the actual publication of the book, more interesting facts will be uncovered. This book is one stepping stone on our way, and the nicest compliment one could get is a lot of critical and constructive remarks. We can only learn from them and, as A. H. Knoll put it, 'The absence of a definite punch line is why I get up in the morning'.

WINDOWS OF OPPORTUNITY

MTC's biggest distinction, compared to manual therapy in adults, is its excessive effectiveness at certain points in time. We know today that the maturation and differentiation of the central nervous system depends on the correct quantity and quality of the stimuli at certain pivotal 'critical periods'. Complex coordinative capabilities can best be acquired at rather narrow windows in time and depend crucially on the social interaction and the quality of the environment (Goldberg 2001, Goldstein et al 2003, Teuchert-Noodt and Dawirs 2001, Wolf and Bruhn 1997).

A smoothly functioning craniocervical junction plays an important part in this. On a lower level, it enables the correlation of optical and vestibular information with the whole body, on a more complex level – to give but one example – a tense baby in fixed retroflexion triggers a different emotional response from a care-giver than an infant that is able to cuddle into the arms of its mother.

These two observations may hint at how complex this interaction is. We do not yet know for sure how to define those phases in which the development of the child is especially sensitive. Our experience indicates that the first year up to verticalization is one of them. The patterns laid down by the interaction between genetic makeup and individual fate determine the sensorimotor development for years and decades similar to the influence of the intrauterine environment for the long-term development of the individual (Lopuhaa et al 2000, Roseboom et al 2001).

A vast area of research lies in front of us, far too big for one team (and one lifetime). A deeper understanding of these long-term influences should help us to maximize the impact of our therapies while minimizing the time and effort invested.

KEEP IT STRAIGHT AND SIMPLE

Having worked with this KISS concept for more than 15 years now, we are convinced that this taxonomy improves our understanding of the functional pathology of vertebrogenic origin. It helps get to grips with the astounding complexity of symptoms which dominate the clinical picture at a given moment, and it aids in predicting the likely outcome of our interventions, making the preparations for additional therapy easier.

It is easy to be carried away by such a potent concept and we have to keep reminding ourselves that KISS *and* KIDD are but two factors in the life of a young child.

For us they are very much in the center of attention, whereas the situation seen from the child's point of view may have other priorities. Apart from all the other diseases and medical problems, there is the entire environment of the child. A youngster in a functioning and supportive family can handle a lot more pressure than one who has to cope with quarreling parents, an unsafe neighborhood and dire financial straits.

Keeping these constraints in mind, it is good to know that MTC does not depend on any external factor to have a positive influence. In a little pilot study we checked the effect of MTC on neurodermatosis. The skin did indeed look better in all those cases where there were signs of functional vertebrogenic disorders – not because we were able to administer a specific treatment, but because the general stress level was lowered a little bit. Schoolchildren in a class of children with learning difficulties improved after MTC if their case history showed signs of KISS at an early age – regardless of whether they were living in a happy or dysfunctional family.

So, MTC functions sometimes like the 'magic bullet' and it is comprehensible that some begin to overestimate the therapeutic possibilities. Maybe it helps to remember how some management consultants define KISS: 'Keep it simple, stupid!'

With this cold shower for the over-eager we will close this book and hope that it will encourage some readers to try the amazing possibilities of manual therapy in the treatment of children and adolescents.

References

Bengtson S 2003 Beneath the great divide. Nature 423:481–482

Dunning A 1990 Uitersten Beschouwingen over menselijk gedrag. Meulenhoff, Amsterdam

Goddard Blythe S, Hyland D 1998 Screening for neurological dysfunction in the specific learning difficulty child. Journal of Occupational Therapy 61(10):459–464

Goldberg E 2001 The executive brain. Oxford University Press, Oxford

Goldstein M, King A, West M J 2003 Social interaction shapes babbling: Testing parallels between birdsong and speech. Proceedings of the National Academy of Sciences USA; online

Hülse M 1998 Klinik der Funktionsstörungen des Kopfgelenkbereiches, In: Hülse M, Neuhuber W L, Wolff H D (eds) Der kranio-zervikale Übergang. Springer, Berlin, p 43–98

Kunert W 1963 Wirbelsäule und Innere Medizin. Enke, Stuttgart

Lopuhaa C E, Roseboom T J, Osmond C et al 2000 Atopy, lung function, and obstructive airways disease after prenatal exposure to famine. Thorax 55(7):555–561

Payer L 1988 Medicine and culture. Varieties of treatment in the United States, England, West Germany and France. H Holt, New York

Roseboom T J, van der Meulen J H, Osmond C et al 2001 Adult survival after prenatal exposure to the Dutch famine 1944–45. Paediatric and Perinatal Epidemiology 15(3):220–225

Ruse M 1999 Mystery of mysteries: is evolution a social construction? Harvard University Press, Cambridge, MA

Teuchert-Noodt G, Dawirs R 2001 Malfunctional reorganization in the developing limbo-frontal system in animals: implications for human psychoses? Zeitschrift für Neuropsychologie 12:8–14

Wilkinson R G 1996 Unhealthy societies: the afflictions of inequality. Routledge, London

Wolf S, Bruhn J G 1997 The power of clan: the influence of human relationships on heart disease. Transaction, New Brunswick

Index

Printed and bound by CPI Group (UK) Ltd, Croydon, CR0 4YY

03/10/2024

01040360-0005